Atlas of
RADIOLOGY
of the
CHEST

EDITORS

Professor Dame Margaret Turner-Warwick
DBE, DM, PhD, DSc. (Hon), FRCP(E), FRACP, FACP, FFOM, PRCP
President
Royal College of Physicians
London

Dr Margaret E. Hodson MD, MSc, FRCP, DA
Reader in Respiratory Medicine
National Heart and Lung Institute
The Royal Brompton Hospital
London

Professor Bryan Corrin MD, FRCPath
Professor of Thoracic Pathology
National Heart and Lung Institute
The Royal Brompton Hospital
London

Dr Ian H. Kerr MA, MBBChir, FRCP, FRCR
Honorary Consulting Radiologist
The Royal Brompton Hospital
London

Gower Medical Publishing • London • New York

Distributed in the USA and Canada by:
J B Lippincott Company
East Washington Square
Philadelphia
PA 19105
USA

Distributed in the UK and Continental Europe by:
Gower Medical Publishing
Middlesex House
34–42 Cleveland Street
London W1P 5FB
UK

Distributed in Australia and New Zealand by:
Harper and Row (Australia) Pty Ltd
PO Box 226
Artarmon
NSW 2064
Australia

Distributed in Southeast Asia, Hong Kong, India and Pakistan by:
Harper and Row (Asia) Pte Ltd
37 Jalan Pemimpin 02-01
Singapore 2057

Distributed in Japan by:
Nankodo Co Ltd
42-6 Hongo 3-chome
Bunkyo-ku
Tokyo 113
Japan

Publisher:
Fiona Foley

Project Manager:
Alison Whitehouse

Design and Layout:
Lee Riches
Mark Willey

Index:
Susan Ramsey

Production:
Susan Bishop

British Library Cataloguing in Publication Data:
Atlas of radiology of the chest.
 I. Turner-Warwick, Professor Margaret
 616.2

Library of Congress Cataloging in Publication Data:
Atlas of radiology of the chest / editors, Dame Margaret
 Turner-Warwick ... [et al.].
 Includes index.
 1. Chest--Radiography--Atlases. 2. Chest--Diseases--
 Diagnosis--Atlases. 3. Diagnosis, Differential--Atlases.
 I. Turner-Warwick, Margaret, 1924–
 [DNLM: 1. Thoracic Radiography--atlases.
 WF 17 A8813]
 RC941.A78   1991
 617.5′407547--dc20

ISBN 0 397 44837 6

Typesetting by M to N Typesetters, London
Text set in Century Schoolbook; captions set in Gill Sans
Illustrations originated in Hong Kong by Imago
Productions Limited
Text origination and page make up by Hilo Offset
Limited, Colchester
Produced by Mandarin Offset Limited
Printed in Hong Kong

Print number: 1 2 3 4:94 93 92 91

Preface

This *Atlas of Radiology of the Chest* is based on the plain chest radiograph, for this remains the easiest, most convenient and cheapest form of chest imaging, providing the most information for the amount of effort and hazard involved. It is used universally by physicians as part of the clinical evaluation of patients with chest disease. Other methods of imaging, which include arteriography, bronchography, conventional and computed tomography, and nuclear medicine, are mentioned where appropriate. Some of the exciting newer modalities, such as magnetic resonance imaging, not yet established in everyday practice in diseases of the chest, have not been included.

The Atlas is not a textbook. Its aim is to present radiographs of a wide range of chest conditions as examples for both trainee and practising physicians. The material is intended to be of interest to consultant radiologists and chest physicians as well as those studying for examinations. The written descriptions are inevitably incomplete and are intended to complement the many more exhaustive and excellent recent textbooks on chest disease by presenting a fuller range of images than such books are able to provide.

We wish to thank all those who have provided material for this Atlas and we hope that our acknowledgements are complete. We apologist humbly if there are any omissions.

Finally we would like to thank Gower Medical Publishing and the Project Editors for all their help and forbearance in the production of the Atlas.

Contributors

The editors wish to thank the following authors for their
contributions to Chapters 4 to 7.

Dr M. Green DM FRCP (Chapter 7)
Consultant Physician, Brompton Hospital, and
Director of the Respiratory Muscle Laboratory.

Dr M.D.L. Morgan MD FRCP (Chapter 4)
Consultant Physician, Glenfield Hospital.

Dr A.J. Newman Taylor FRCP FFOM (Chapters 6 and 7)
Consultant Physician, Brompton Hospital, and Director,
Department of Occupational Medicine, National Heart
and Lung Institute.

Dr I.D. Starke MD MSc MRCP (Chapter 5)
Consultant Geriatrician, Lewisham and Hither Green
Hospitals and Senior Lecturer in Geriatric Medicine,
United Medical and Dental School, Guy's Hospital.

Dr A. Woodcock BSc MD MRCP (Chapter 4)
Consultant Physician, Regional Cardiothoracic Centre,
Wythenshawe Hospital.

Contents

1

The Normal Chest Radiograph

The chest radiograph is a two-dimensional image of a three-dimensional structure and is produced by the differential absorption of X-rays by the tissues of the body. The tissues can be divided into four groups depending on their density: the most dense are calcified bones; second are the soft tissues and body fluids, which include cartilage, muscle, connective tissue and blood; third is fat; and least dense are gases. Where an interface between these absorption bands occurs, an edge is visible on the radiograph and thus the structures become identifiable. When there is no interface between these absorption bands, where two structures of the same density are adjacent, no edge is visible and the two structures appear as one. The image of a chest on the radiograph is therefore produced by the absorption of the X-rays by calcium in the ribs, by soft tissues and blood in the heart, mediastinum and chest wall, by fat in the chest wall and the mediastinum and by air in the airways and lungs.

Clear understanding of the anatomy of the normal structures of the chest is essential to the interpretation of the radiograph; familiarity with normal appearances is therefore immensely important. Radiographs should be examined in the same planned and local manner as a patient is examined clinically.

The Frontal Radiograph

When examining the frontal radiograph (Fig. 1.1) the observer should first make certain that the patient is straight. This is done by ensuring that the medial ends of the clavicles are equidistant from the pedicles of the dorsal spine, provided there is no scoliosis.

The effect of rotation (Fig. 1.2) is to accentuate or mask mediastinal shift, make one hilum more prominent than the other, and to increase the general density of the lung which is closest to the film.

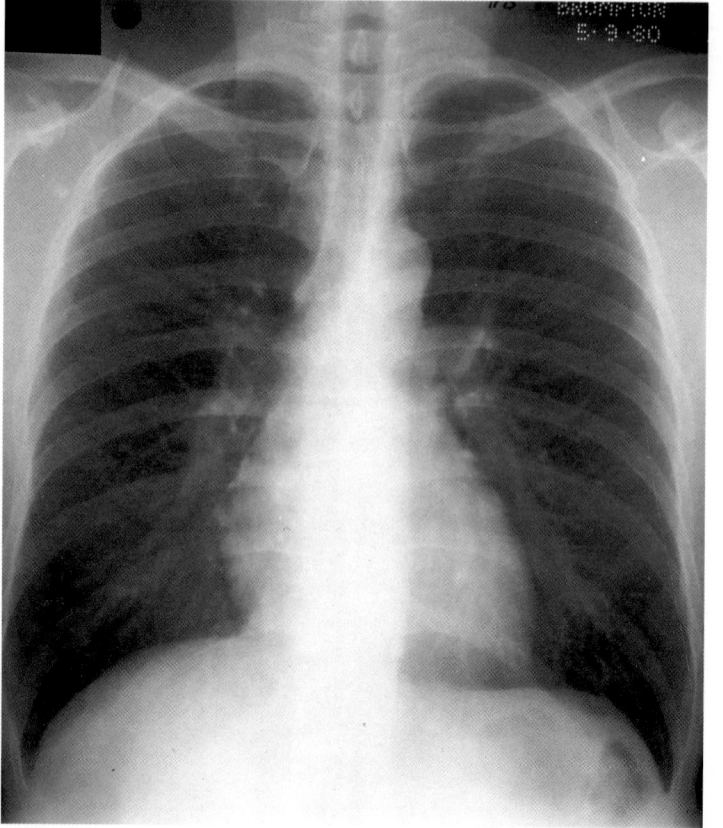

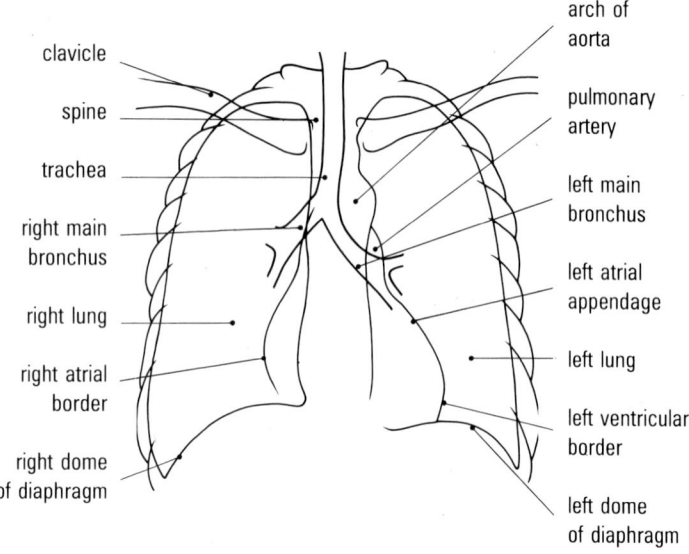

clavicle
spine
trachea
right main bronchus
right lung
right atrial border
right dome of diaphragm

arch of aorta
pulmonary artery
left main bronchus
left atrial appendage
left lung
left ventricular border
left dome of diaphragm

Fig. 1.1 A normal frontal radiograph.

The observer should follow a regular pattern of inspection: chest wall first, followed by soft tissues, diaphragm, heart and mediastinum, and finally the lungs. The search should not be terminated prematurely, even when an abnormality is discovered, otherwise information present elsewhere on the radiograph may be overlooked. A meticulous search should be directed towards the presence or absence of changes related to the original observation and also to clinical information. The possible presence of unrelated abnormalities should also be sought.

It has been shown that the accuracy with which a given edge sharpness is perceived decreases as the angle that the lesion subtends from the eye increases. In other words, the closer the lesion is to the observer the more difficult it is to see. It is therefore suggested that, in ideal circumstances, all radiographs at some stage of the examination should be viewed at a distance of 2–3m, or through a diminishing lens. Special care should be exercised when examining the 'hidden areas' (see below). The radiograph should be correctly illuminated on a viewing box; background lighting, such as sunlight, should be reduced to a minimum so that abnormalities are not missed.

The skeleton and soft tissues

The configuration of the bone should be examined to exclude such deformities as a depressed sternum. A search should be made for specific lesions in the spine, ribcage (Fig. 1.3) and shoulder girdle, such as metastases.

Increases in soft tissue shadowing are usually due to obesity or breast tissue. Normal soft tissue outlines include the axillary folds of pectoralis major (Fig. 1.4). An erroneous diagnosis of intrapulmonary hypertranslucency may be made if the absence of these folds is not observed in cases where the soft tissues of the chest wall including the pectoralis muscle are absent (Fig. 1.5). Nipple shadows,

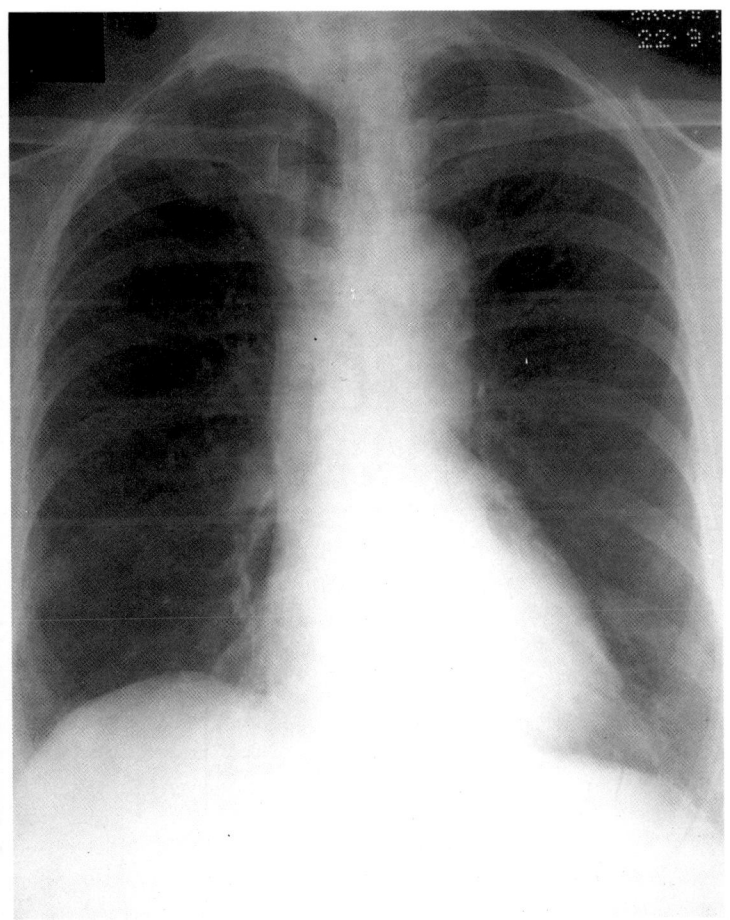

Fig. 1.2 The normal frontal radiograph with the patient slightly rotated to the right. Note the position of the clavicles in relation to the spine. The left lung, nearest to the film, is more dense (whiter) than the right lung, moved away from the film as a result of rotation.

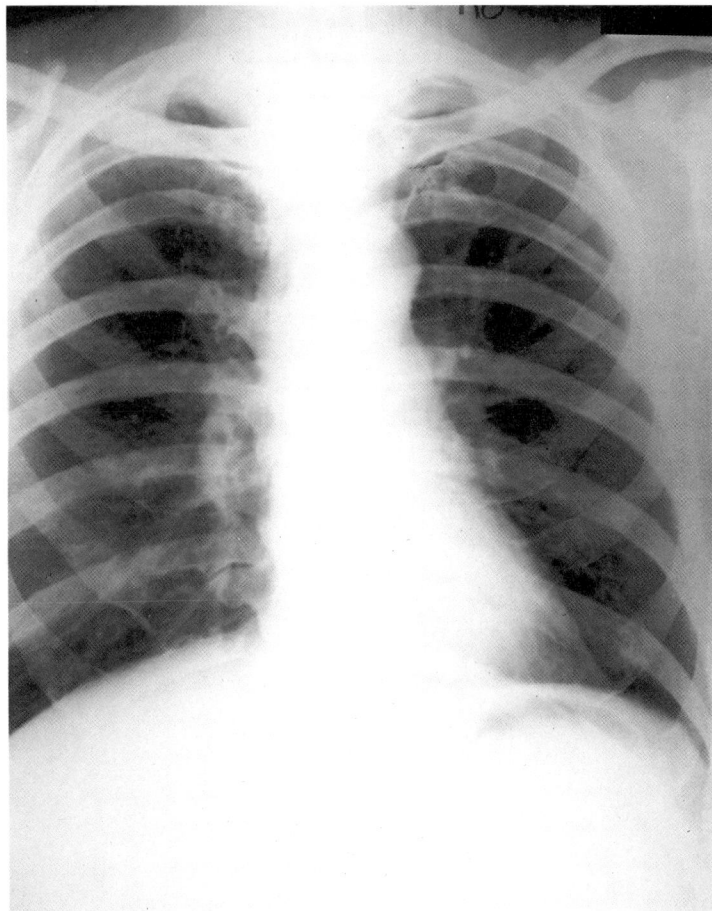

Fig. 1.3 Normal chest radiograph showing bifid anterior end of the left first rib. Such a defect could be mistaken for a cavity in the lung.

when visible, are usually seen on both sides and in males lie over the fifth interspace anteriorly. In females their position is variable. They should not be confused with intrapulmonary lesions and it may be necessary to mark the nipple and repeat the radiograph if there is doubt. Papillomata, warts and other skin tumours may masquerade as intrapulmonary space-occupying lesions. Other artefacts include hair, particularly if plaited, which may

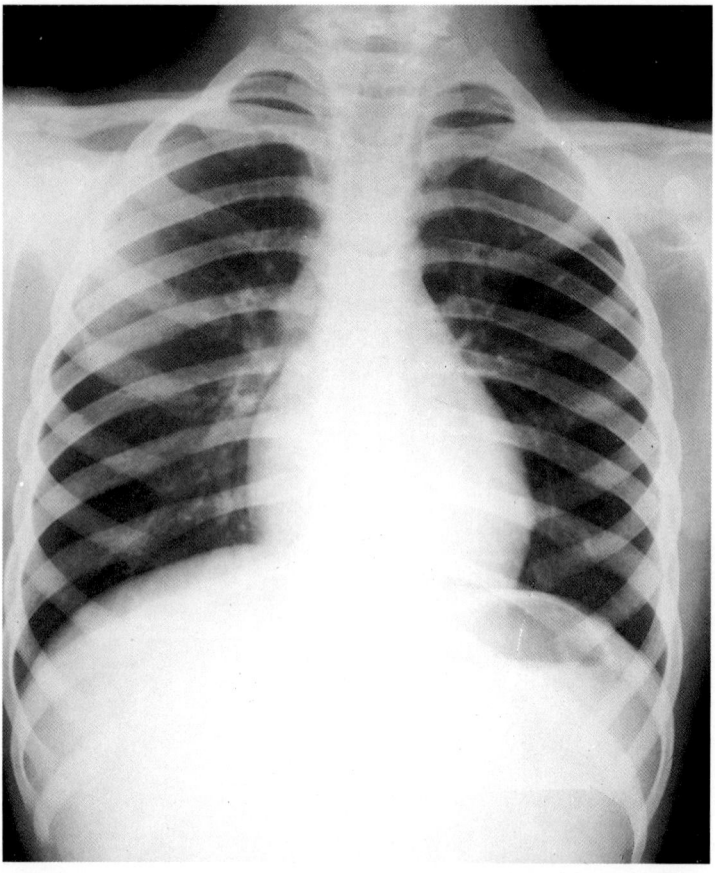

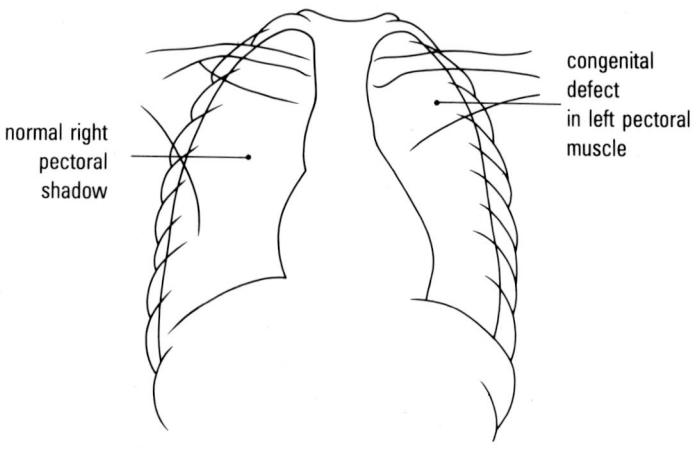

Fig. 1.4 Congenital absence of left pectoralis major. The right pectoral muscle is normal, but the shadow cast by the left pectoral muscle is much smaller.

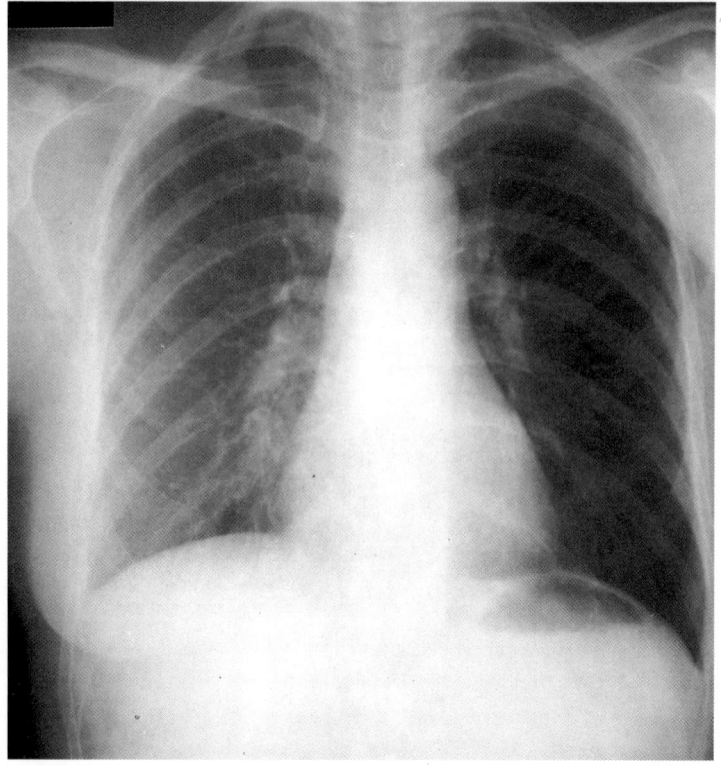

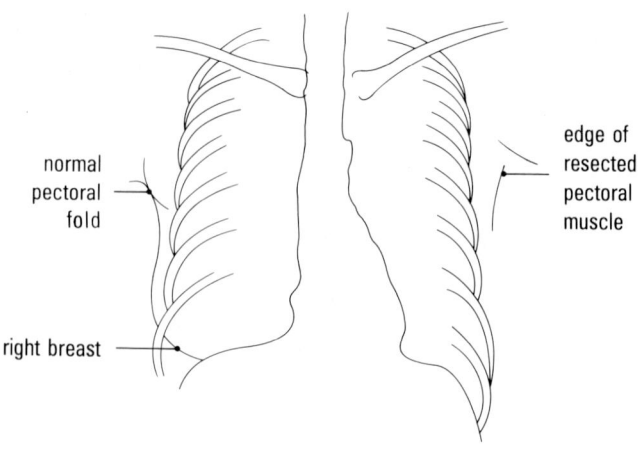

Fig. 1.5 Absence of the left breast and pectoral muscle shadows following radical mastectomy. Note apparent difference in density of the lung fields.

overlie the apices of the lungs (Fig. 1.6). Clothing may produce line shadows. These are usually identified by noting that they pass outside the lung field and overlie the soft tissues. Prostheses in the breasts after mammoplasty produce symmetrical opacification over the lower lung fields (Fig. 1.7).

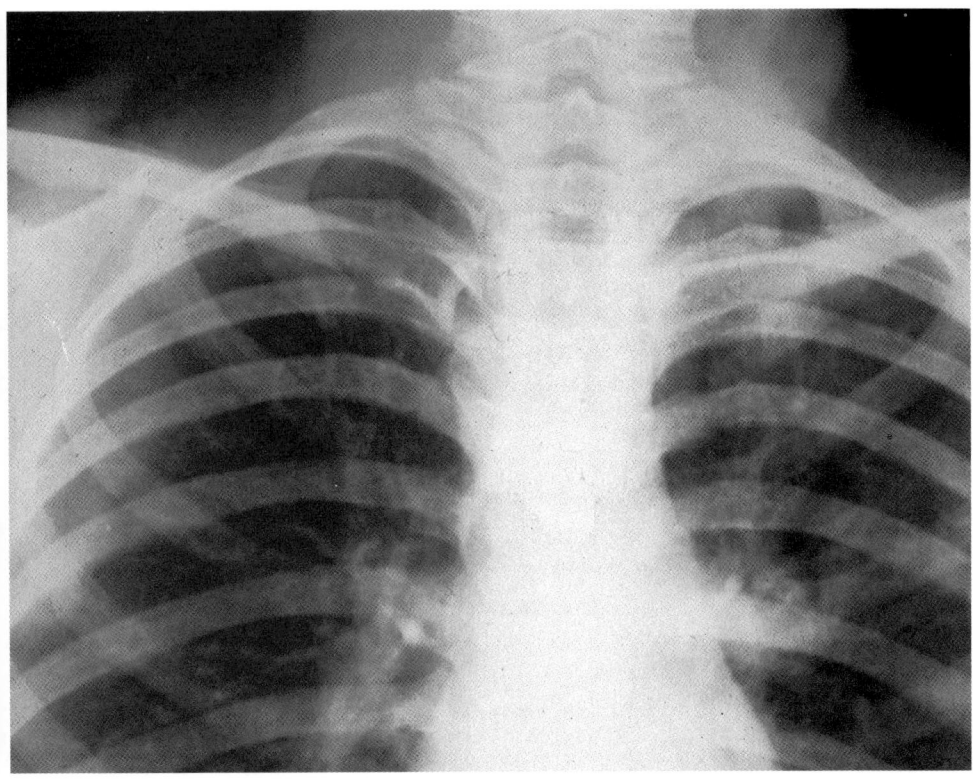

Fig. 1.6 Hair plaits causing opacities overlying the apices of the lungs. The shadows can be traced outside the lung fields into the lower part of the neck.

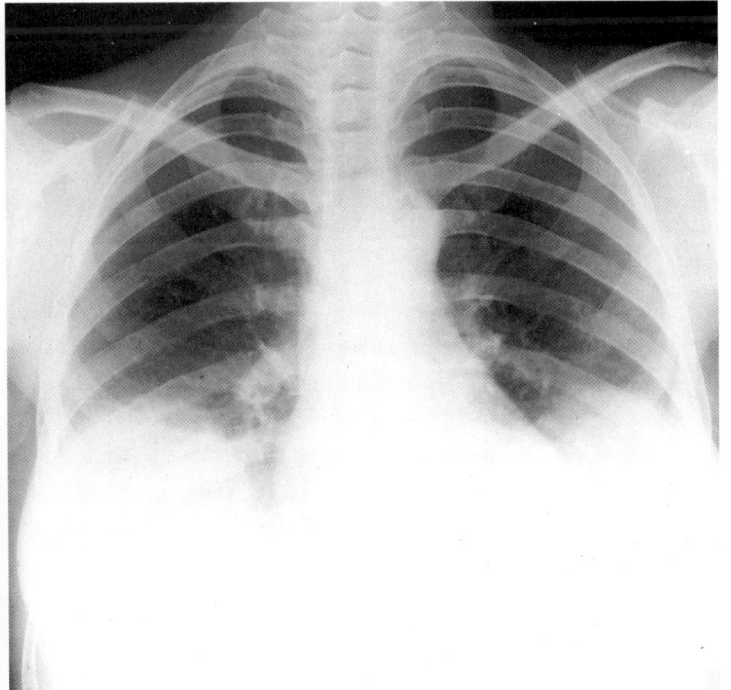
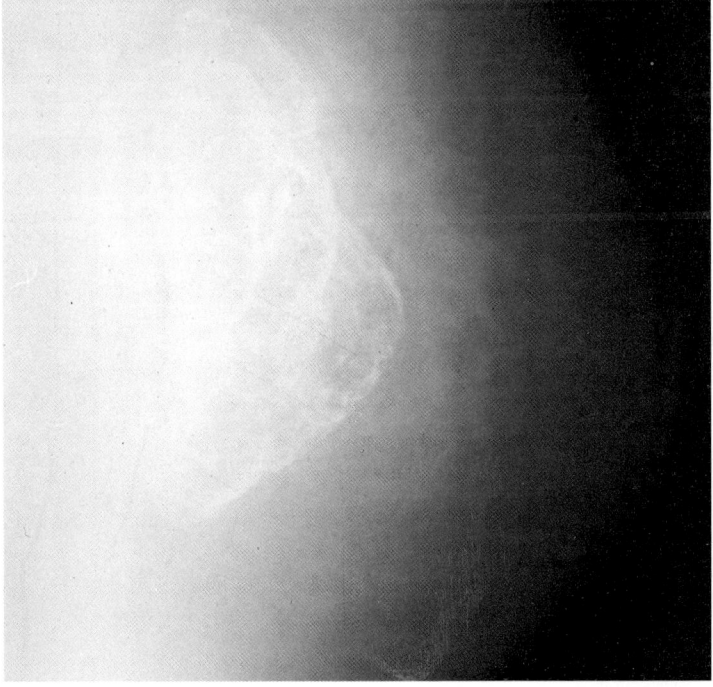

Fig. 1.7 Mammoplasties causing well circumscribed opacities over the lower lung fields (left). A lateral view of the breast (right) shows a prosthesis within the soft tissues.

The diaphragm

The right side of the diaphragm should normally be 1–2cm higher than the left.

The mediastinal shadow

When assessing heart size and configuration, the presence of fat pads in the cardiophrenic angles must not be mistaken for an enlarged heart or tumour. Deviation of the mediastinum is indicated by a shift in position of the heart or trachea. The normal right heart border projects just to the right of the spine. The area behind the heart should be carefully examined to exclude a left lower lobe collapse, or a paravertebral or mediastinal lesion. The position of the aortic knuckle should be noted; its site can be determined by the position of the trachea. The tracheal wall on the opposite side from the arch can be seen following the right mediastinal border. The configuration of the aorta, including its descending portion, should then be determined. An aortic lesion may masquerade as a mediastinal or intrapulmonary mass. The outline of the upper mediastinum should be a narrow pedicle ranging in width from approximately 3cm at the level of the clavicles to about 5cm just above the main pulmonary artery. Apart from the aortic knuckle, the margins should be straight and merge smoothly into the soft tissues of the neck.

The hila

The normal hilar shadows consist of radiodense vascular structures and the bronchi which, being air-filled, may be seen as radiolucent areas. The right hilum is formed by the right pulmonary artery and the right upper pulmonary vein. The shape of the left is almost completely formed by the shadow of the left pulmonary artery.

The lung fields

The lung fields are traversed by the normal pulmonary vessels. These vessels are distributed evenly to all areas and there is a uniform reduction in the calibre of the vessels from the centre outwards. The chest radiograph is, however, normally exposed with the patient in the erect position and there is thus greater flow through the lower zones compared with the upper. The vessels in the lower zones appear larger. The arteries in the upper lobes run upwards from the hila and the veins lie on the lateral side of their corresponding arteries.

In the lower lobes the arteries take a more vertical course than the veins which pass almost horizontally towards the left atrium. Changes in the size and pattern of the vessels indicate pathological processes. The lung fields should be searched carefully for the presence of opaque regions, taking care than none is obscured by overlying ribs and, in particular, that none is lying in the 'hidden areas', behind the heart, below the crests of the domes of the diaphragm, and at the apices of the lungs. The horizontal fissure normally lies on the right side between the third rib and fourth anterior interspace. Its position and configuration should be observed, as deviation may indicate a localized loss of lung volume.

The Lateral Chest Radiograph

The lateral chest radiograph (Fig. 1.8) should be examined in a logical manner in the same way as the frontal radiograph. The degree of rotation may be assessed by observation of the posterior ends of the ribs which should be superimposed or nearly superimposed, assuming there is

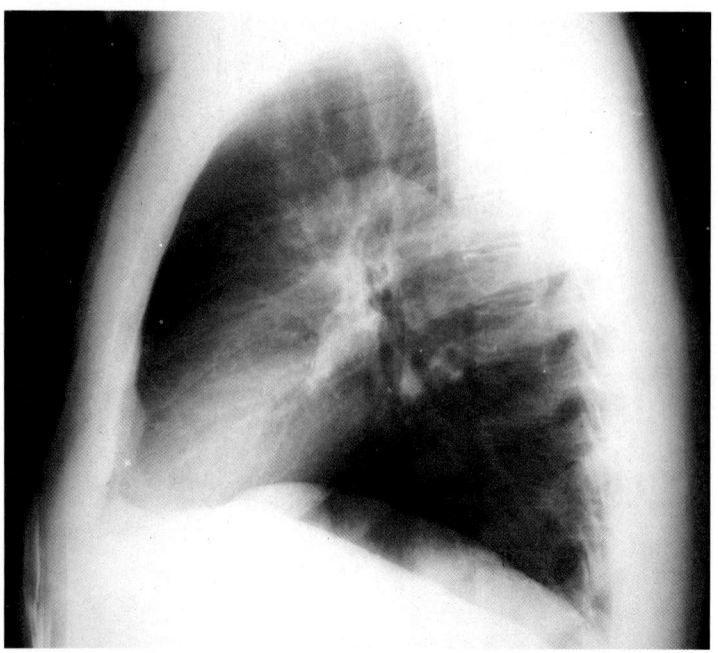

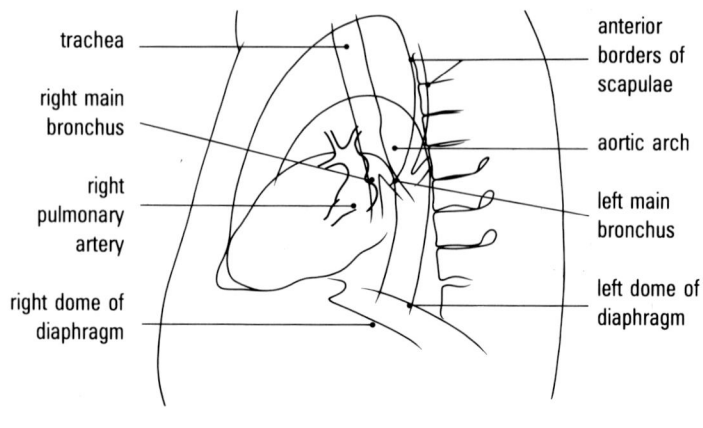

Fig. 1.8 A normal lateral projection of the chest.

trachea

right main bronchus

right pulmonary artery

right dome of diaphragm

anterior borders of scapulae

aortic arch

left main bronchus

left dome of diaphragm

no asymmetry of the chest wall. Anteriorly the sternum should be in profile.

The heart shadow usually meets the anterior chest wall about 4cm above the diaphragm. The trachea and main bronchi should be identified and the aortic arch and pulmonary arteries may be seen. The two domes of the diaphragm should also be identified. The anterior end of the left dome of the diaphragm blends with the inferior margin of the heart shadow and frequently the gastric air bubble can be seen just under this dome. The overall density of the lung above the heart shadow and behind the sternum should be approximately the same as that of the lung behind the heart just above the diaphragm.

In the lateral view one may also examine the dorsal vertebrae. Anterior margins of the scapulae can be seen as vertical lines overlying the vertebral bodies in the upper part of the chest. The maximum width of the retrosternal space is normally 3.5cm when measured horizontally from the posterior margin of the sternum, 3cm below the manubriosternal angle to the anterior margin of the ascending aorta.

The right pulmonary artery may be seen as an oval opacity lying in front of the right intermediate and the middle lobe bronchi. It should not be mistaken for a hilar mass. The left pulmonary artery passes backwards over the left main bronchus, seen end on as an oval translucency. The left main bronchus may frequently be mistaken for the bifurcation of the trachea which is usually not well-defined and lies slightly higher. The anterior border of the ascending aorta is usually visible, but its posterior margin blends with the pulmonary artery and the hilar shadows. The superior outline of the arch may be seen distal to the origin of the head and neck vessels. Part of the inferior wall of the arch can be identified and a small transradiant window is generally seen between this and the left pulmonary artery. Visualization of the outline of the descending aorta is variable: as the vessel becomes more tortuous with age, it becomes more easily seen and may produce an opacity behind the heart, thus simulating a tumour.

The oblique and horizontal fissures are frequently visible on the lateral radiograph. The oblique fissures run from the diaphragmatic surface of the visceral pleura, commencing 2–4cm behind the sternum. They pass upwards and backwards, overlying the hilar shadows, to reach the posterior pleura at the level of the fifth dorsal vertebra. The horizontal fissure runs forwards from the oblique fissure overlying the hilum towards the anterior chest wall. The fissures may be displaced by a loss of volume of part of the lung or, less frequently, deviated by a space-occupying lesion.

The diaphragm is seen in profile. If there is uncertainty regarding the identification of the domes of the diaphragm, the posterior ends of the two domes can be identified by the size of the ribs to which they are attached, the ribs nearest the film being smaller. This observation necessitates knowing whether the radiograph is a left or right lateral view, that is, which side of the patient was nearest to the film.

Depression of the sternum can be confirmed on the lateral projection (Fig. 1.9) and the anteroposterior diameter of the chest can also be assessed.

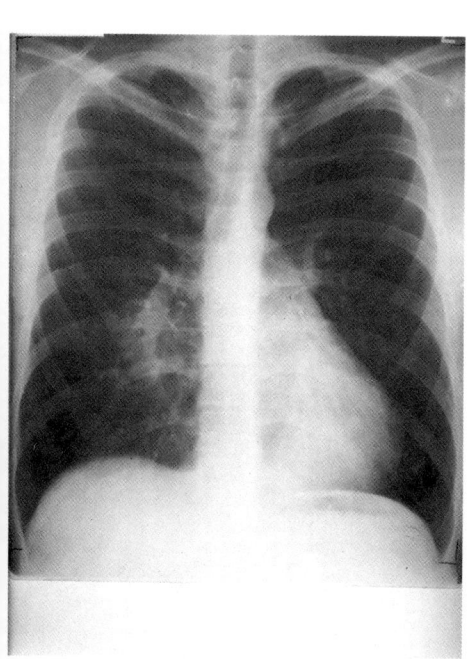

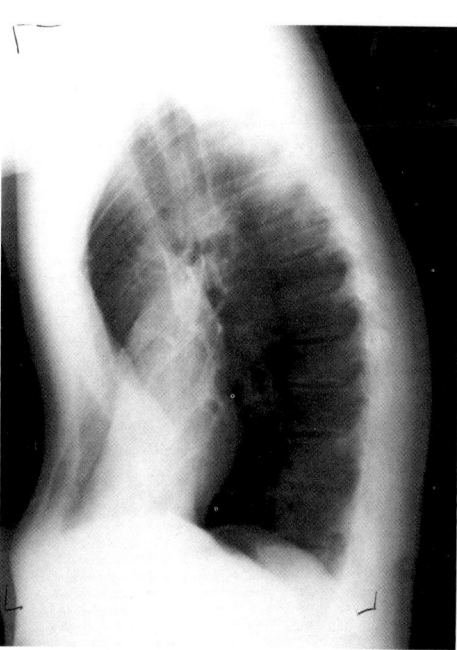

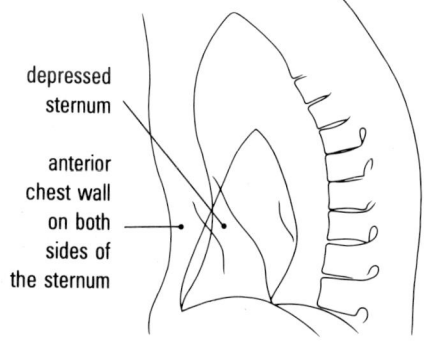

depressed sternum

anterior chest wall on both sides of the sternum

Fig. 1.9 Pectus excavatum (depressed sternum). The frontal view shows displacement of the heart to the left and a relative translucency in the centre of the lower part of the chest. The lateral view confirms the severe depression of the lower end of the sternum, which can be seen through the heart shadow.

Oblique Radiographs

A 50° oblique projection is often of value in showing lesions in the mediastinum and in the hila and major bronchi (Figs 1.10 and 1.11). Oblique views are essential in demonstrating lesions in the ribs and chest wall. It is often of great help to obtain views in different degrees of obliquity, by using a fluoroscopic machine and taking spot films to demonstrate lesions in the ribs and also in the lung or pleura, close to the chest wall.

Lateral Decubitus Views

Lateral decubitus radiographs are taken using a horizontal X-ray beam with the patient lying on his side. In these views free fluid can be demonstrated in the pleural space or cavities, shifting with change of position.

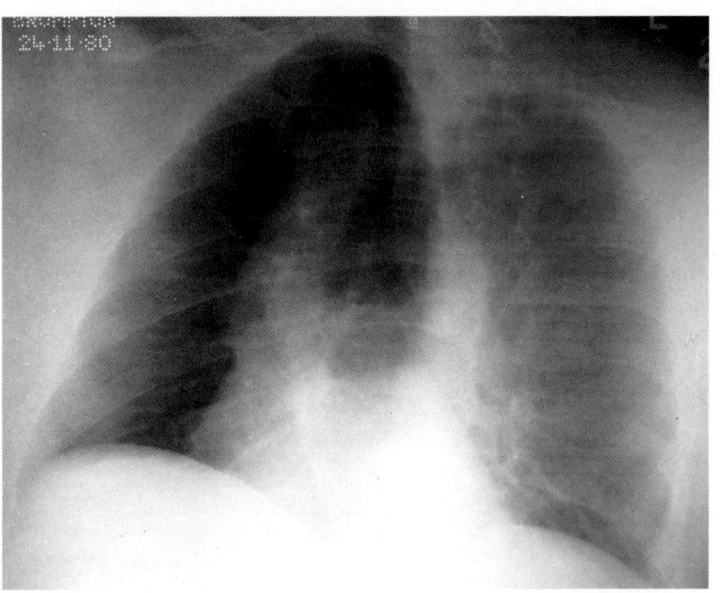

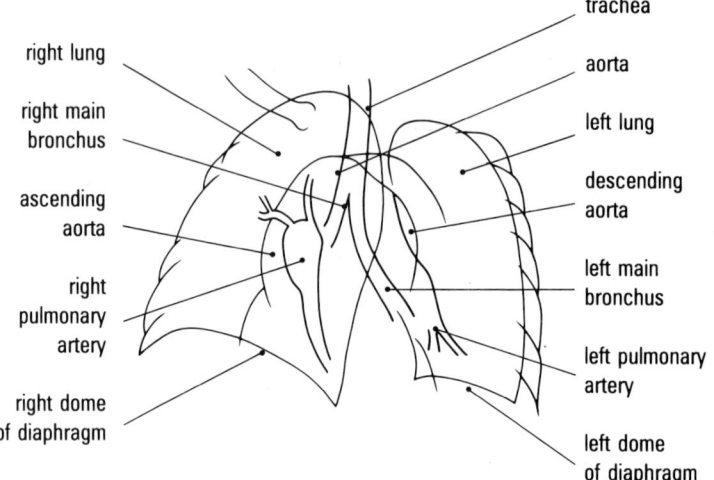

Fig. 1.10 Left anterior oblique projection.

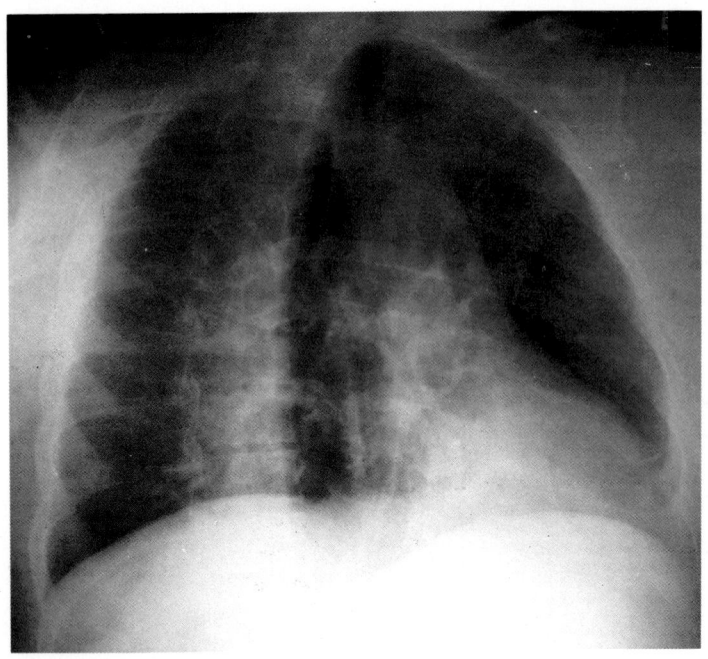

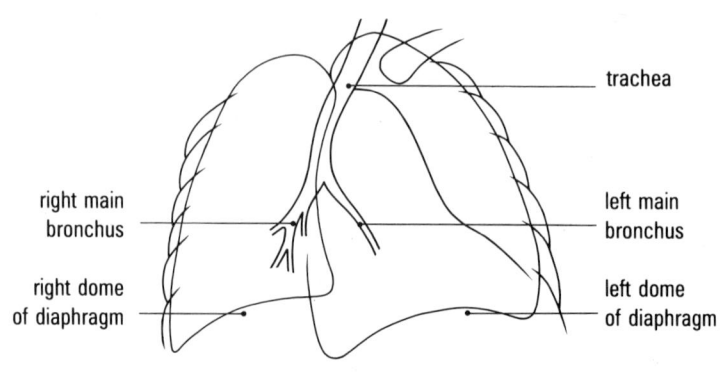

Fig. 1.11 Right anterior oblique projection.

8

Apical Views

The apices of the lungs are often obscured on the frontal radiograph by the upper ribs and clavicle, but may be seen by angling the X-ray tube by 30°, or by placing the patient in the lordotic position. The clavicle is then projected outside the lung field (Fig. 1.12).

Inspiration and Expiration Radiographs

A frontal radiograph taken on full expiration may be compared with that taken on full inspiration to show diaphragmatic movement (Fig. 1.13). Air trapping may also be demonstrated in the lungs or in a pneumothorax by this technique.

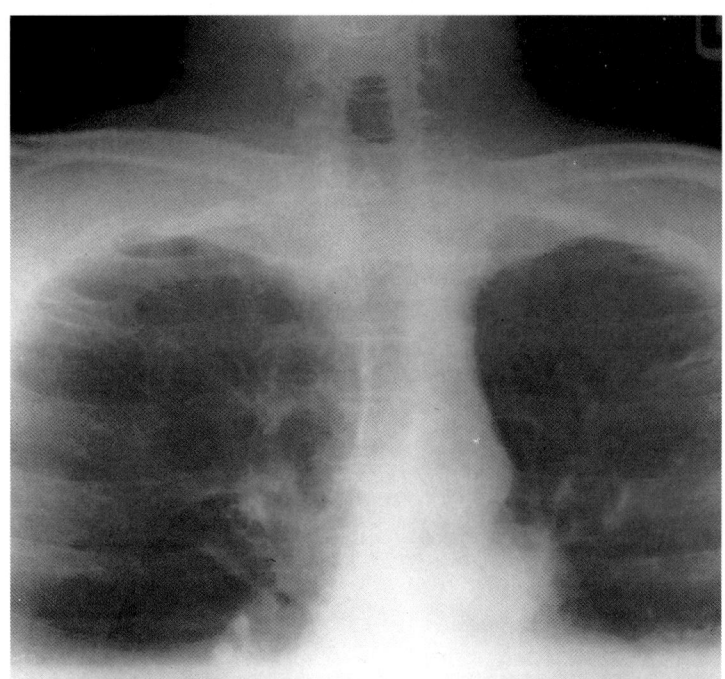

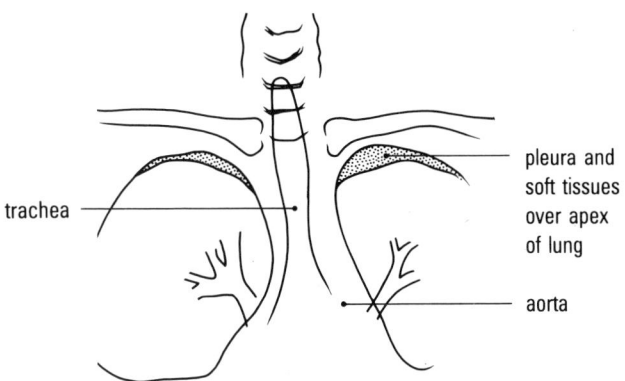

Fig. 1.12 Apical view. The patient is in a lordotic position, so that the clavicles are projected over the soft tissues of the neck rather than the apices of the lungs.

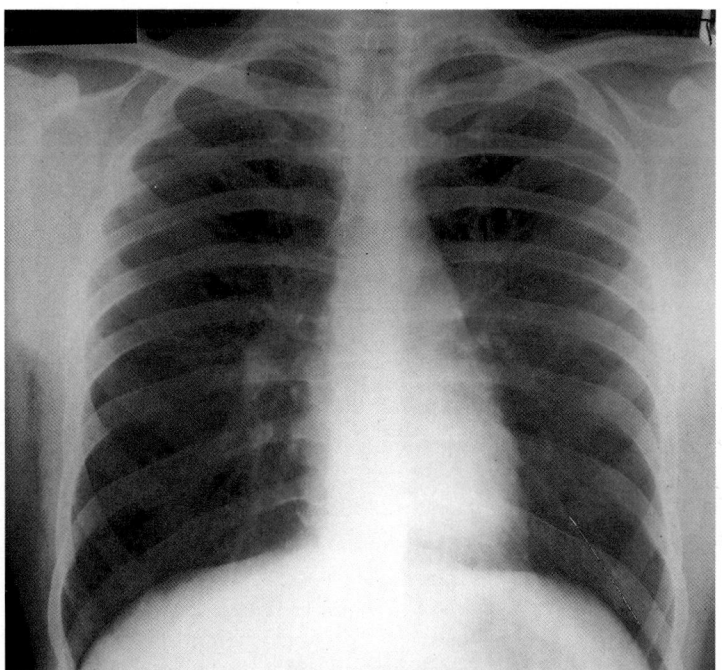

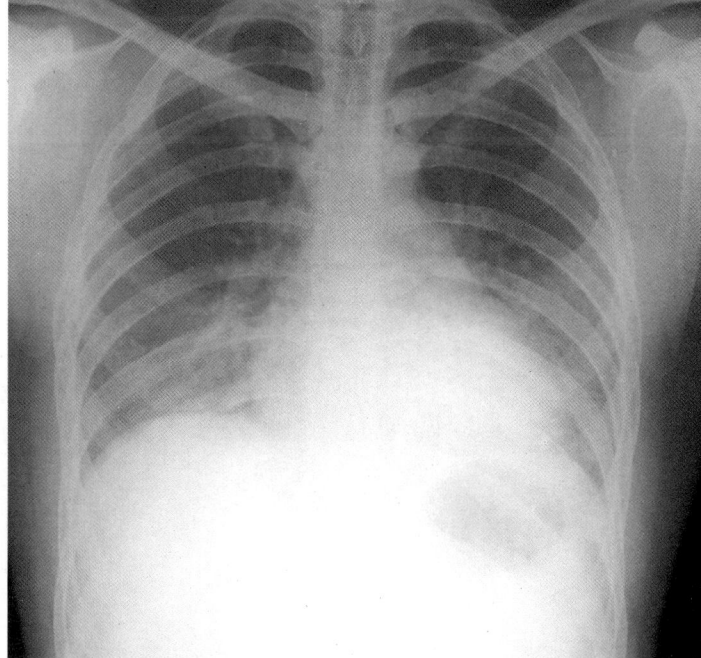

Fig. 1.13 Inspiration (left) and expiration (right) radiographs of the chest. Note the change in heart shape.

Barium Swallow

Lesions in the mediastinum may displace the oesophagus; their extent and position can be assessed by a barium swallow with radiographs taken in frontal, lateral and oblique positions (Fig. 1.14). The normal oesophagus is deviated to the right by the arch of the aorta and then passes gently forward and to the left, around the posterior border of the heart. It reaches the oesophageal hiatus slightly in front and to the left of the aorta as they both pass through the diaphragm. Tumours in the mediastinum, or congenital anatomical variants such as a right-sided aortic arch (Fig. 1.15), cause deviation and displacement of the barium column. Abnormalities within the oesophagus itself, achalasia and hiatus hernia, may also be revealed by a barium swallow.

Tomography

By a coordinated movement of the X-ray tube together with movement of the film in an appropriate direction and distance, an image of a plane within the body can be obtained. Objects in front of and behind this plane are blurred. By this simple method, images of slices of the lung and mediastinum may be obtained without their being obscured by the chest wall. The motion of the tube and radiograph provides a pivot. The position of the pivot determines the level of the layer to be examined and the angles at which the tube moves determines the thickness of the layer examined: the larger the angle, the thinner the layer of clarity. By positioning the thorax, tomograms in the coronal or sagittal plane or oblique slices through the chest (Figs 1.16–1.20) can be obtained.

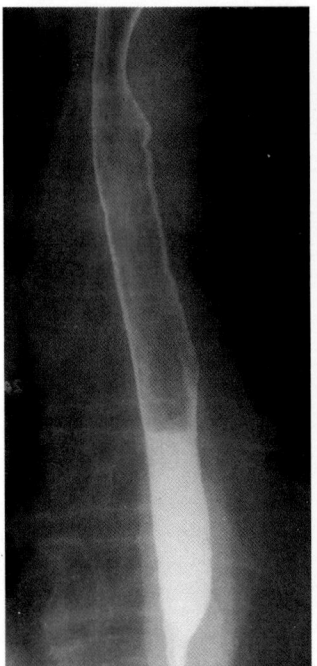
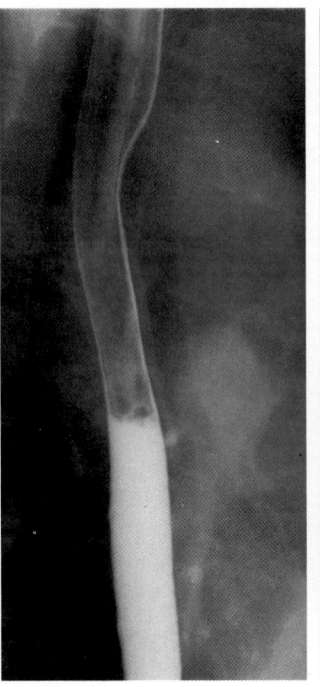
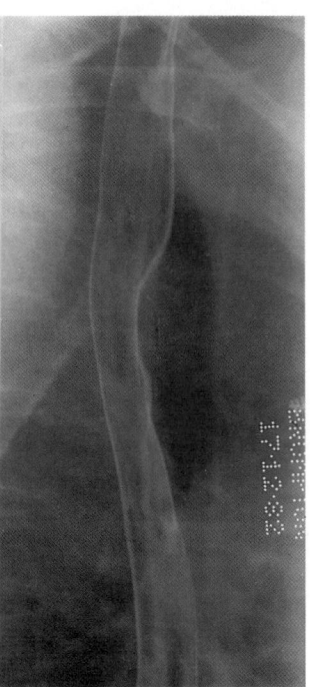
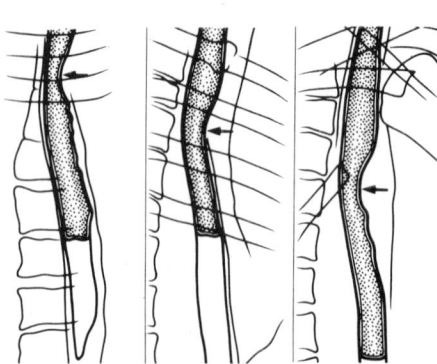

impression of aorta

Fig. 1.14 Normal oesophagus shown by barium swallow: frontal (left), right anterior oblique (middle), lateral (right) projections.

The image produced in tomography is affected by the type of movement. The simplest and most commonly used type is linear tomography, when the tube and the film move in a straight line, usually in the long axis of the patient. Lesions in the lung are shown clearly by this method but opacities lying in the plane of movement are not blurred and are reproduced at many levels. Thus the shadow produced by the dorsal spine causes a density overlying the mediastinum, for the dorsal spine, although blurred, always remains in the line of tube movement. Rotational movement of the tube blurs superimposed shadows in all directions.

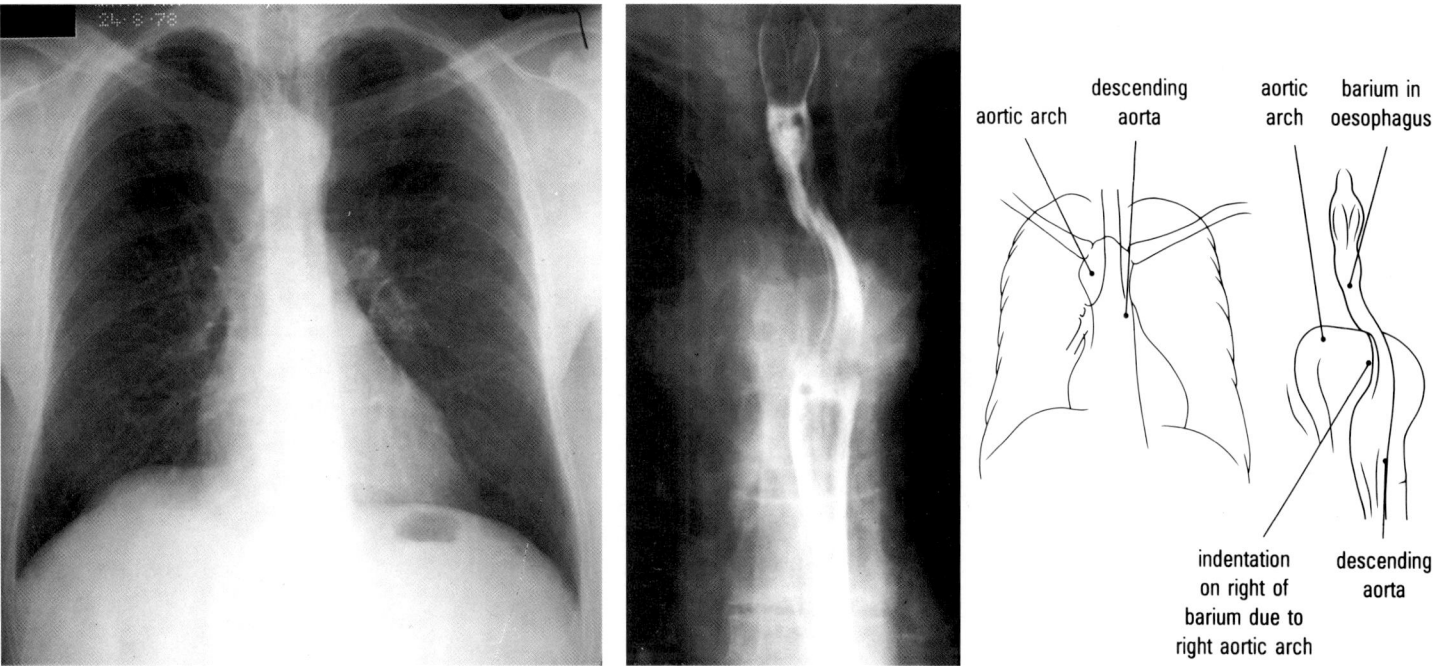

Fig. 1.15 Right-sided aortic arch. Plain frontal radiograph (left); barium swallow (right). The descending aorta is on the left, so that the arch passes to the right and then behind the oesophagus. In many instances the arch and descending aorta are both on the right.

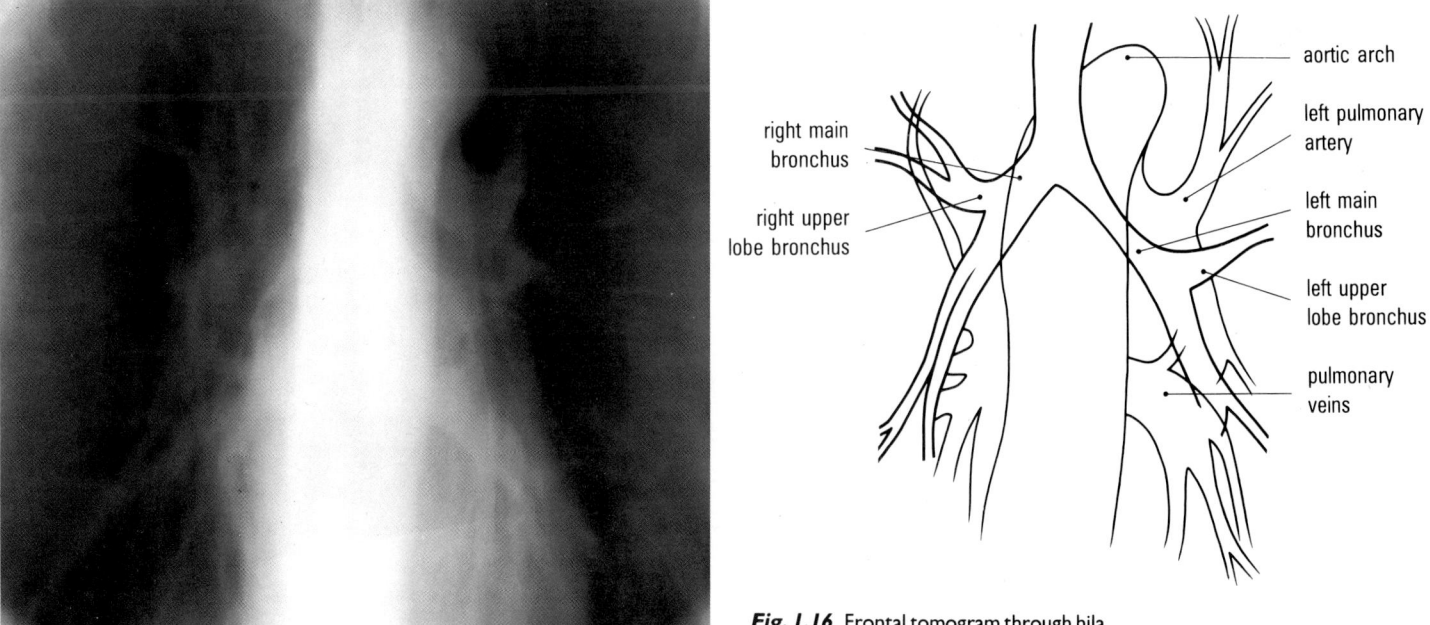

Fig. 1.16 Frontal tomogram through hila.

11

Computed tomography

Computed tomography (CT) again involves the principle of movement of the X-ray beam around the patient, although in this case the detector of radiation is not an X-ray film but a scintillation crystal. The signals received by this detector are processed by a computer and depend upon variations in absorption of the X-ray beam as it passes through the subject. The image is reconstructed by the computer, forming a picture which represents a cross-sectional slice of the body. CT provides the third dimension to the frontal and lateral views. Again, images are formed because of the different absorption of calcium, soft tissues,

fat and air, but the technique is much more sensitive to minor differences in density than conventional methods. The great advantage of CT is the ability to manipulate the image stored in the computer, so that one may visualize the structures in the spine, the mediastinum or the lungs after examination of the patient has been completed. This manipulation is called 'window setting'.

The interpretation of CT of the thorax, as elsewhere in the body, depends on knowledge of the normal anatomy, now in cross-section. CT is ideal for demonstrating the mediastinum. Above the level of the aortic arch, the head, neck and upper limb vessels are seen in front of the trachea (Fig. 1.21). Behind the trachea lies the oesophagus.

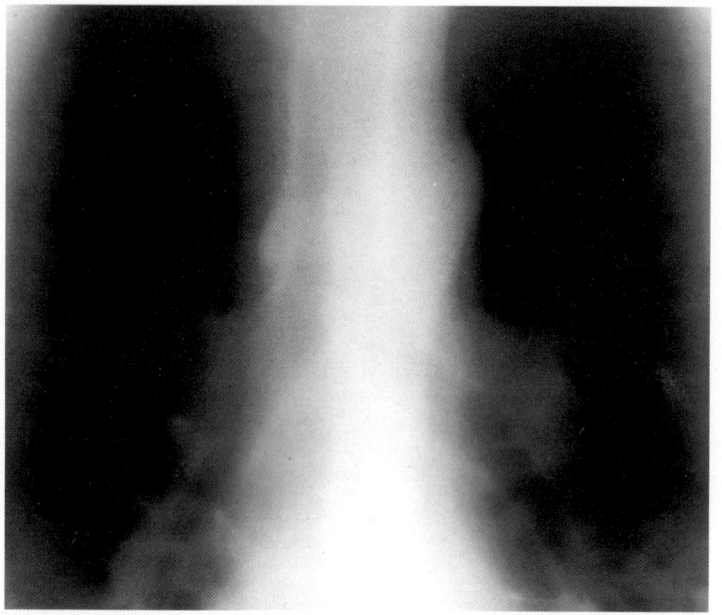

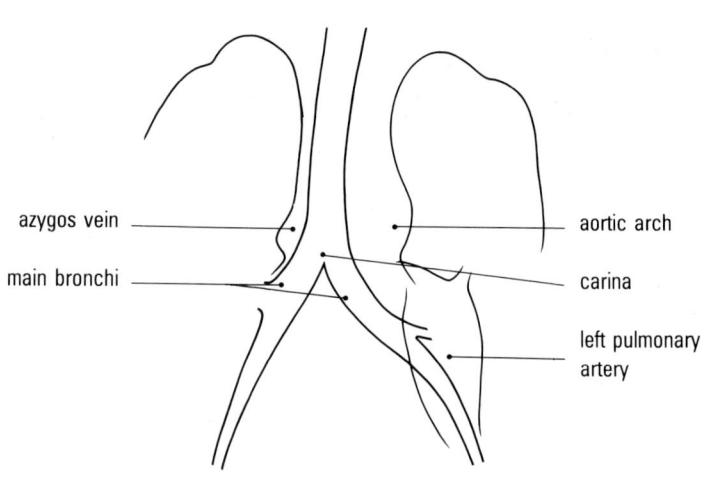

Fig. 1.17 Frontal tomogram through hila but just behind Fig. 1.16.

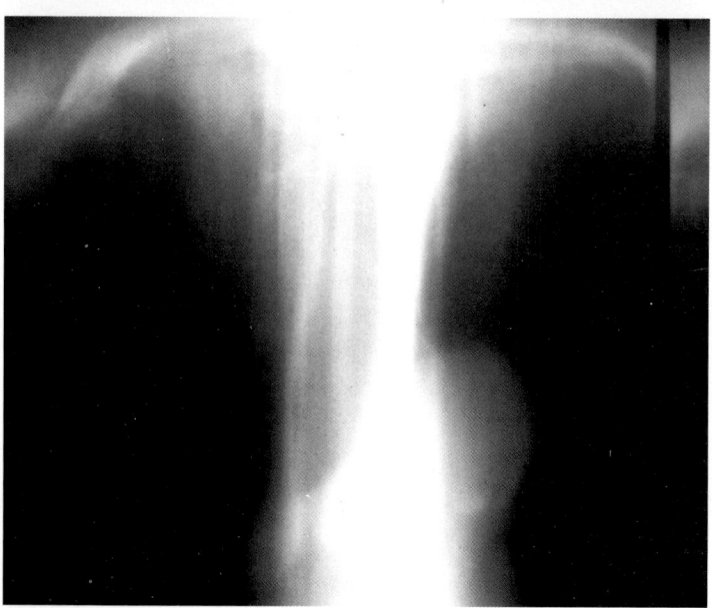

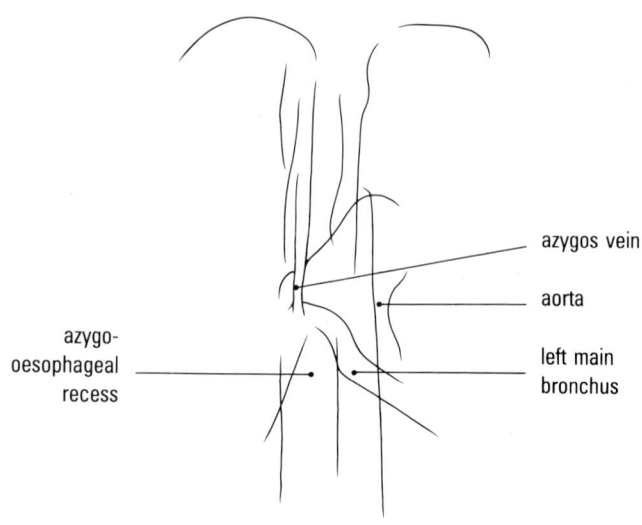

Fig. 1.18 Frontal tomogram behind hila.

At the level of the tracheobronchial angle, the azygos vein can be identified arching forward to join the superior vena cava. The bifurcation of the trachea is seen below the level of the arch of the aorta. Above the left main bronchus, the left pulmonary artery is seen passing backwards to lie just in front and to the left of the descending aorta (Fig. 1.22, upper). Just below this level the right pulmonary artery passes to the right in front of the right main bronchus (Fig. 1.22, lower). The left main bronchus lies just in front of the oesophagus and descending aorta. Below the right pulmonary artery the left atrium is seen at the back of the heart, with the pulmonary veins entering from each lung. The superior vena cava lies to the right, at first in front of the trachea, and in front of the right pulmonary artery, before reaching the right atrium.

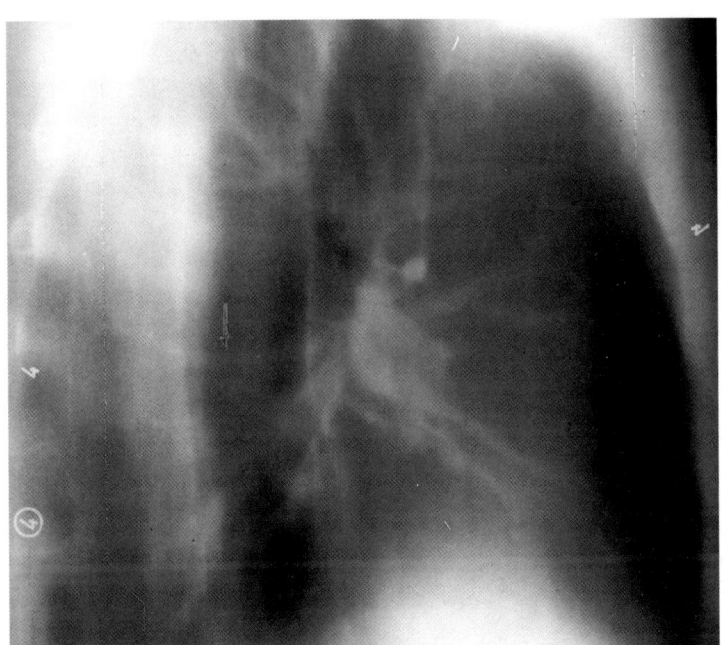

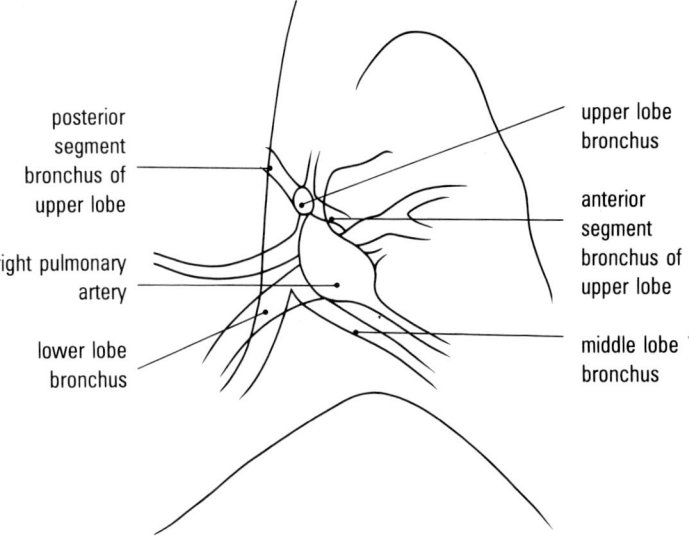

Fig. 1.19 Lateral tomogram through right hilum. The pulmonary artery lies in front of the bronchus.

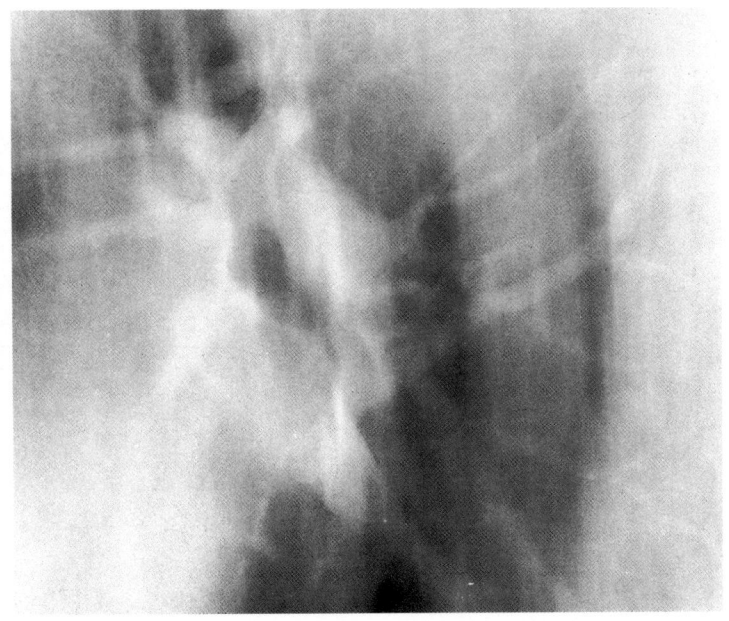

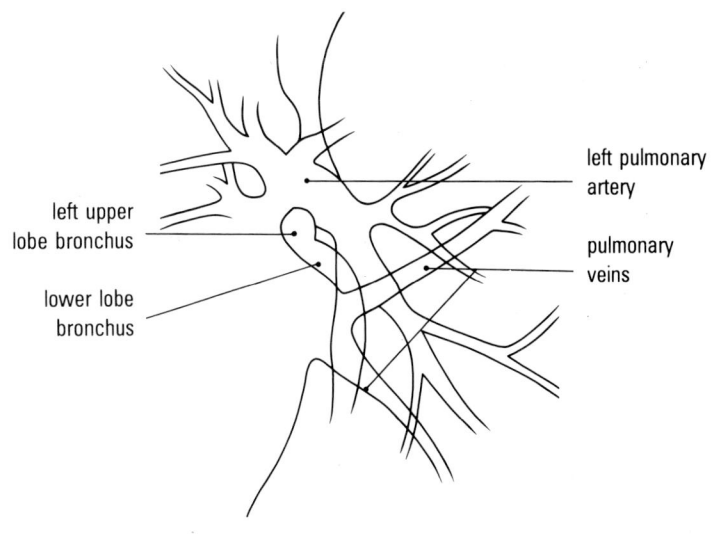

Fig. 1.20 Lateral tomogram through left hilum. The pulmonary artery lies behind the bronchus.

13

The pericardial fat often clearly outlines the pericardium and, at the level of the diaphragm, the inferior vena cava can be seen running upwards to the right atrium (Fig. 1.23).

The mediastinal structures are outlined by fat, but the vessels can be enhanced by intravenous injection of contrast medium. Lymph nodes can be seen in the mediastinal fat, and are normally less than 1cm in diameter. Injection of contrast medium helps in distinguishing vessels from lymph nodes.

Different window settings give images on which the structures in the lungs are seen (Fig. 1.21, lower). The vessels are visible, and any pathological process occurring in the lung can be seen. As on the plain radiograph, bronchi are not normally visible for more than 2–3cm from the hila. The pleura may be seen to be separated from the chest wall by extrapleural fat. Pleural lesions including effusions are readily demonstrated. Lesions in the ribs may be more difficult to see, as each rib, being oblique to the transverse plane, is only partly seen in each section.

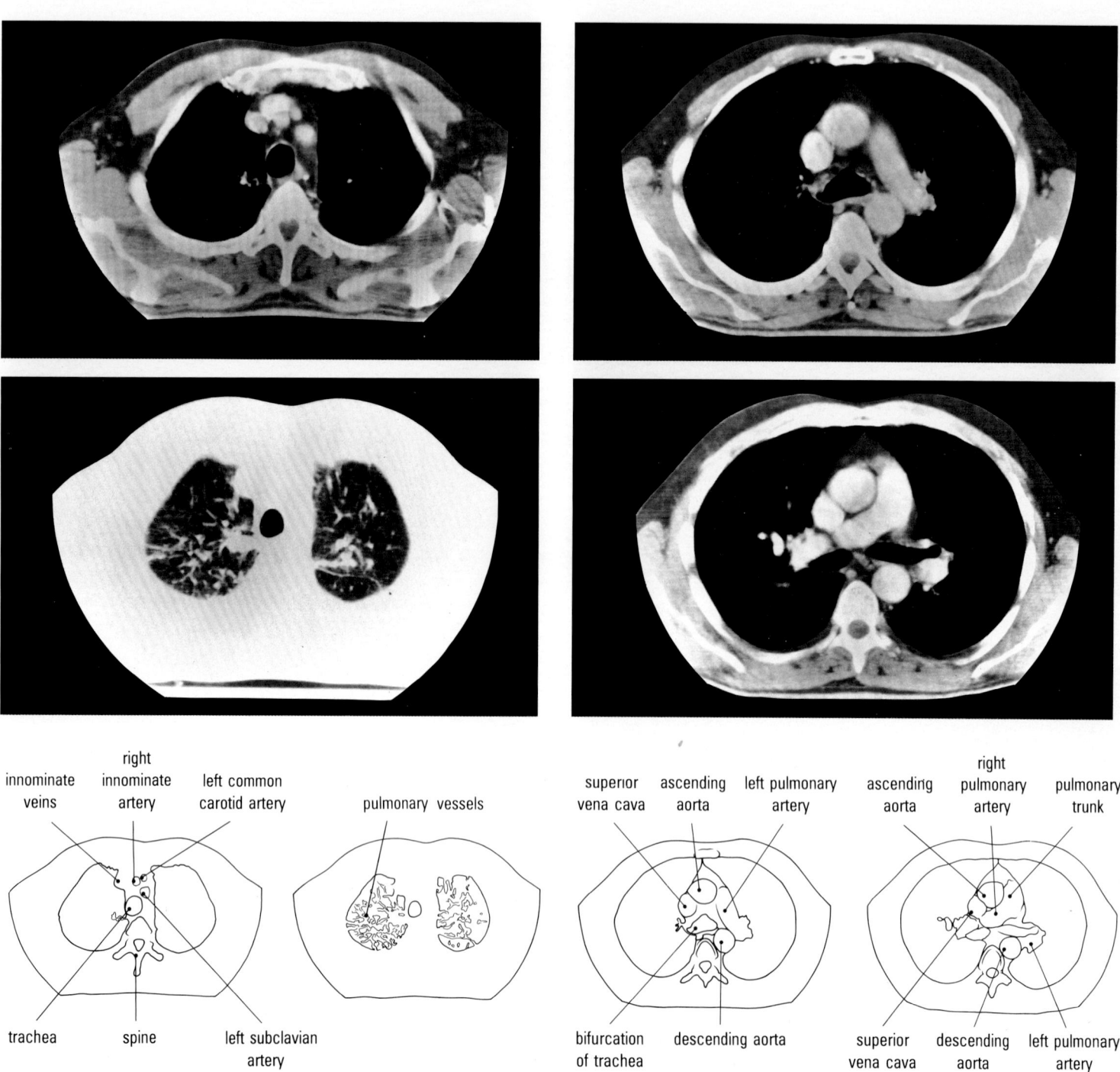

Fig. 1.21 CT scan of superior mediastinum above the aortic arch (upper) and with window setting to show lungs (lower).

Fig. 1.22 CT scan at level of the carina showing left pulmonary artery (upper). At a lower level the right pulmonary artery is shown (lower).

Bronchography

Injection of radiographic contrast material into the trachea outlines the trachea, major bronchi and bronchial tree (Fig. 1.24). The trachea begins at the larynx and passes downwards in the midline, to enter the thorax just behind the manubrium sterni. In the upper part of the mediastinum the trachea lies in the midline or just to the right of it, and passes slightly backwards at an angle of about 15° to the coronal plane. As the trachea enters the chest it is related on either side to the common carotid arteries and posteriorly to the oesophagus. Anteriorly it is separated from the manubrium by the pretracheal fascia in which lie the inferior thyroid veins. In the upper part of the mediastinum the left innominate vein and, below this, the arch of the aorta pass in front of the trachea.

The innominate vein and left common carotid artery arising from the arch of the aorta lie in front of the trachea as they diverge to ascend into the neck. The oesophagus separates the trachea from the vertebral column. The trachea is indented on the left side at its lower end by the arch of the aorta and slightly on the right side and posteriorly by the azygos vein. The recurrent laryngeal nerves ascend one on each side between the trachea and the oesophagus. The trachea ends by bifurcating at the level of the fourth dorsal vertebra, just below the level of the aortic arch. The right main bronchus descends in the same line as the trachea, deviating only 20–30° to the right. The left main bronchus, however, passes to the left at an angle of 45–55° with the median plane and also inclines slightly backwards. The carinal angle varies with the build of the patient, being widest in the short thick-set and narrowest in the asthenic person. The carinal angle may vary from 50° to 100°. The right main bronchus is about 2.5cm long and 1.5cm in diameter. The left main bronchus is approximately 5cm long and 1.3cm in diameter. The longer and narrower left main bronchus is thus more vulnerable to occlusion by compression from surrounding lesions.

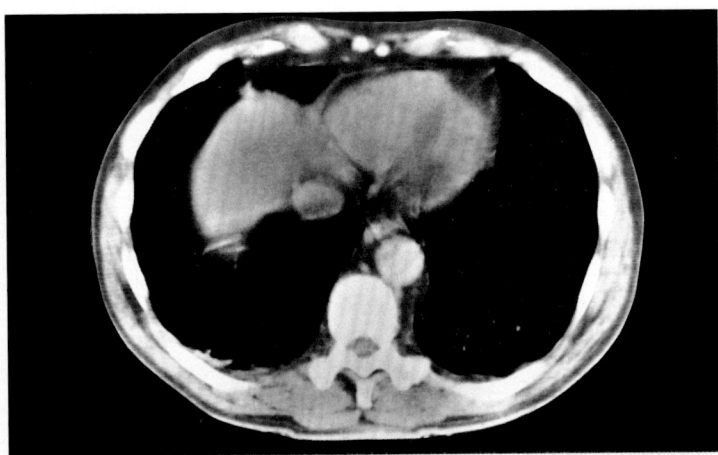

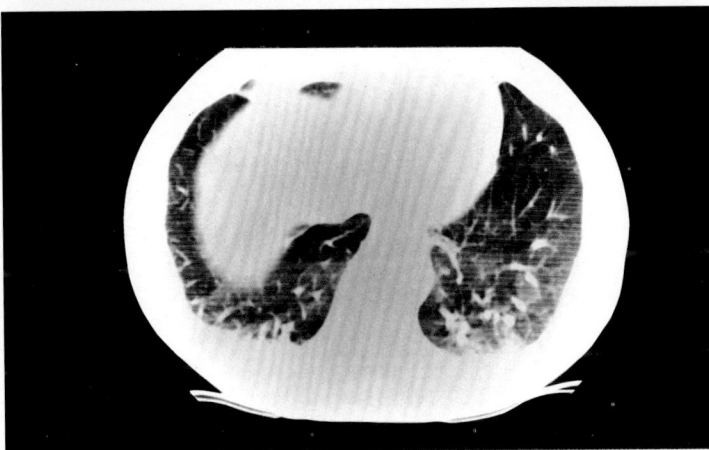

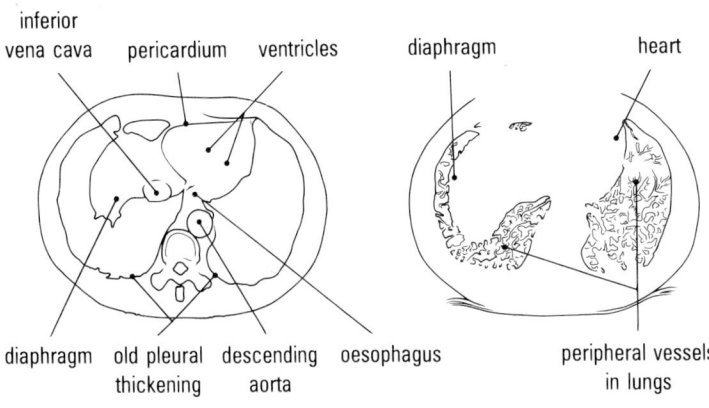

Fig. 1.23 CT scan of chest just above the diaphragm: mediastinal window setting (upper) and lung window setting (lower).

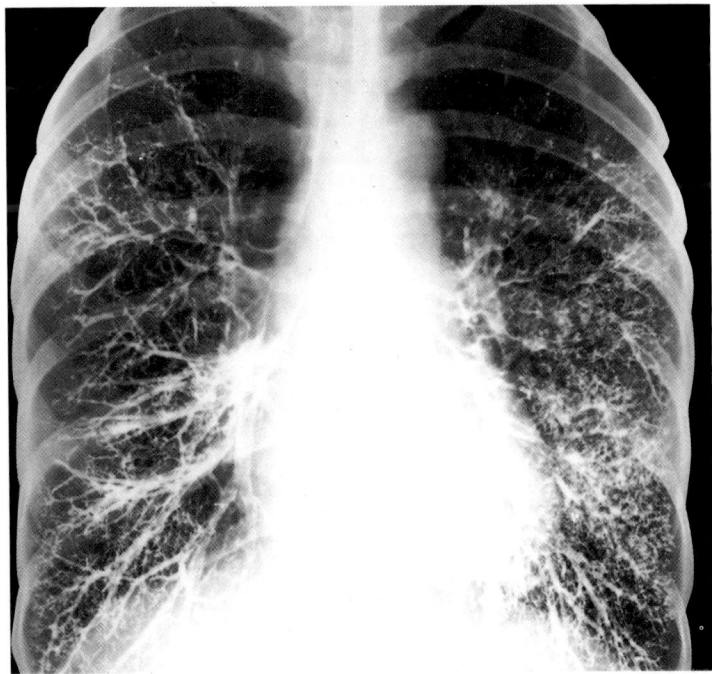

Fig. 1.24 Normal bronchogram: frontal view.

15

Right bronchial tree

The right upper lobe bronchus arises from the right main bronchus just where the airway enters the lung. The right upper lobe bronchus passes laterally in the coronal plane and is approximately 1cm long, ending by dividing into three segmental bronchi (Fig. 1.25). There is occasional variation in the branching but, in general, the apical bronchus arises first and passes vertically upwards to supply the apical segment of the lung. The anterior segmental bronchus passes forwards and slightly laterally to supply the anterior segment and, lastly, the posterior segmental bronchus passes laterally backwards and upwards to the posterior segment. The upper lobe arteries lie anterior to the right main bronchus and the upper lobe bronchus. After the origin of the upper lobe bronchus, the right main bronchus continues in a straight line as the intermediate bronchus. This is approximately 2–3cm long and lies behind the right pulmonary artery. Just below the right pulmonary artery the middle lobe bronchus passes forwards and slightly laterally. Within 1–2cm, the middle lobe bronchus divides into medial and lateral segmental branches. Proximity of the right pulmonary artery to the middle lobe bronchus often gives rise to the impression on lateral tomograms and in bronchograms of compression and narrowing of the first part of the middle lobe bronchus. Directly opposite the middle lobe bronchus and passing posteriorly in the sagittal plane is the bronchus of the apical segment of the lower lobe. The lower lobe bronchus below this divides into four basal segmental bronchi: viewed from the front, these lie in the order anterior,

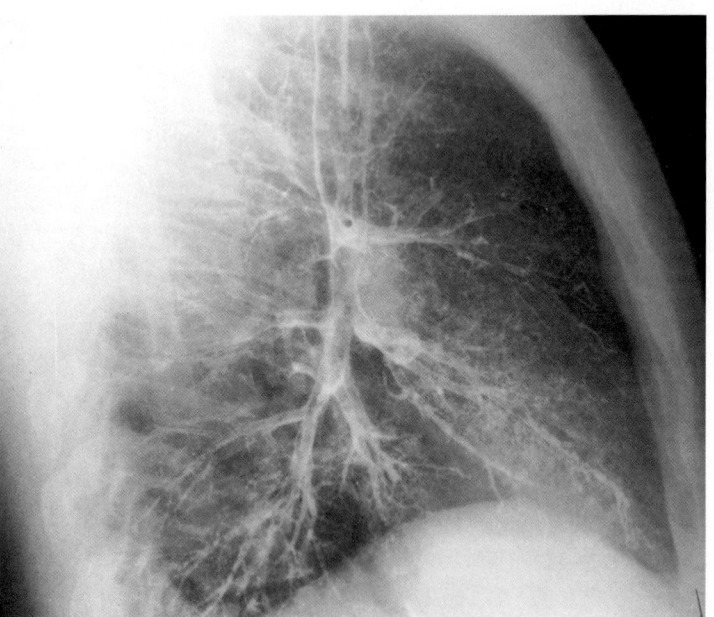

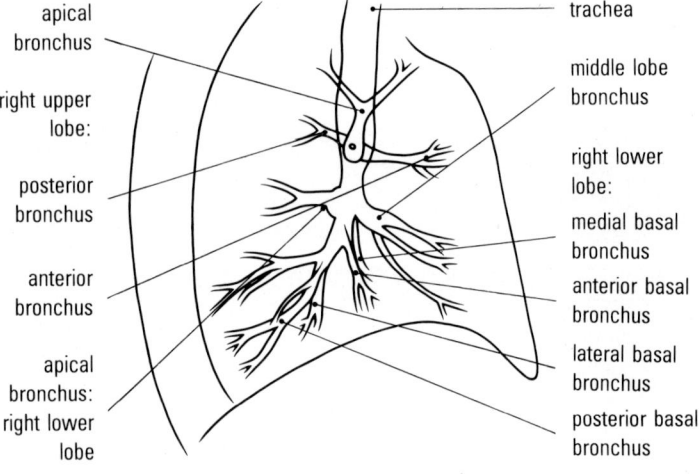

Fig. 1.25 Normal bronchogram of right lung: lateral view.

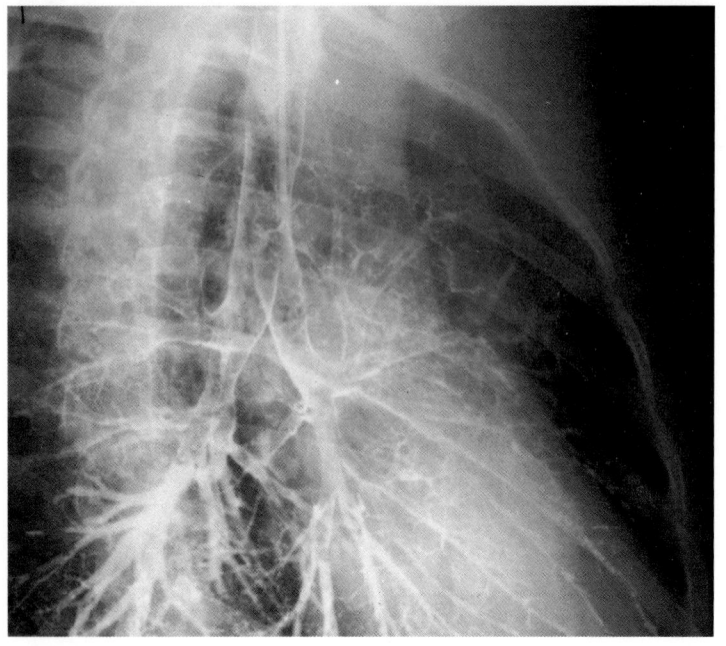

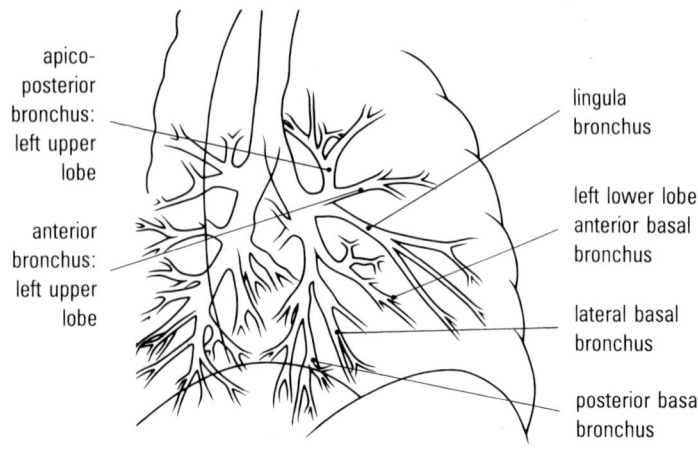

Fig. 1.26 Normal bronchogram: left posterior oblique position.

lateral, posterior and medial; viewed from the side, they are anterior, medial, lateral and posterior.

Left bronchial tree

The left main bronchus is narrower and longer than the right and passes below the arch of the aorta to the root of the left lung, which it enters opposite the sixth dorsal vertebra. Here the left pulmonary artery loops over the bronchus to lie behind it. The upper wall of the left atrium lies inferiorly and medially to the left main bronchus (Fig. 1.26). The upper lobe bronchus arises from the lateral aspect of the left main bronchus. After 1cm it divides, giving rise to the lingular bronchus. The lingular bronchus runs forwards, downwards and laterally, branching into two divisions: superior and inferior. After giving off the lingular bronchus, the lobar bronchus bifurcates into: the anterior segmental bronchus, which runs forwards and slightly laterally, and the apicoposterior bronchus, which runs vertically and slightly posteriorly. The left lower lobe bronchus continues downwards, laterally and backwards. Immediately after its origin the bronchus of the apical segment of the lower lobe arises and passes directly backwards. The lower lobe bronchus then divides into anterior, lateral and posterior segmental branches. Variations of this normal pattern of the bronchial tree are not infrequent.

In the lung the airway divides into two sorts of pathways: the axial pathway, which runs the longest course within the segment, passing directly from the hilum of the lung to the most distal pleural surface; and the collateral pathway, which supplies the regions between the hilum and the distal pleural surface. In the axial pathway the bronchi divide regularly at a relatively acute angle but in the collateral pathway the bronchi divide roughly at right angles. Towards the periphery, in the region of the small bronchi and the larger bronchioli, the airway divides at intervals of 0.5–1cm until near the end where the branches cccur nearly every 2 or 3mm. These appearances on bronchography have been called, respectively, the centimetre and millimetre patterns. The distal limit of the bronchial tree is represented by the respiratory bronchiole, but on bronchography contrast medium is not usually seen beyond the terminal bronchiole, which is the airway immediately before the respiratory bronchiole.

Pulmonary Arteriography

Contrast medium injected through a catheter into the main pulmonary trunk outlines the pulmonary arterial tree and the pulmonary veins (Fig. 1.27). The pulmonary trunk arises from the infundibulum of the right ventricle, and the pulmonary valve lies behind the left third costal cartilage near the left border of the sternum. The pulmonary trunk runs upwards and backwards in front and to the left of the ascending aorta. It then divides under the aortic arch at the level of the fifth thoracic vertebra into left and right pulmonary arteries. Throughout its length the pulmonary trunk lies within the pericardium.

The right pulmonary artery (Fig. 1.27) reaches the lung by passing horizontally to the right above the upper margin of the left atrium, behind the ascending aorta and in front of the oesophagus. It reaches the lung anterior to the right intermediate bronchus between the upper and middle lobe bronchi. It gives rise to its largest branch, the truncus anterior which supplies the upper lobe, and then lies on the lateral aspect of the bronchus as the pars interlobaris until the arteries of the middle lobe and apical segments of the lower lobe take origin. From this point the artery

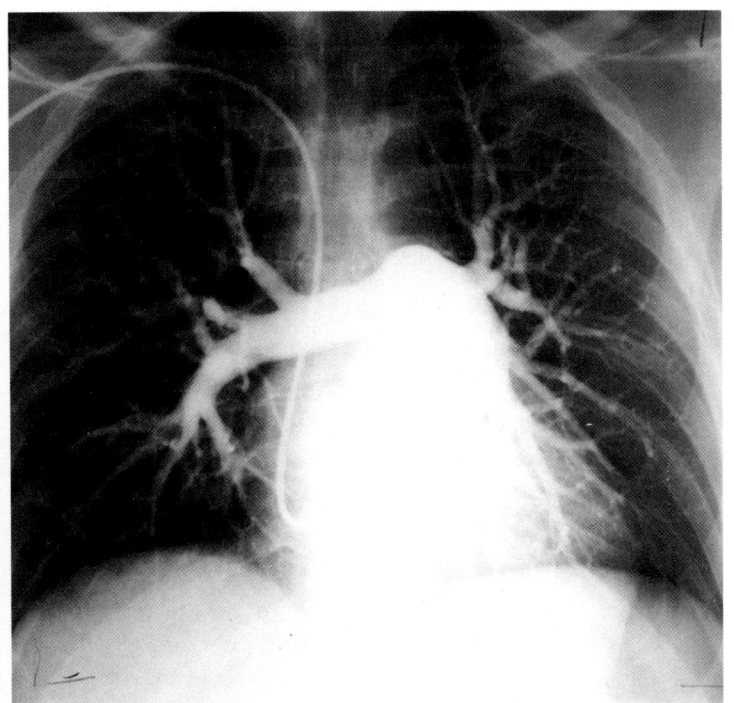

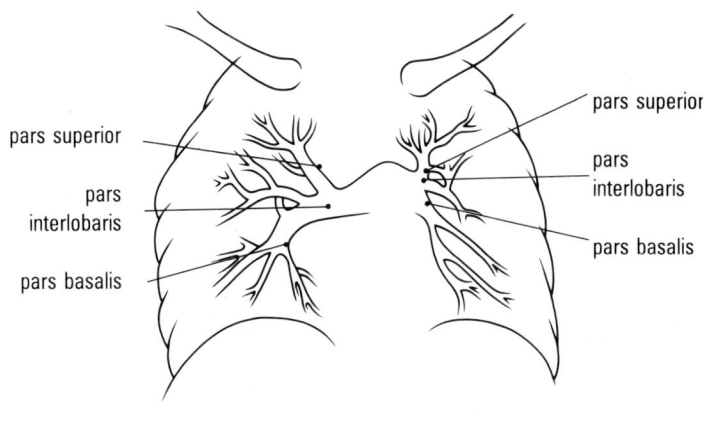

Fig. 1.27 Normal pulmonary arteriogram: arterial phase.

continues to descend as the pars basalis on the antero-lateral side of the bronchus, to supply the basal segments of the lower lobe.

The left pulmonary artery is shorter than the right. It arches backwards over the left main bronchus as the pars superior and pars interlobaris to reach the left lung. It then descends, lying posterolateral to the bronchus as the pars basalis to reach the lower lobe. There is no definite truncus anterior on the left side, the upper lobe being supplied by a variable number of small branches arising from the outer aspect of the pulmonary artery as it curves posteriorly and downwards over the left main bronchus.

The hilar shadows of the lung obtain their characteristic shape on the plain frontal radiograph from these arteries, though on the right side the hilum is also partly composed of the descending upper lobe veins. The right hilar shape is that of a wide-angled V, with the apex pointing to the left; the pars interlobaris and par basalis form the inferior arm and the truncus anterior and descending upper lobe vein form the superior arm. On the left side the hilum is shaped like a long flat comma produced by shadows of the pars superior, the pars interlobaris and the pars basalis. The small upper lobe arteries arise from the outer curve of the comma.

In the lung the arteries accompany the bronchi and branch together with the airways. Arteries gradually diminish in calibre, in proportion to their distance from the hilum. Vessels are normally straight or gently curved and not tortuous. At any equivalent level of generation of branching, lower lobe arteries are wider than those in the upper lobes. Any branch has a diameter less than the stem, but the sum of the diameters of all the branches exceeds the stem diameter.

Two types of arterial branches are visible: bifurcations, where the stem divides into two branches of almost equal size at an angle of 10–60°; and collateral branching, where the stem divides into two unequal branches, one of which is almost as large as the stem and the other much smaller. The larger branch runs in the same direction as the stem, but the smaller leaves the stem at an angle of 30–80°. The pattern of branching of arteries follows that of the bronchial tree in that each bronchus is accompanied by a branch from the artery. However, studies of injected post-mortem lungs have shown that there are many more pulmonary artery branches than there are branches from the bronchial tree. These extra arterial or 'supernumerary' branches occur throughout the length of the artery, but are more numerous towards the periphery and at all levels they are more numerous than accompanying airways.

The pulmonary veins (Fig. 1.28) run in a different direction from the arteries and bronchi to reach the left atrium. On the right side the segmental veins from the middle and lower lobes join to form the inferior pulmonary vein which passes horizontally and medially into the left atrium. This is often identifiable in a plain radiograph below the hilar shadow of the right pulmonary artery. The veins of the right upper lobe vary in number, but descend in the medial direction crossing the pars interlobaris of the right pulmonary artery at the hilum and joining to enter the upper border of the right side of the left atrium just below the right hilum. On the left side the venous drainage is similar to that on the right, with segmental vessels joining to form a superior pulmonary vein and an inferior pulmonary vein entering the left atrium.

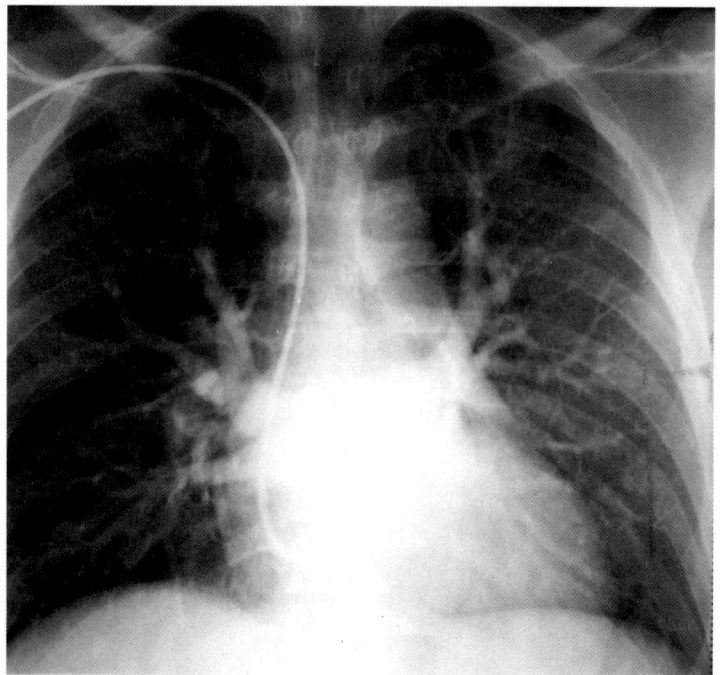

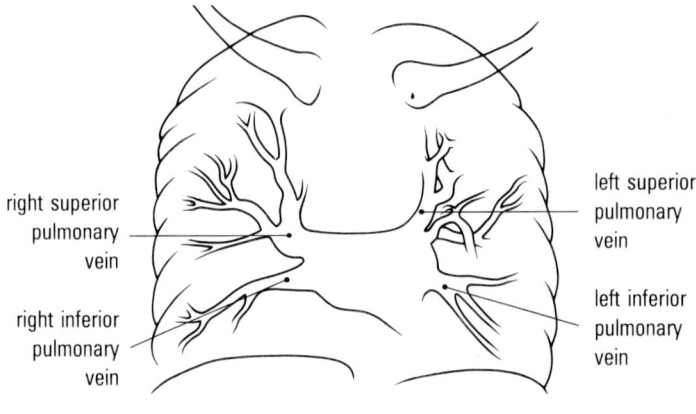

Fig. 1.28 Normal pulmonary arteriogram: venous phase.

right superior pulmonary vein

right inferior pulmonary vein

left superior pulmonary vein

left inferior pulmonary vein

In the segmental and small vessels of the lungs there is always a close relationship between vessels and bronchi. Normally the artery, bronchus and vein are found in that order proceeding anticlockwise from the vertical in the right lung and in the same order but clockwise in the left, when viewed from the front. As with the arteries, when the subject is in the erect position the veins of the upper lobe are smaller than those of the lower lobes, but in the supine position the upper lobe veins fill with blood so that there is less difference in size. In the erect position the apex of the lungs is about 15cm above the pulmonary valve; when the subject is resting, the pulmonary arterial pressure is sufficient only to cause flow through the upper part of the lungs during systole. Perfusion through the upper lobes in the normal resting subject when erect is therefore less than through the lower lobes and this is reflected in the size of the vessels as seen in the radiograph.

Aortography

The ascending aorta commences at the aortic valve, which lies behind the left side of the sternum and at the level of the fourth costal cartilage (Fig. 1.29). It passes upwards, slightly forwards and to the right, to the level of the second costal cartilage before it becomes the arch of the aorta. The arch crosses to the left in front of the spine and gives rise to the head and neck vessels. After the origin of the left subclavian artery the aorta descends to the diaphragm where it becomes the abdominal aorta. At the level of the ninth dorsal vertebra the descending aorta which has been lying to the left of the spine passes forwards and to the

right, to lie directly in front of the spine.

In the child the aortic arch is almost in the sagittal plane. With passing years, particularly beyond the ages of forty and fifty years, there is progressive degenerative change with loss of elastic fibres, and the aorta unfolds (Fig. 1.30). Before this takes place the normal aorta does not usually form part of the right side of the mediastinal outline. However, in patients with obstructive lesions in the region of the aortic valve and diseases of the aortic wall, the ascending aorta may be sufficiently dilated to form part of the right side of the mediastinal shadow.

Superior Venacavography

The superior vena cava is formed by the junction of the innominate veins (Fig. 1.31). It descends over approximately 7cm from the level of the first right costal cartilage to the third right costal cartilage where it enters the right atrium. The trachea and right vagus nerve lie postero-medially and the root of the right lung is posterior. The remainder of the superior vena cava is surrounded by the pleura and the right lung. The azygos vein passes forwards at the level of the fourth dorsal vertebra in the right tracheobronchial angle, entering the back of the superior vena cava. In about one percent of the population a small part of the apical segment of the right upper lobe develops between the azygos vein and the mediastinum as the vein loops forward, forming an azygos lobe (Fig. 1.32). The azygos vein is then seen on the frontal radiograph as a comma-like opacity at the lower end and a fissure is formed by the invaginated pleura.

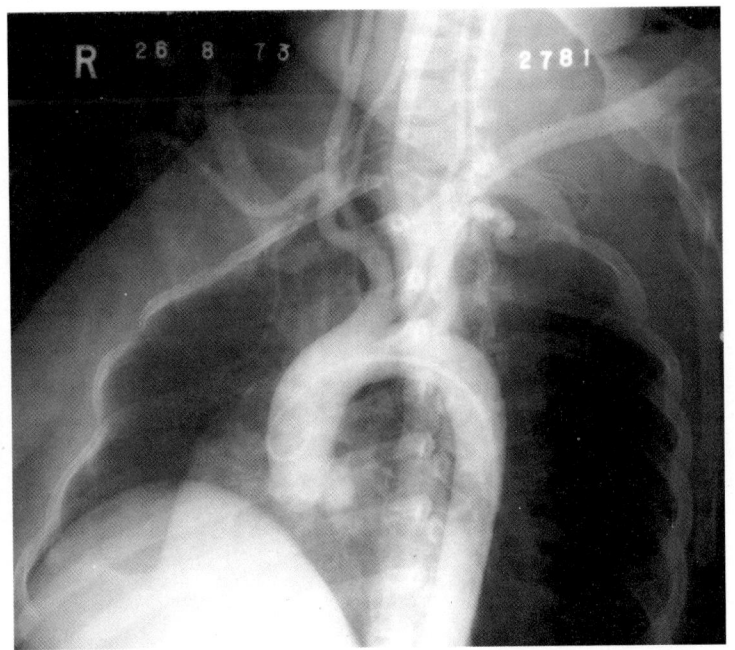

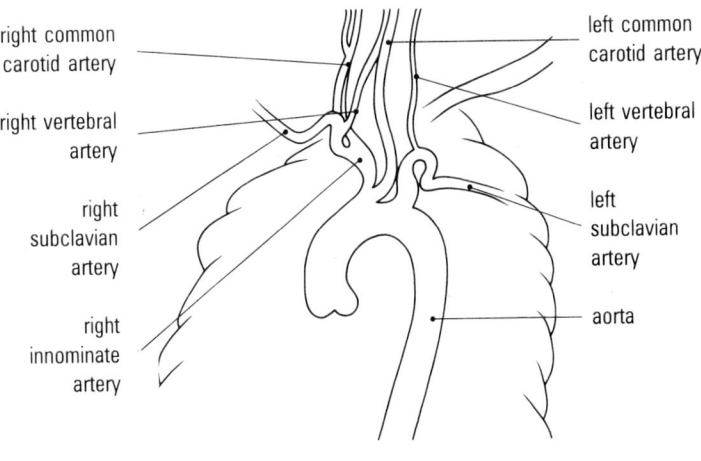

Fig. 1.29 Normal aortogram: left anterior oblique projection.

left common carotid artery

right common carotid artery

right vertebral artery

left vertebral artery

right subclavian artery

left subclavian artery

aorta

right innominate artery

The Thoracic Skeleton

The dorsal spine

There are twelve thoracic vertebrae. The vertebrae increase in size from the top to the bottom, the third vertebra being the smallest. A normal dorsal kyphosis is present and thus in the anteroposterior radiograph there is some overlapping of the vertebral bodies. The vertebral bodies are separated by relatively thin intervertebral discs. Usually the adjacent vertebral surfaces are flat, but a notch, Schmorl's node, may be visible radiologically in up to forty percent of adult spines. On the frontal view the pedicles can be clearly seen as oval rings overlying the vertebral bodies near the lateral margins; the distances between pedicles follow a regular pattern, decreasing down to the level of the fourth or fifth dorsal vertebra, and then the distances remain the same

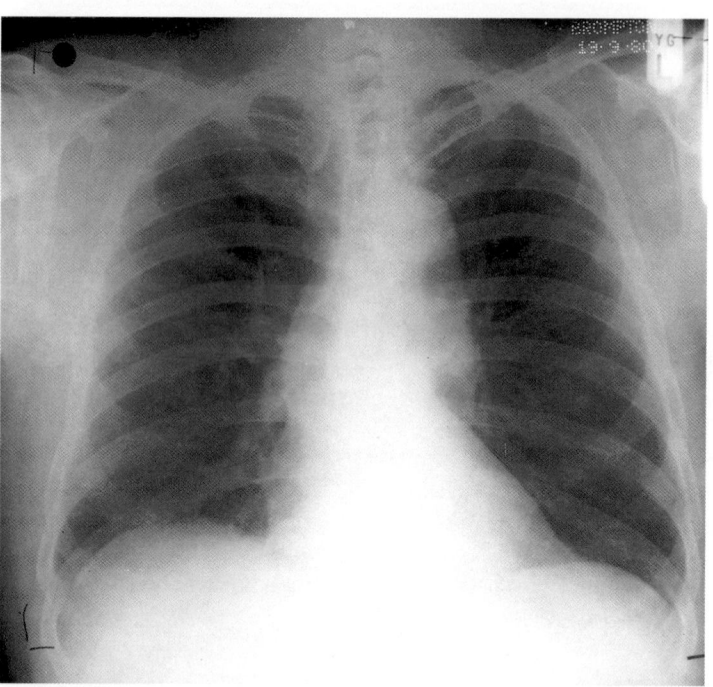

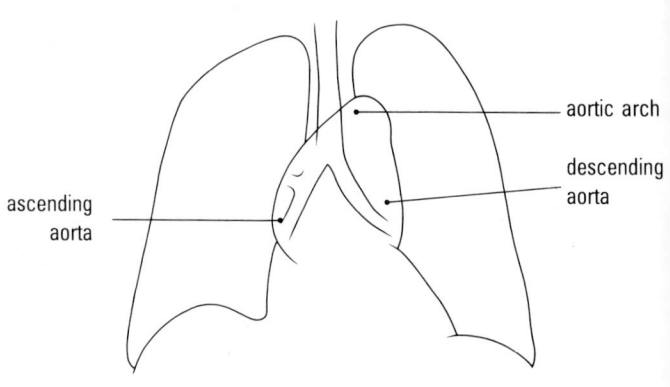

Fig. 1.30 Frontal chest radiograph showing unfolding of the aorta in an elderly patient.

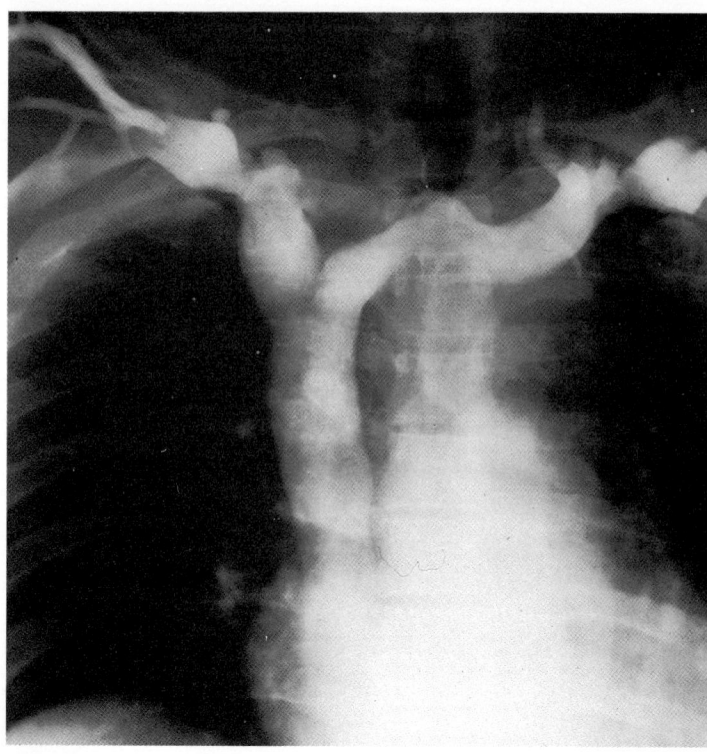

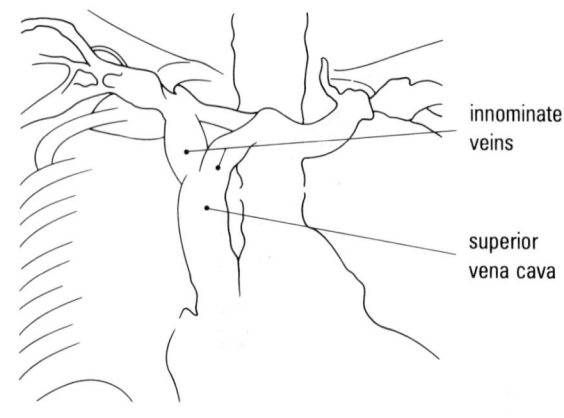

Fig. 1.31 Frontal view of normal superior venacavagram. Contrast medium is injected simultaneously into the arm veins on each side.

until the seventh or eighth vertebra where they gradually increase. The intervertebral foramina are circular and smaller than those in the cervical and lumbar regions.

The ribs

There are normally twelve pairs of ribs. The head of each rib articulates with the body of a vertebra and the tubercle of each rib articulates with a facet on the transverse process. The ribs curve around the posterior chest wall to end anteriorly in the costal cartilages. The first seven costal cartilages are inserted into the manubrium or body of the sternum. The eighth, ninth and tenth costal cartilages unite peripherally with the seventh costal cartilage, whilst the eleventh and twelfth ribs, although having cartilage tips, are not inserted and may be described as 'floating ribs'.

Opacification almost invariably occurs in the costal cartilages with increasing age. Early calcification is usually of no pathological significance and may be seen in normal children. The first costal cartilage calcifies most densely, followed by cartilages associated with the lower ribs. Different patterns of calcification are seen according to sex: in the male the upper and lower borders of the cartilage calcify, whereas in the female the calcification occurs in the centre of the cartilage. Anterior ends of the ribs widen slightly as they unite with the costal cartilages.

Anomalies of the ribs are frequent, the most frequent being a bifid anterior end to a rib (Fig. 1.3) which may be mistaken for a cavity in the underlying lung.

The sternum

On the frontal chest radiograph the upper end of the manubrium is seen, but on the lateral film the whole sternum may be visualized.

Soft tissues

In the thorax the pericardial fat pad is the most common non-pathological soft tissue shadow. It is usually found in the cardiophrenic angle on either or both sides and it can be up to several centimetres in size. Its upper and outer border is usually convex and there is usually a decrease in density from within outwards; on the lateral film it is seen at the junction of the anterior chest wall and diaphragm. The breasts usually have a clear inferior and lateral margin; however, with small or developing breasts there may be no clearly defined margin but a poorly defined opacity may be seen overlying the lower lung fields on each side.

Companion shadows

The most obvious companion shadow is that adjacent to the superior surface of the clavicle and is due to the reflection of the subcutaneous tissues passing over the clavicle into the supraclavicular fossa. It is no longer visible when there is a large mass in the supraclavicular fossa. This companion shadow becomes continuous with the outline of the sternomastoid when this is visible. Similar but less clearly defined companion shadows are visible adjacent to the inferior margins of the ribs on the inside, as they curve around the chest wall.

Diaphragm

In the majority of patients the right hemidiaphragm in inspiration lies between the anterior end of the fifth rib and the sixth anterior intercostal space. In approximately half it lies at the level of the sixth rib anteriorly, and only in a small percentage is the right hemidiaphragm at or below the level of the seventh rib. Excursion of the right

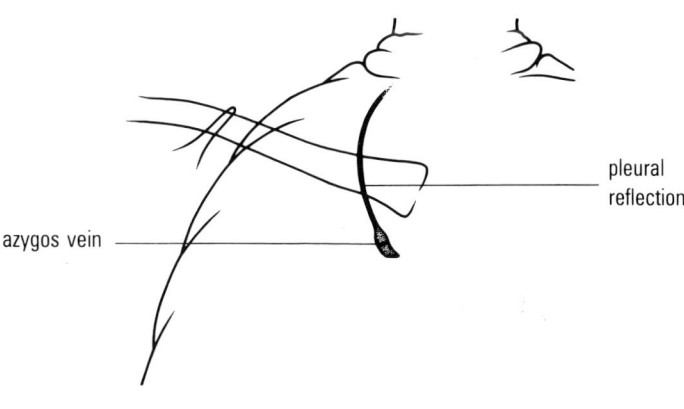

Fig. 1.32 Azygos lobe. The comma-shaped opacity of the azygos vein is at the lower end of the fissure.

hemidiaphragm in fifty percent of normal subjects is approximately 0.75cm greater than the left hemidiaphragm. In twenty-five percent of subjects the excursions are equal and in the remaining twenty-five percent the left hemidiaphragm moves about 1cm more than the right. The normal range of movement is 3–6cm and in only two to three percent of people is it greater than this. In most persons the right hemidiaphragm lies half an interspace higher (1–2cm) than the left hemidiaphragm. In approximately ten percent of cases the left hemidiaphragm is at the same level or higher than the right: gaseous distension of either the stomach or the colon is the usual cause of the elevated left dome.

Mediastinum

On the plain frontal chest radiograph the mediastinal structures form the central opacity. Alteration in shape or position of these contours usually indicates a pathological process. The heart forms a large structure within the mediastinum and its shape varies with circumstances. The pericardium is attached to the diaphragm, so that the heart takes on a relatively elongated appearance on full inspiration and a relatively transverse position in full expiration (Fig. 1.13). The normal outline of the mediastinal shadows in the postero-anterior view, commencing on the right side superiorly, is formed by the innominate vein and the superior vena cava, although these are frequently not visible in the erect position. The margin of the upper part of the mediastinum on the right is far less clearly defined than that of the left. At the level of the fourth costal cartilage the superior vena cava enters the heart and the right border is now formed by the right atrium which continues as the inferior margin of the mediastinum as far as the spine. However, just above the diaphragm the margin is formed by the extreme right edge of the hepatic veins and inferior vena cava where they enter the heart. Passing to the left from the spine the inferior border is formed by the right ventricle lying on the diaphragm to within 2–3cm of the apex of the heart when the margin becomes the left ventricle. The left ventricle constitutes the left border of the mediastinum from the apex to the fourth costal cartilage; the left atrial appendage forms a border over the next 2cm and above this lies the infundibulum of the right ventricle and the pulmonary trunk. The pulmonary trunk is often quite prominent in normal young persons, probably because of the relatively smaller size of the aorta. The superior border of the pulmonary artery is continuous with the arch of the aorta above which lies the left subclavian artery.

The thymus

The thymus lies in the anterior mediastinum. It extends upwards from the fourth costal cartilage and may reach as far as the lower cervical vertebrae. Anteriorly it is covered by the sternum and posteriorly it lies on the pericardium, the roots of the great vessels and the trachea. At birth the thymus weighs approximately 10g.

There is a steady increase in its weight, to 30–40g at puberty, but it slowly regresses with age. Radiographically the thymus becomes smaller after the end of the first year of life and by three years of age it can usually no longer be identified. It is most commonly seen as a widened upper mediastinum (Fig. 1.33), or increased shadowing on the right side of the cardiac silhouette with a sharp lateral border. In ten percent of young children the radiological appearance of the normal thymus is that of the classical sail shadow. This is most commonly visible on the right but may occasionally be on the left or, least frequently, bilateral.

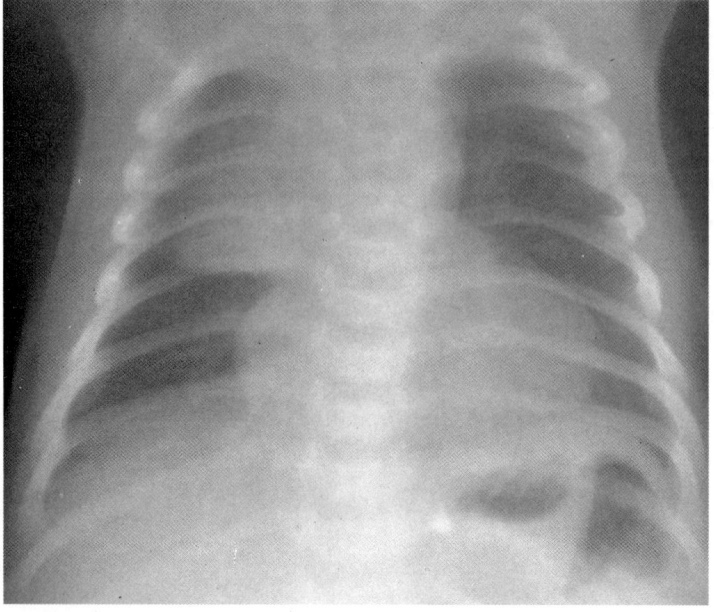

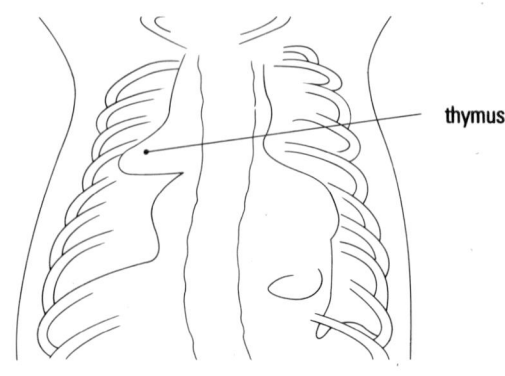

Fig. 1.33 Thymus shadow in an infant causing a clearly defined widened superior mediastinum.

2

Differential Diagnosis of a Mass on the Chest Radiograph

Masses seen on chest radiographs may be diagnosed with some degree of accuracy but it is rare for a lesion to be diagnosed definitively on radiographic appearances alone; examination of bacteriological, cytological or histological specimens usually has to be employed.

There are, however, some helpful general radiological principles which should be employed when a mass is seen on a chest radiograph. The most important investigation when an abnormality is found radiologically is examination of any previous radiographs of the patient; change in appearance of a lesion over a period may provide important evidence as to its nature. Anatomical localization of the lesion should be the first objective, as this will determine the differential diagnoses involved. Is the lesion in the chest wall, pleura, lung or mediastinum? Does the lesion cross anatomical boundaries such as the pleura? If in the lung, is the lesion segmental?

Extrapulmonary Masses

Tumours of the skin overlying the lungs appear as clearly defined opacities, outlined by air in the same way as are lesions in the lung. If an opacity cannot be seen in the lung in two projections, examination of the skin and chest wall may elucidate the cause (Fig. 2.1). Artefacts, such as buttons on clothing, hair plaits or dressings outside the patients, may sometimes cause opacities over the lung fields. Tumours of the chest wall that cause a mass on a chest radiograph often involve the ribs, and expansion, destruction or displacement of the ribs should be observed (Fig. 2.2). Some extrapleural tumours such as lipomas and neurofibromas (Fig. 2.3) expand inwards, frequently not involving the ribs, and are indistinguishable from pleural tumours. In general, both pleural and extrapleural tumours have smooth medial borders which blend with the adjacent pleura at an obtuse angle.

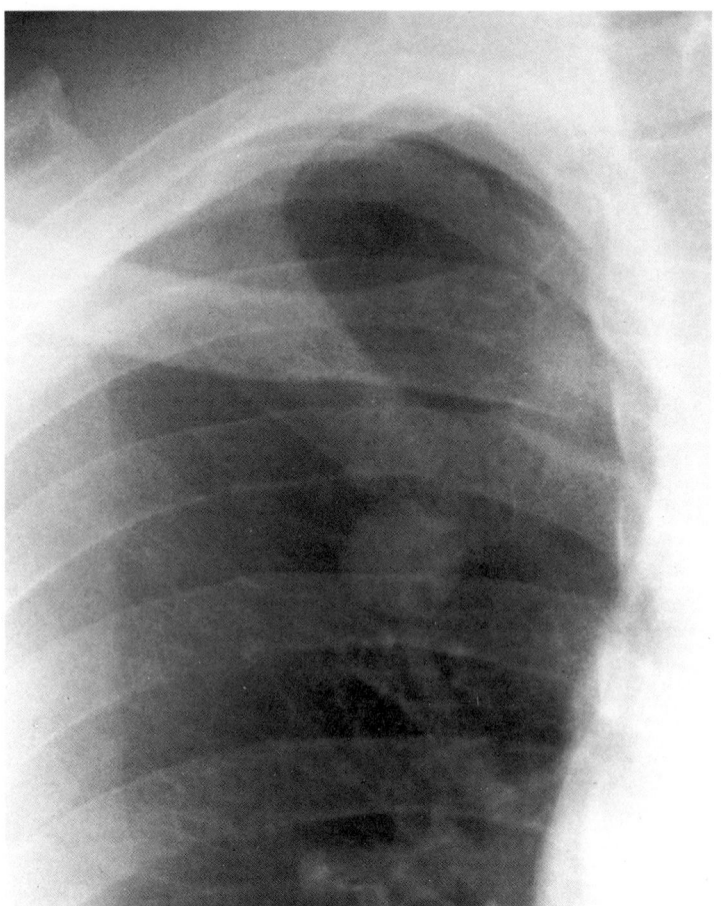
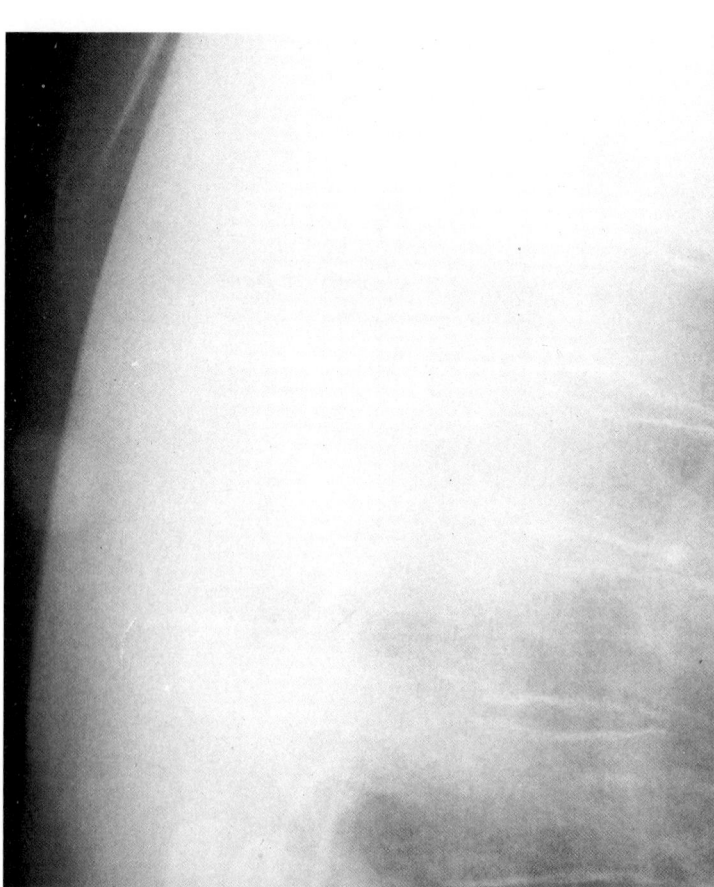

Fig. 2.1 Skin tumour. A well-defined round opacity, apparently in the right upper lobe on the frontal view is seen on lateral view to be due to a small papilloma of the skin on the back.

Pleural Tumours

Pleural tumours causing localized opacities are rare. Fibromas of the pleura may become very large before discovery. Mesotheliomas spread along the pleura and do not often produce localized pleural masses, though lobulation of greatly thickened pleura is frequently seen (Fig. 2.4). Loculated interlobar pleural effusions, in either the

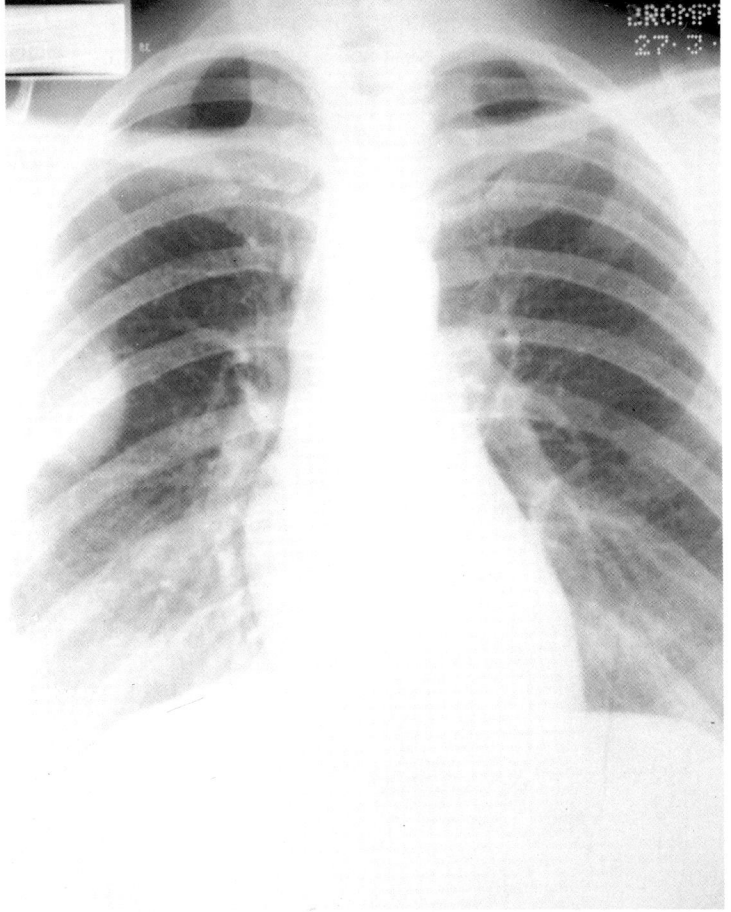

Fig. 2.2 Multiple chondromas of the ribs. The opacity on the right side clearly involves the anterior end of the fifth rib, which is expanded. On the left side, destruction of the anterior ends of the fourth and fifth ribs associated with a mass was due to malignant changes in a chondroma.

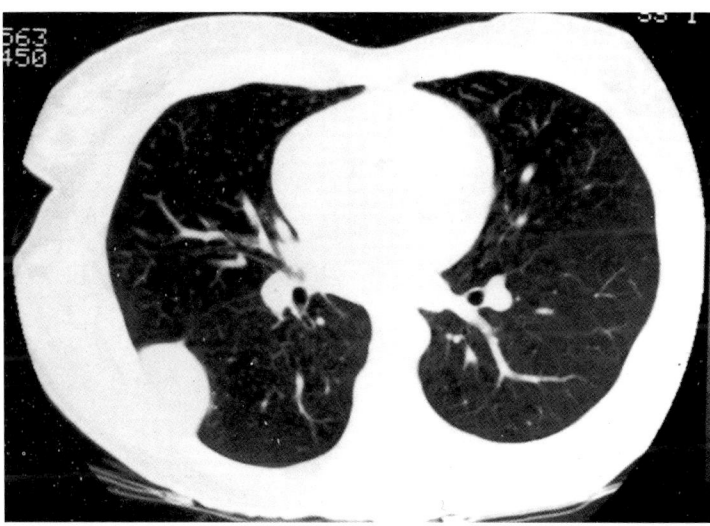

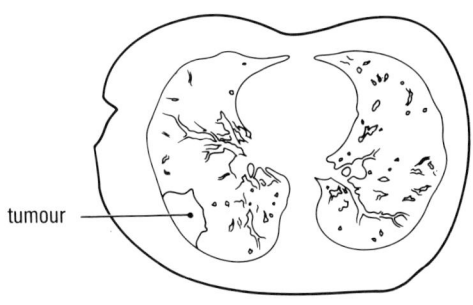

tumour

Fig. 2.3 Neurofibroma of the chest wall. The opacity in the right mid-zone (left) shows the characteristic well-defined border on one side but a poorly defined outer border of a pleural or extrapleural lesion. The CT scan clearly shows that the lesion is of the pleura or extrapleural tissues.

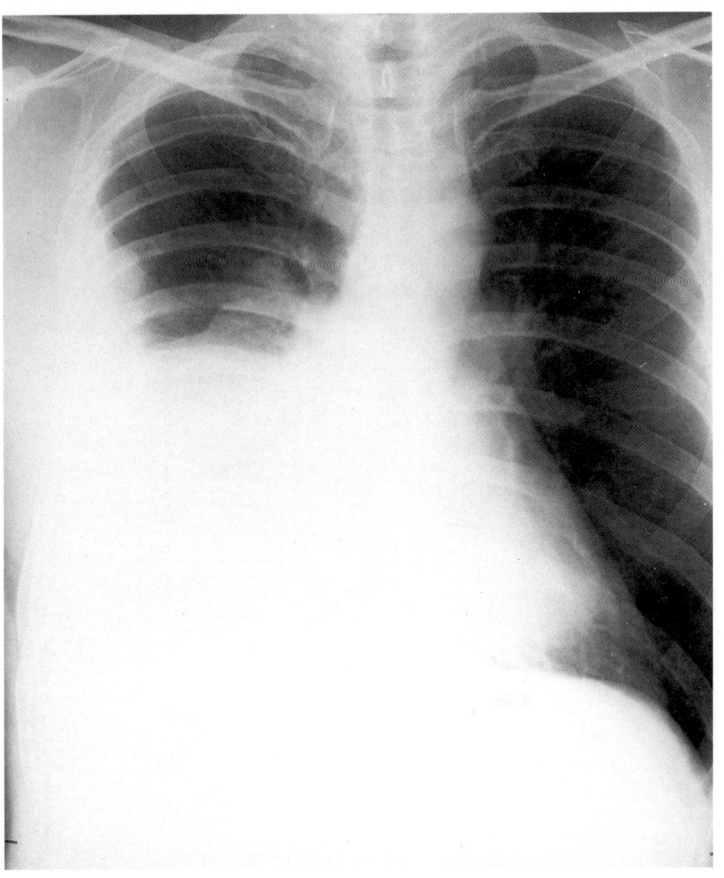

Fig. 2.4 Mesothelioma. There is a lobulated mass attached to the chest wall, with extensive involvement of the lower part of the right hemithorax.

oblique or horizontal fissures, produce an opacity which may be mistaken for a pulmonary mass. In the frontal view a loculated pleural effusion in the horizontal fissure appears as a round, clearly defined opacity. In the oblique fissure the opacity is clearly defined on its lower margin but is less dense and less well-defined in its upper part (Fig. 2.5, left). Lateral projection shows the lesion to lie in the appropriate fissure. In each case it is oval in shape, with its long axis in the line of the fissure and a 'tail' at each end blending with the fissure (Fig. 2.5, right).

Intrapulmonary Masses

An intrapulmonary mass on a chest radiograph is an opacity caused by a circumscribed lesion which is not usually confined to normal anatomical boundaries. The causes include congenital and acquired cysts, benign and malignant tumours, and inflammatory lesions, usually chronic. The mass may occlude a bronchus and then be associated with a secondary segmental or lobar infection. Thus, opacities with a segmental distribution are not usually termed masses, but they may be associated with them.

When the air in the alveoli is displaced by an inflammatory exudate, fluid or tumour, a homogeneous or 'ground-glass' opacity occurs. The airspace opacification is of the same density as water and thus obliterates the normal vascular pattern. If the bronchi are patent and still contain

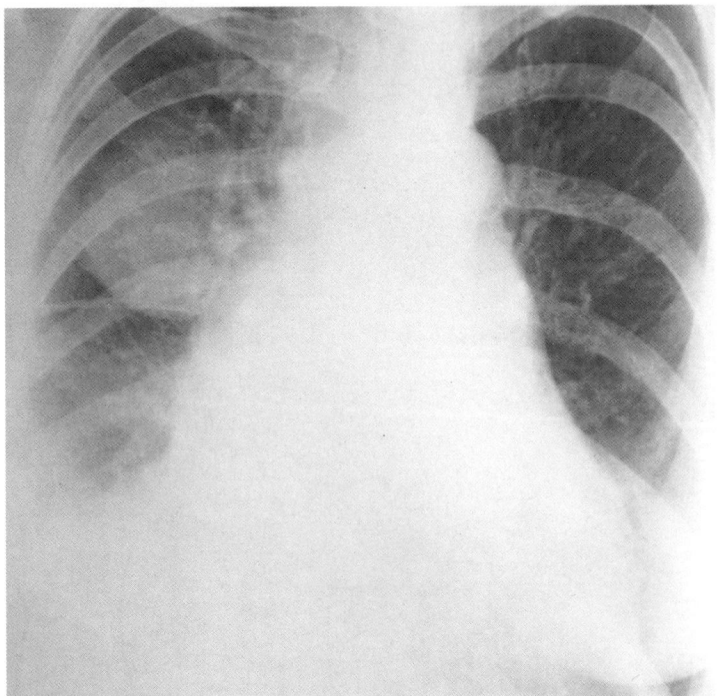

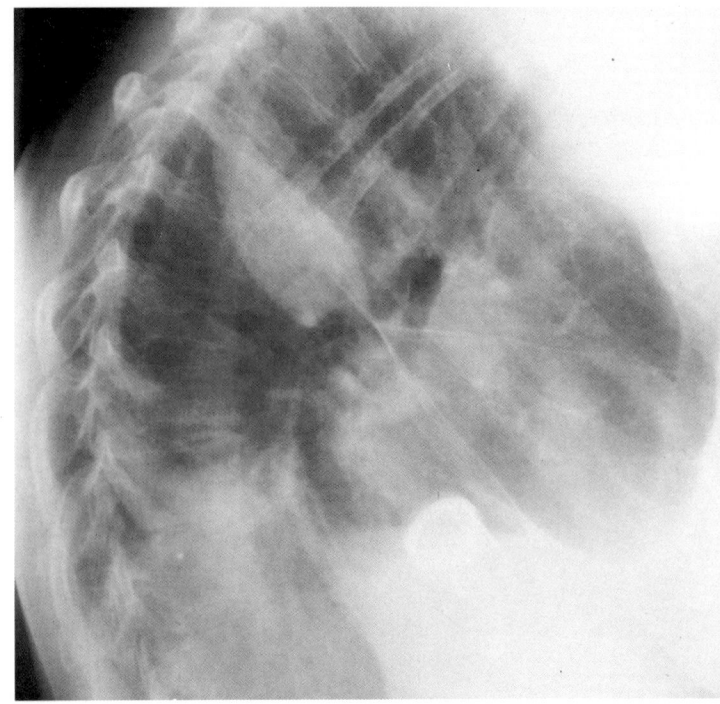

Fig. 2.5 Loculated interlobar effusion. This patient, in heart failure, has a right pleural effusion. The round opacity in the right mid-zone has a sharp lower margin and ill-defined upper margin on frontal view. The lateral view shows the elliptical opacity in the upper end of the oblique fissure.

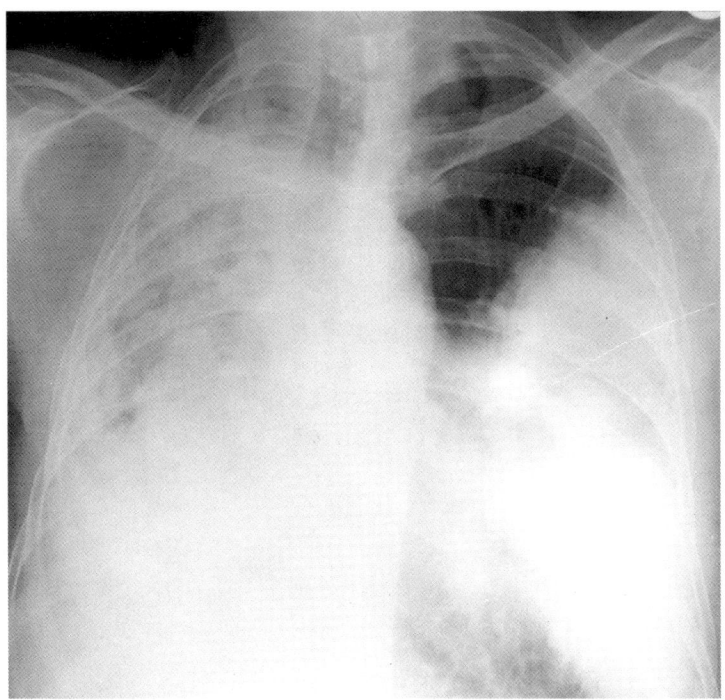

Fig. 2.6 Bronchiolar (alveolar) cell carcinoma. This patient had a lobectomy for carcinoma of the right lung two years previously. Tumour has recurred in the remaining portion of the right lung and also throughout the periphery of the

air, they can be seen within the opacification; this is termed an air bronchogram. Airspace opacification with an air bronchogram generally indicates an inflammatory condition or alveolar oedema, with the rare exception of a few infiltrating tumours such as bronchiolar cell carcinoma (Fig. 2.6).

Displacement of surrounding structures, such as vessels and fissures, may occur in association with some masses. Displacement away from the lesion is seen in benign lesions, such as cysts; malignant lesions which rapidly infiltrate cause no displacement. Displacement towards the lesion indicates collapse or fibrosis; for example, progressive massive fibrosis (Fig. 2.7).

Calcification

Calcification is seen radiologically in inflammatory masses, and in slow-growing benign tumours. It is a fairly reliable sign of the benign nature of the lesion, though one must remember that both tuberculosis and carcinoma are common diseases and a calcified old tuberculous lesion may be the site of a carcinoma, so-called 'scar cancer'. In the United Kingdom a tuberculoma is the most common calcified granuloma (Fig. 2.8). Other inflammatory granulomas which calcify include those due to histoplasmosis and, rarely, coccidioidomycosis, blastomycosis and ruptured hydatid cysts; the calcification in these cases is laminated or densely punctate, and a small central nidus may be present. Irregular 'popcorn' or punctate calcification is seen in hamartomas (Fig. 2.9). Amyloid nodules may calcify (Fig. 2.10) but calcification is virtually never seen in

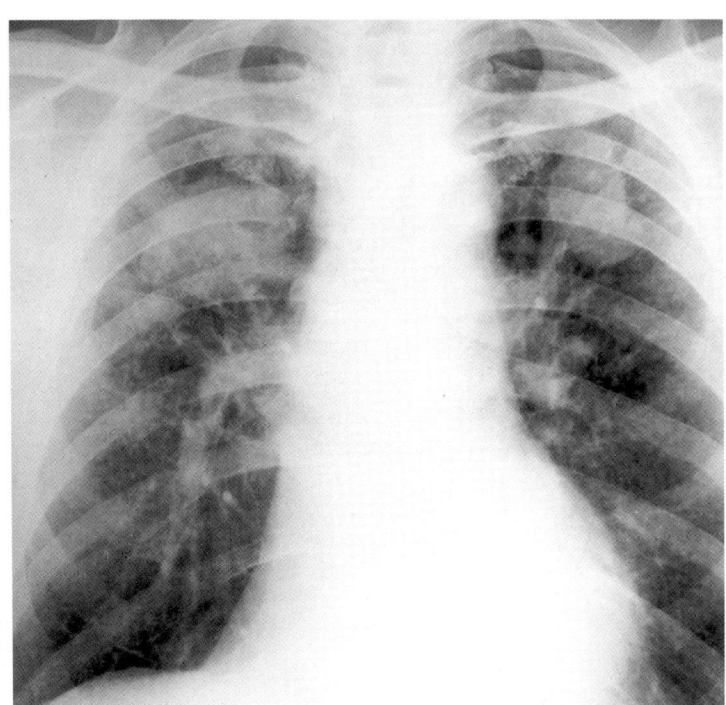

Fig. 2.7 Progressive massive fibrosis. This coalminer, with widespread nodular opacities, developed massive conglomerate shadows in the mid and upper zones due to massive fibrosis. The displacement of the hilar vessels on the right indicates contraction of the lung.

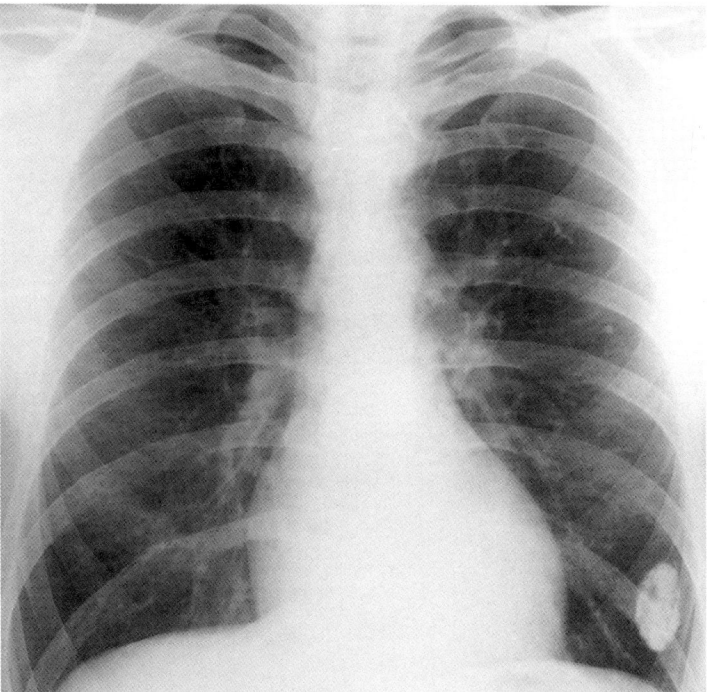

Fig. 2.8 Tuberculoma. Irregular calcification is seen throughout the lesion at the left base. Smaller calcified lesions are also present in the left lung, and there is some calcification of the hilar nodes.

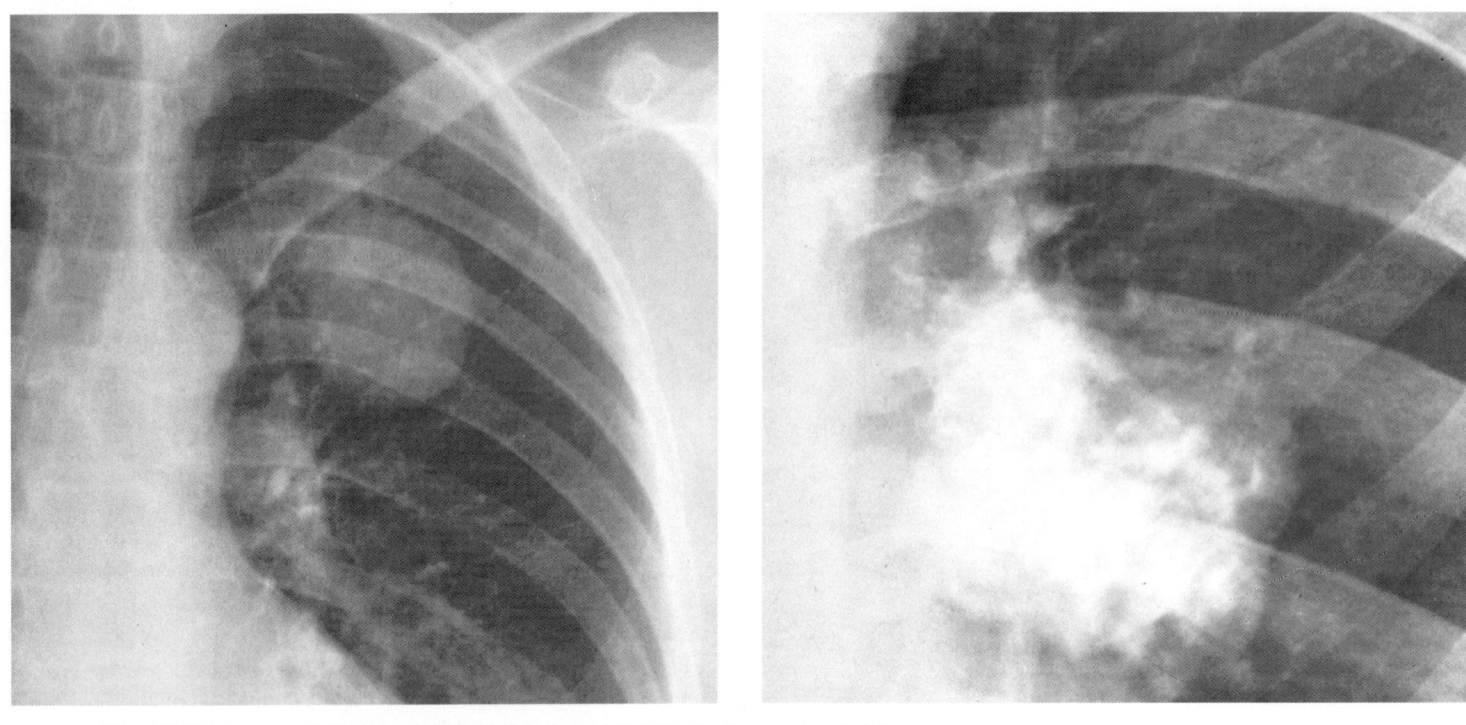

Fig. 2.9 Hamartomas: (left) non-calcified; (right) calcified. Calcification is central and of the popcorn type.

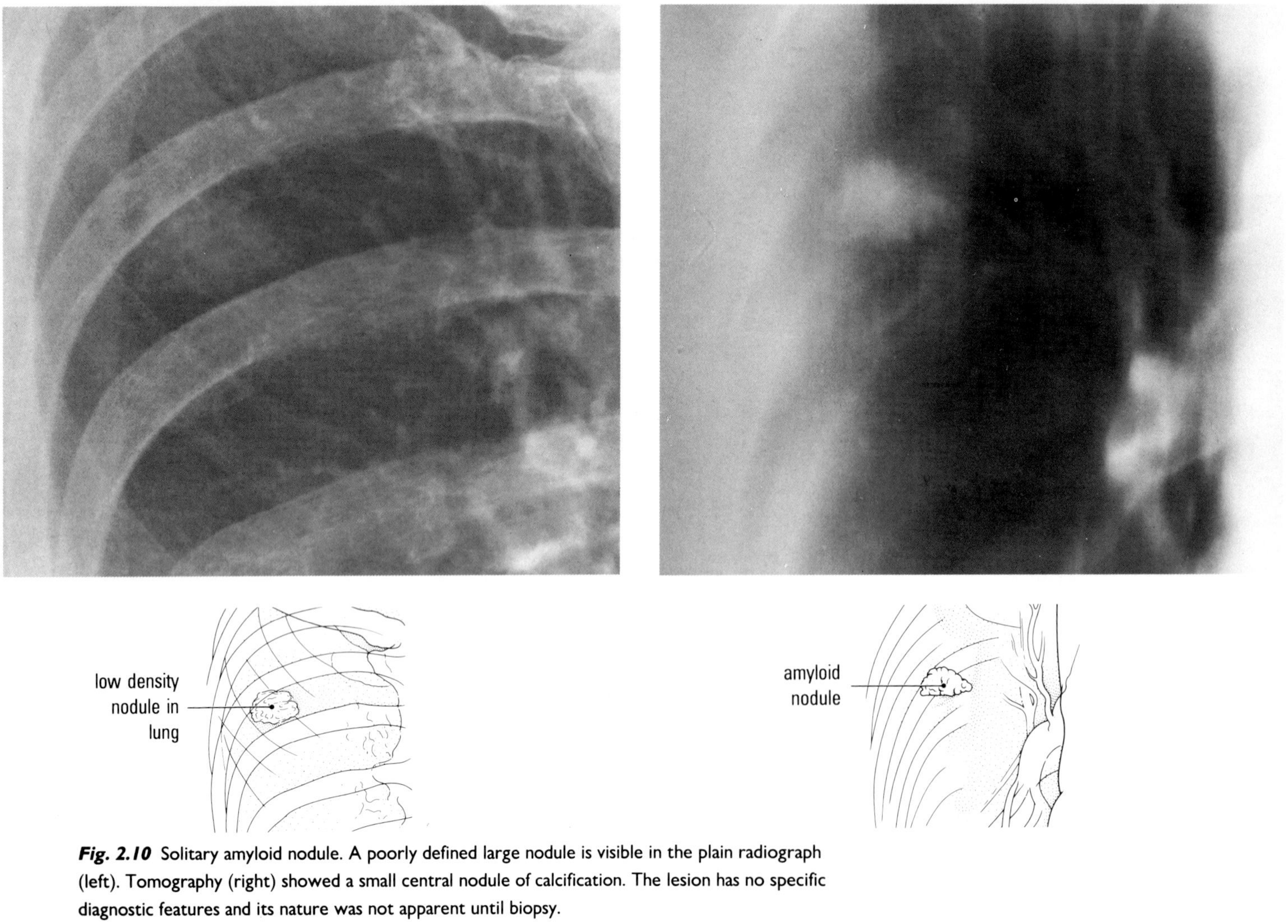

low density nodule in lung

amyloid nodule

Fig. 2.10 Solitary amyloid nodule. A poorly defined large nodule is visible in the plain radiograph (left). Tomography (right) showed a small central nodule of calcification. The lesion has no specific diagnostic features and its nature was not apparent until biopsy.

rheumatoid nodules (Fig. 2.11) or in Wegener's granulomatosis (Fig. 2.12). Occasionally calcification, or bone, is seen in carcinoid adenoma, and metastases from osteogenic sarcomas may contain calcified osteoid tissue.

Cavitation

Cavitation is seen in any mass which undergoes central necrosis. It occurs in lung abscesses, tumours, tuberculosis, histoplasmosis, coccidioidomycosis, blastomycosis, rheumatoid nodules, Wegener's granulomatosis, post-traumatic pneumatocele and progressive massive fibrosis, and following pulmonary infarction. Of the tumours which cavitate, squamous cell carcinoma does so most often, though any rapidly growing carcinoma may outgrow its blood supply and undergo central necrosis (Fig. 2.13). The cavity in the

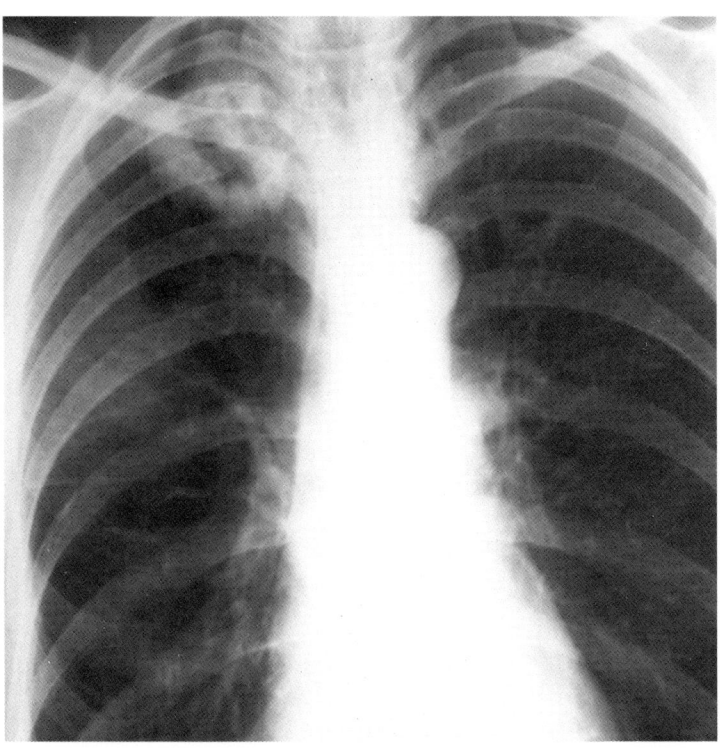

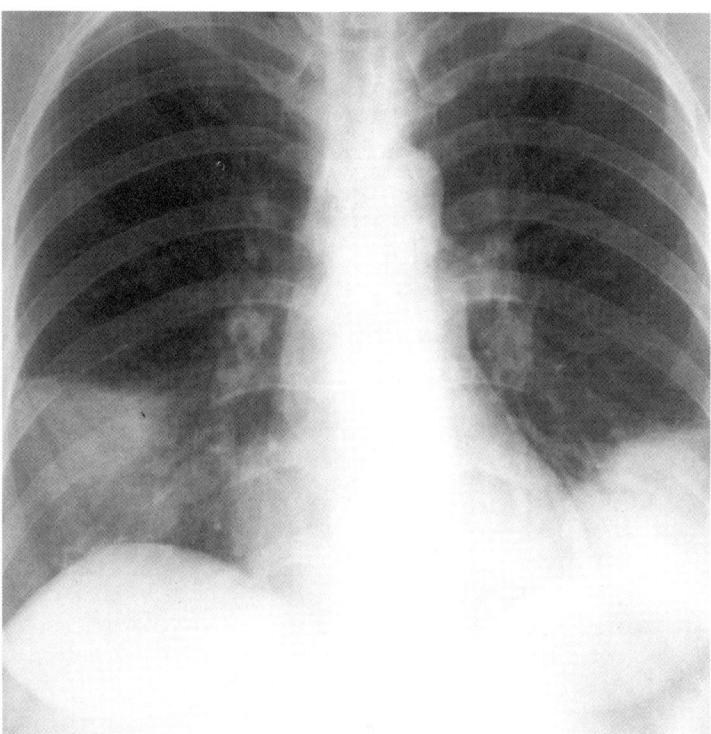

Fig. 2.11 Necrobiotic nodule in rheumatoid disease. In this atypical case, a large cavitating nodule is present in the right upper lobe. Nodules are commonly smaller and may be multiple.

Fig. 2.12 Wegener's granulomatosis. Ill-defined areas of consolidation are seen in the right middle and left lower lobes.

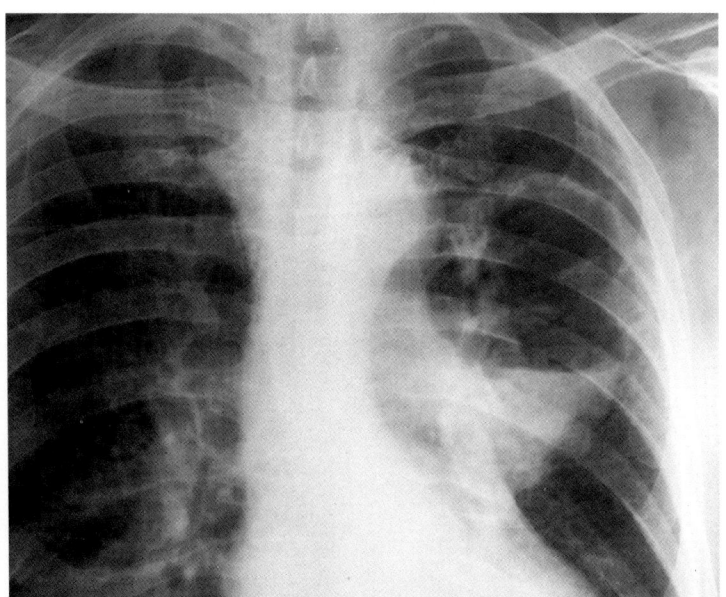

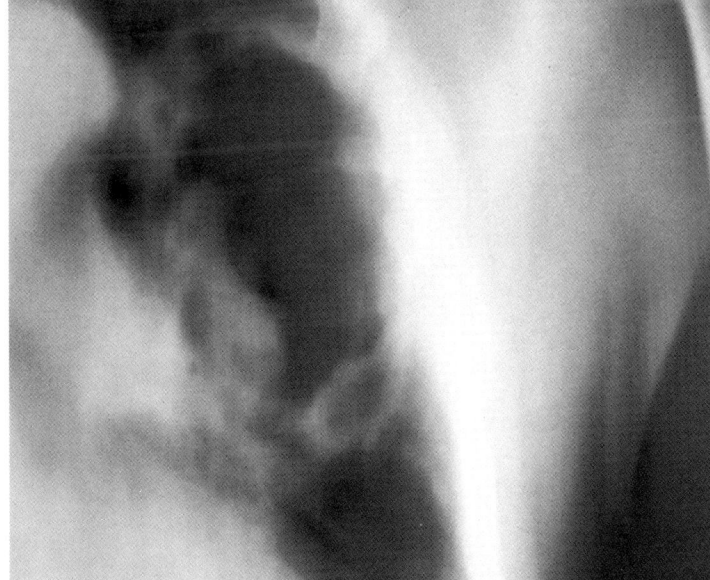

Fig. 2.13 Cavitating squamous cell carcinoma. The erect plain radiograph shows a large irregular cavity with a fluid level in the left upper lobe. Tomography (right) shows an irregular cavity with a mass near the hilum; the fluid level is not seen as the patient is supine.

neoplasm is often eccentric and irregular, though this is not a reliable differential sign.

Cavities may contain fluid when there is liquefaction of necrotic material; this occurs particularly in acute abscesses (Fig. 2.14) but also in some granulomas, such as in tuberculosis. Post-traumatic pneumatoceles often contain fluid. Ruptured cysts may have an air/fluid level; in ruptured hydatid cysts, remnants of the endocyst are seen floating

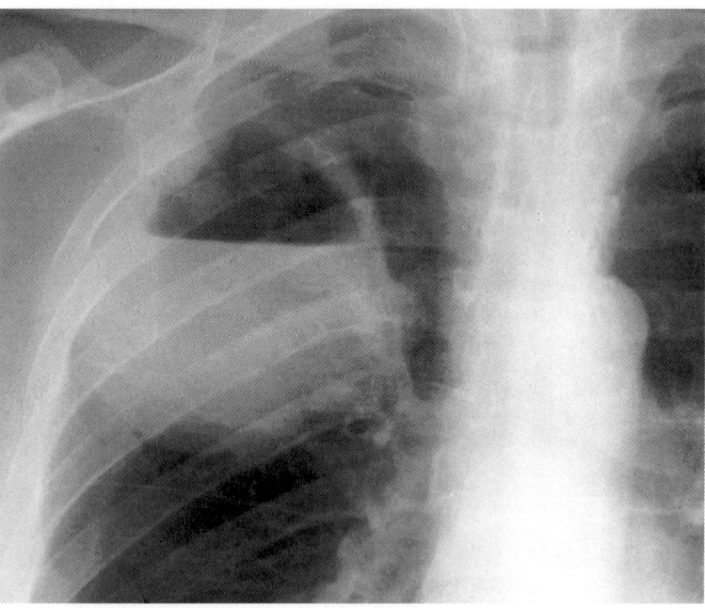

Fig. 2.14 Lung abscess. The radiograph shows a round cavity with a fluid level and a slightly irregular wall. Staphylococci were abundant in the purulent sputum.

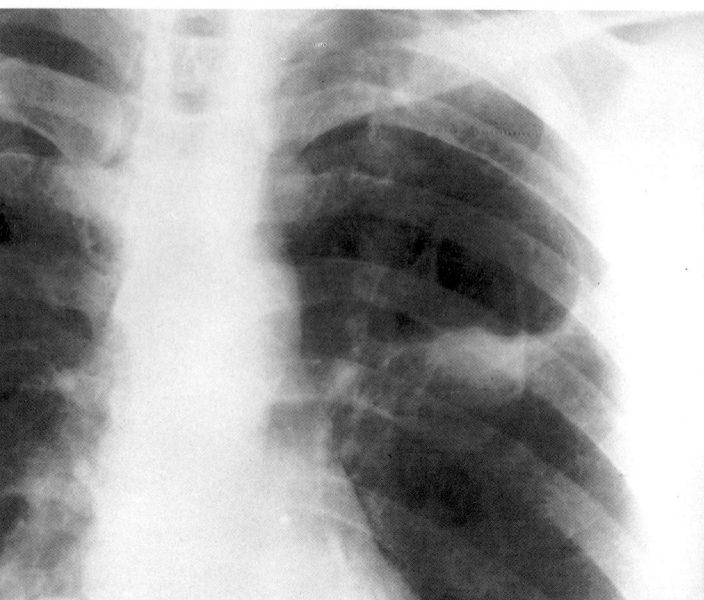

Fig. 2.15 Ruptured hydatid cyst. A thin-walled cavity with a fluid level contains remnants of the ruptured cyst, giving the characteristic 'water-lily' sign.

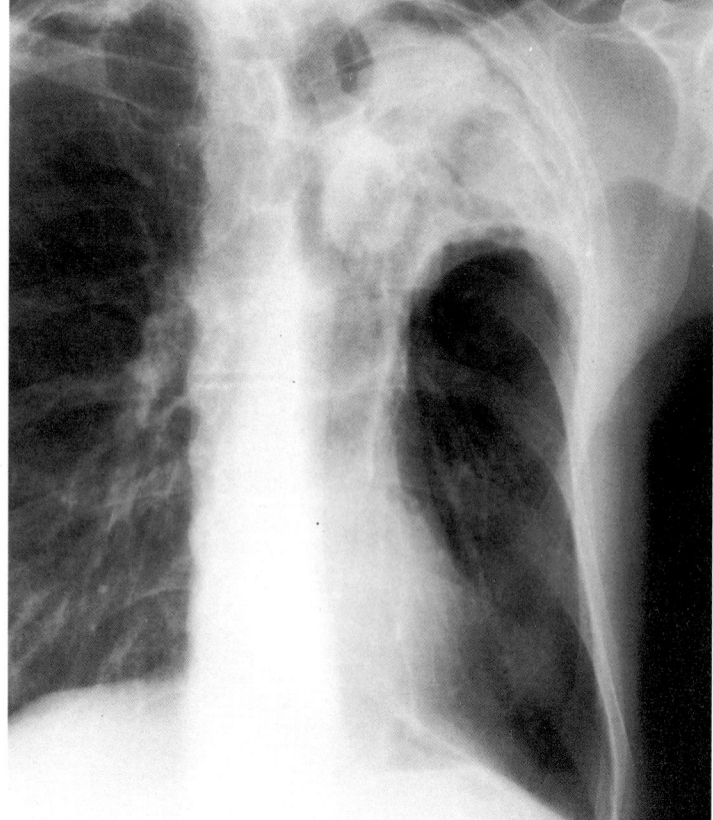

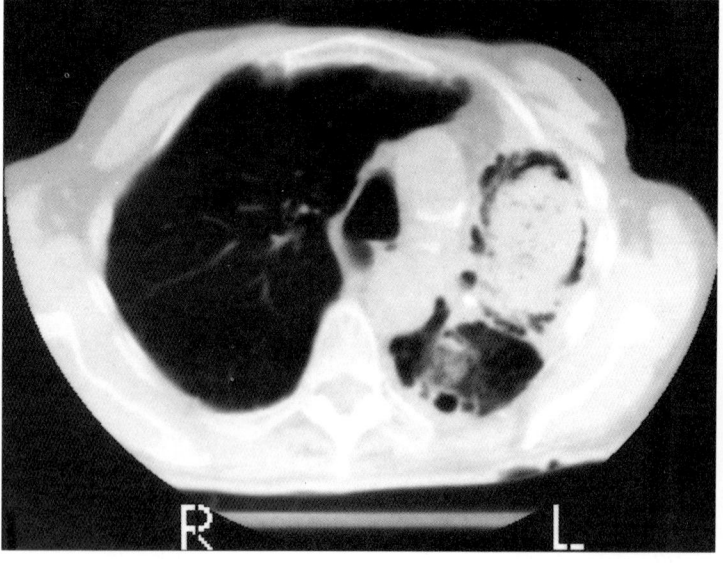

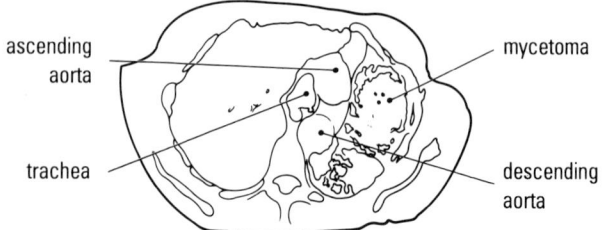

Fig. 2.16 Mycetoma. A cavity at the left apex, the site of previous tuberculosis, contains a 'fungus ball' of *Aspergillus*. The radiograph and CT scan show a crescent of air around the fungus ball.

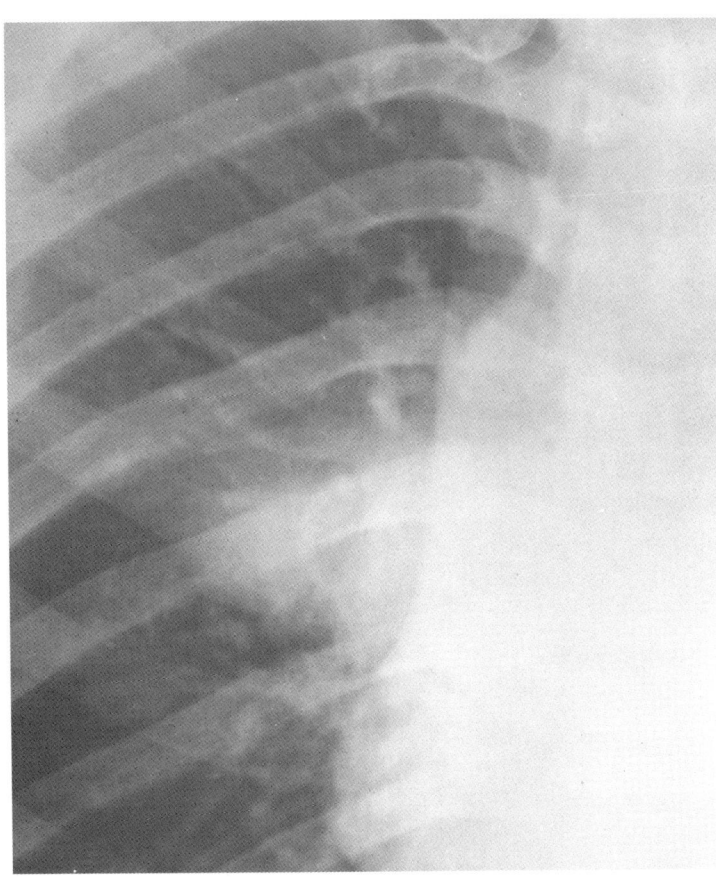

in the fluid — the 'water lily' sign (Fig. 2.15). Necrotic material or blood clot may fill a cavity, and infection by fungus, particularly aspergillosis, produces a central ball of mycelia and fibrin, a mycetoma (Fig. 2.16).

Position

The position of the mass in the lung may suggest a possible diagnosis. Tuberculous infection is commonest in the apex of the upper lobes posteriorly or in the apical segment of the lower lobes, but can occur anywhere in the lungs. Hamartomas (Fig. 2.9) are equally common in the upper and lower lobes but are usually within 2cm of the pleural surface. Carcinoid tumours are more frequently central and arise from the larger bronchi (Fig. 2.17). Bronchogenic cysts are also usually central and occur more commonly in the mediastinum (Fig. 2.18). Intralobar sequestrated segments, deriving their blood supply from the aorta and not the pulmonary artery, are seen posteriorly and medially at the lung base and are twice as common in the left than the

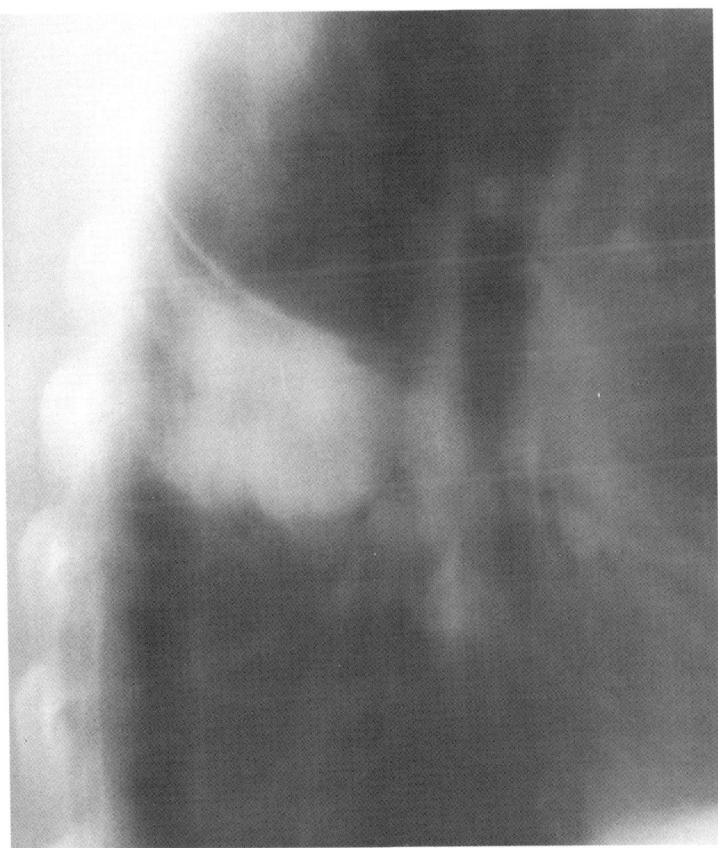

Fig. 2.17 Carcinoid tumour. A lobulated mass is seen in the apical segment of the right lower lobe, behind the right hilum, in the frontal radiograph (upper) and is clearly defined below the oblique fissure in the lateral tomogram (lower).

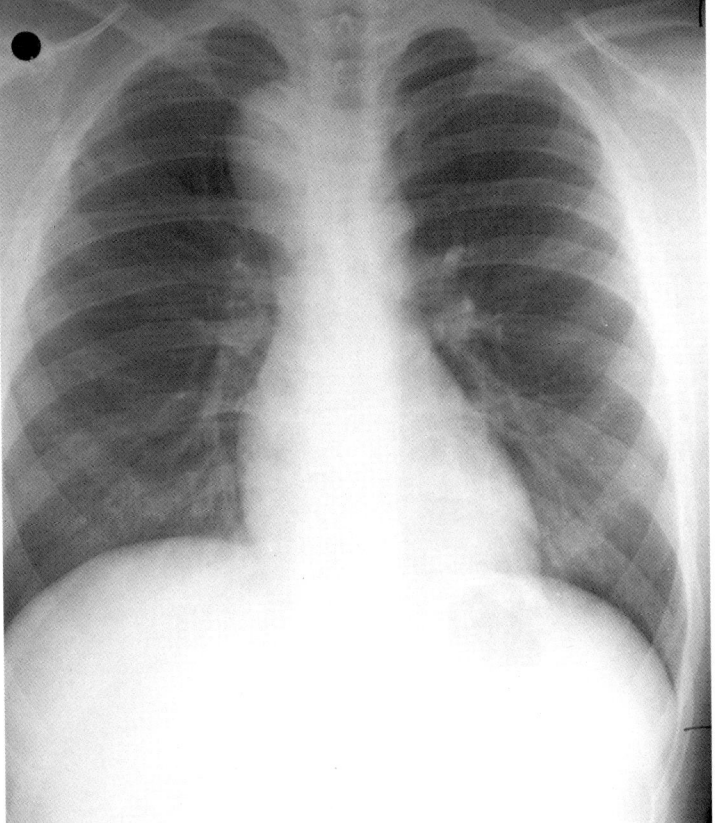

Fig. 2.18 Bronchogenic cyst. This well-defined round smooth opacity on the right of the superior mediastinum is in a typical site, though a retrosternal thyroid would produce the same appearances.

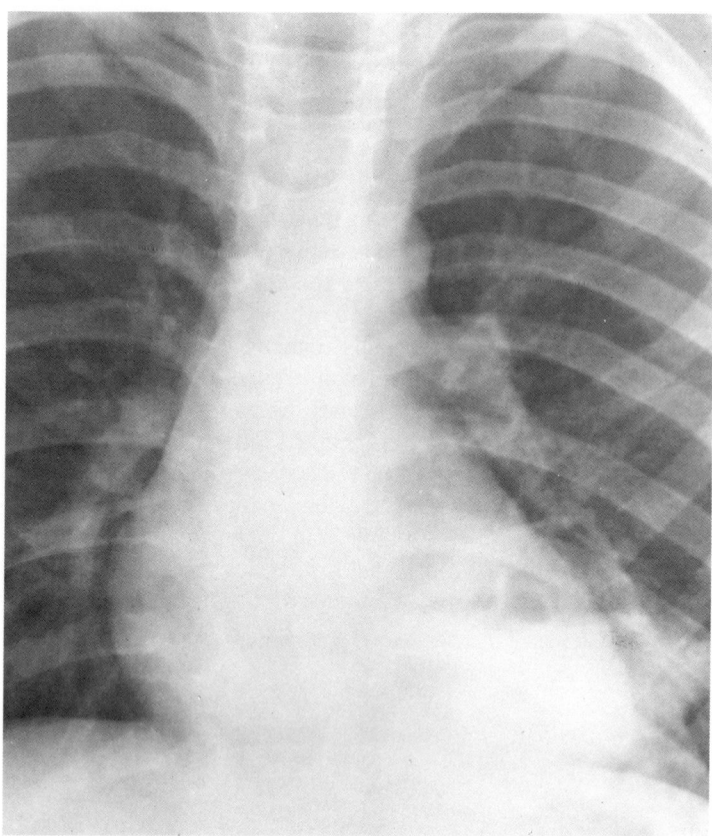

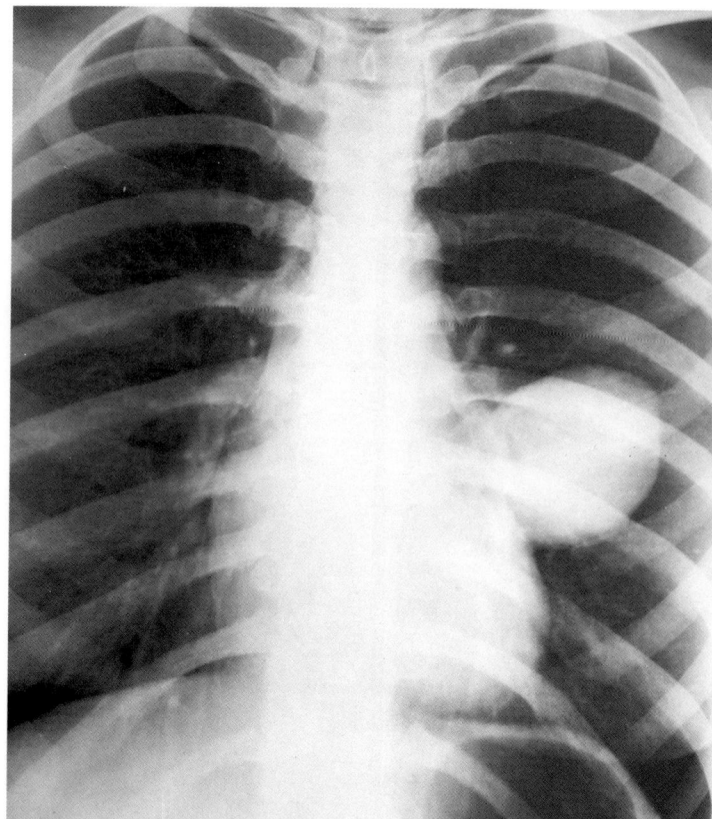

Fig. 2.20 Hydatid cyst. There is a clearly defined smooth round opacity in the upper part of the lingular segment of the left upper lobe. Hydatid cysts are more usually found in the lower lobes.

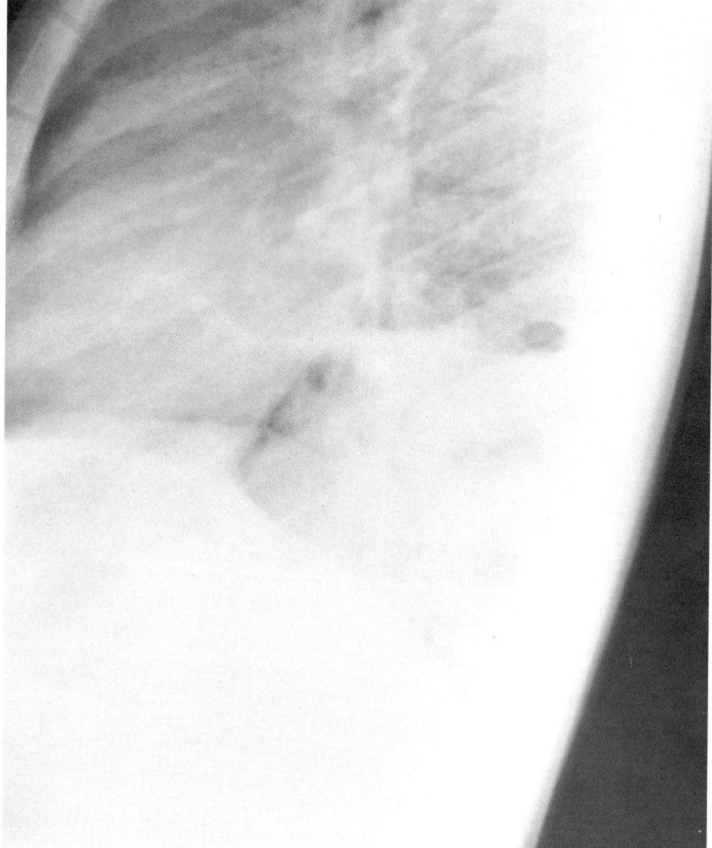

Fig. 2.19 Intralobar sequestrated segment in a child. A cystic lesion with a fluid level is seen in the left lower lobe behind the heart. Some patchy areas of consolidation due to infection are present in the adjacent lung.

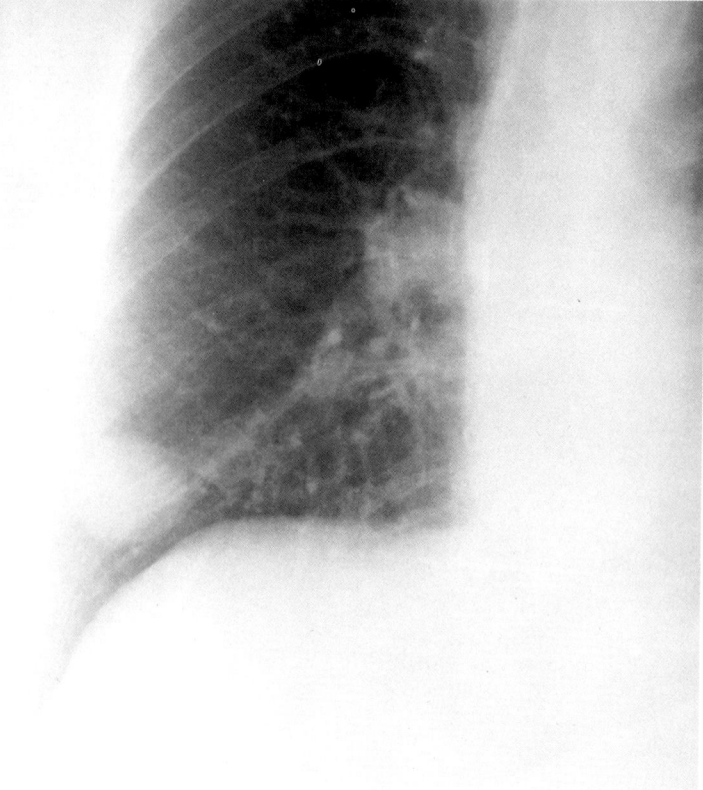

Fig. 2.21 Arteriovenous malformation (fistula). The draining vein and feeding artery cause band shadows between the hilum and heart and the lesion.

right lung (Fig. 2.19). Hydatid cysts are more common in the lower lobes than the upper (Fig. 2.20), as are arteriovenous malformations (Fig. 2.21). Mycetomas, in contrast, are more common in the upper than the lower lobe, since they frequently develop in old tuberculous cavities (Fig. 2.16). Inflammatory lesions are usually confined by the pleura and do not cross fissures or invade the chest wall by direct extension. Actinomycosis (Fig. 2.22) and blastomycosis are the exceptions and may involve the pleura, ribs and intercostal structures or vertebral bodies when there is infection in the lung periphery; the ribs show destruction and periostitis. Malignant disease frequently crosses the pleural boundaries and involves adjacent lobes of the lung, ribs and vertebrae (Fig. 2.23).

Changes in the normal vessel pattern

These are seen in association with some masses in the lungs. In arteriovenous fistula (Fig. 2.21) a large feeding artery and a large draining vein can be identified running to the hilum. Tomography may be necessary to visualize these vessels well and their position can be confirmed by pulmonary arteriography. In malignant disease the pulmonary artery may be invaded by tumour and occluded so that an area of relative avascularity is seen; such an area may also be seen when the bronchus is narrowed, partially blocked by the lesion, due to the reflex constriction of the pulmonary vessels resulting from hypoxia of the affected lung.

Rate of development

Knowledge of the rate of development or growth of a lesion is of considerable value in the differential diagnosis. Lesions which develop over several days are almost certainly inflammatory; lesions which grow only very slowly over several years are more likely to be benign than malignant.

Shape

The shape and margin of a mass are often not as helpful in diagnosis as one might hope. In general, lesions which are clearly defined, smooth, and round or oval are benign (Fig. 2.24), whereas malignant lesions tend to be lobulated with an irregular or spiculate edge. Umbilication of the margin of a round mass has been described as a sign of malignancy, but no one sign is absolutely reliable.

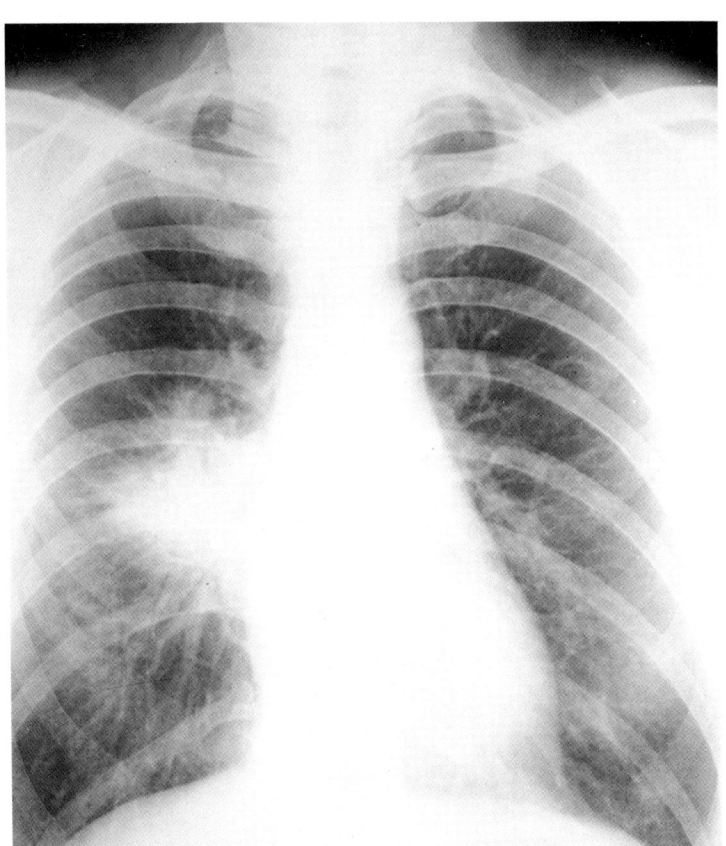

Fig. 2.22 Actinomycosis. An irregular mass at the right hilum, simulating a bronchial carcinoma, is seen to involve all three lobes, crossing the fissures.

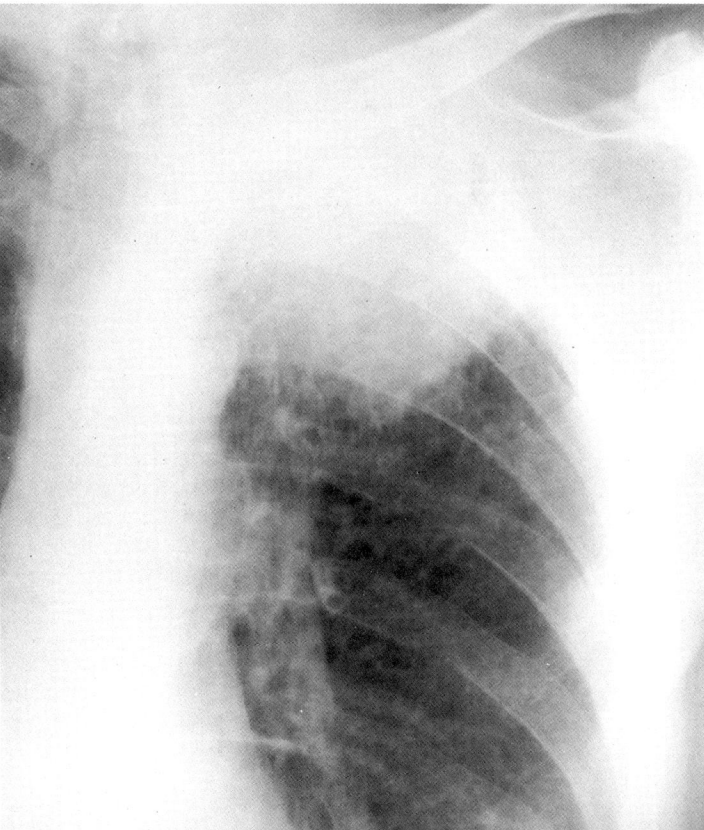

Fig. 2.23 Carcinoma of bronchus. A large mass in the upper part of the left upper lobe has destroyed the posterior parts of the upper five ribs. The tumour has also infiltrated the brachial plexus, giving pain and weakness in the left arm (Pancoast's tumour).

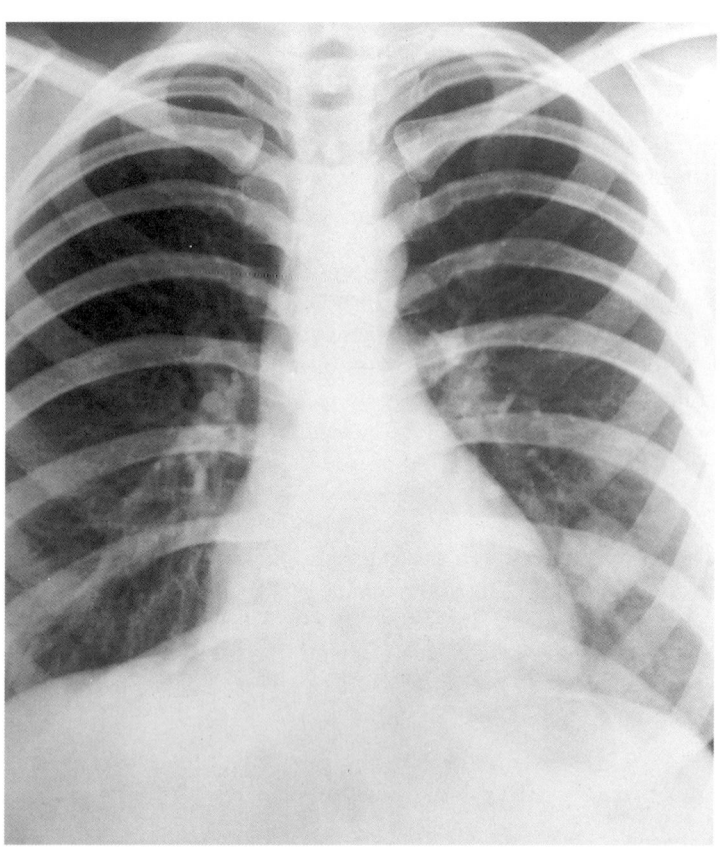

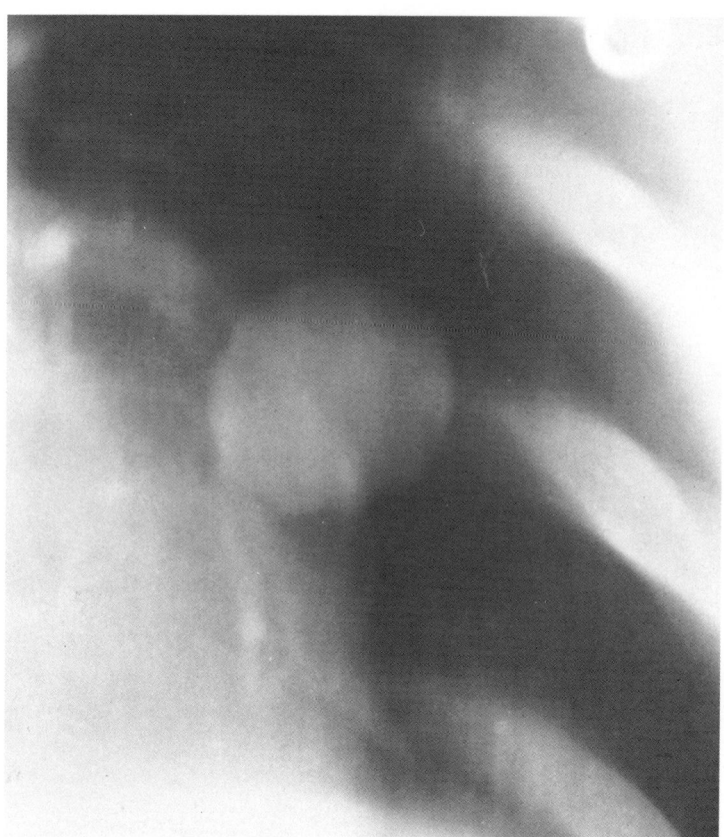

Fig. 2.24 Lymphangioma. This rare benign tumour in the lung has a clearly defined margin and is smooth and round.

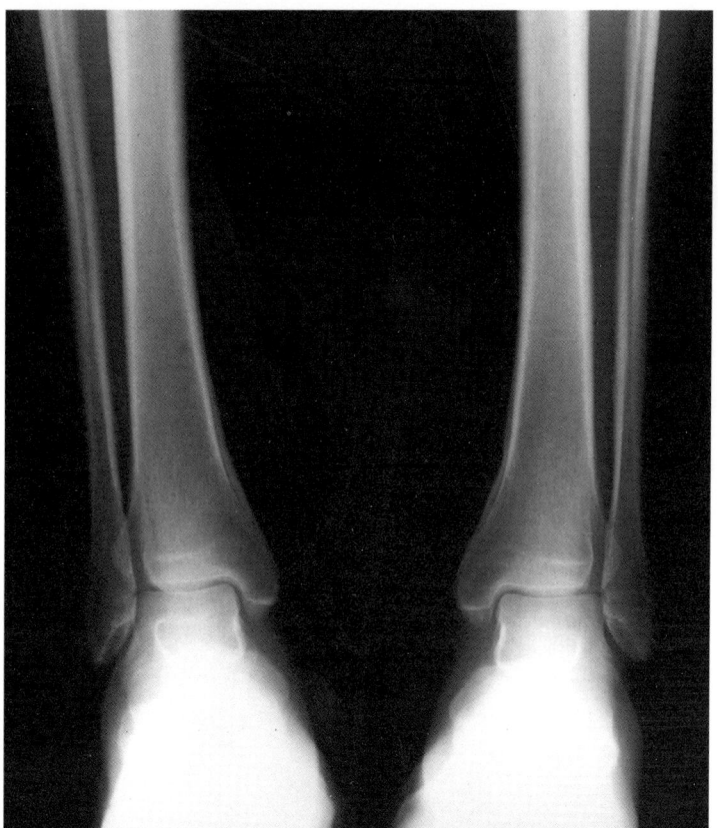

Fig. 2.25 Hypertrophic pulmonary osteoarthropathy. There is periosteal new bone on the medial aspects of both tibias.

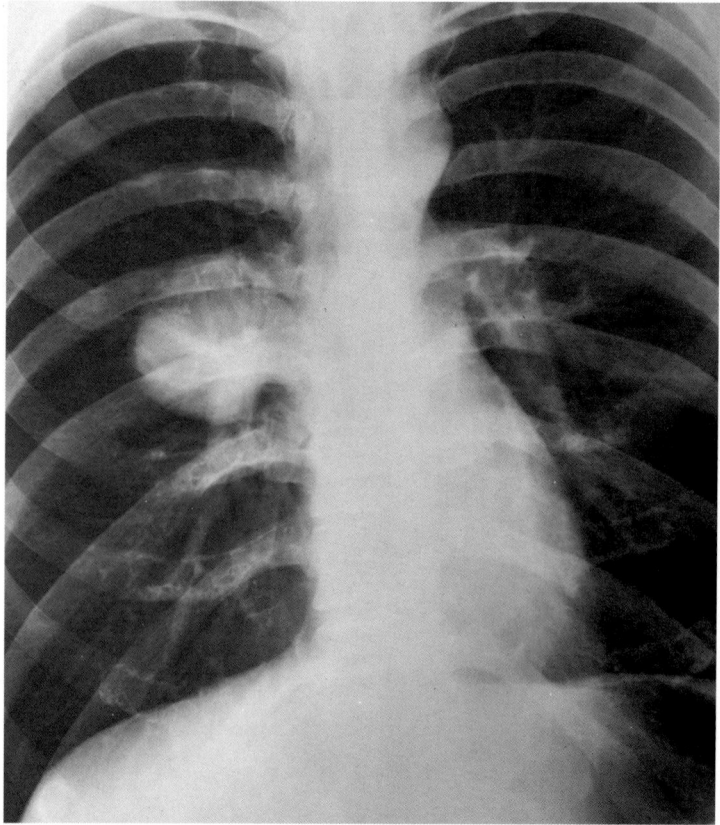

Fig. 2.26 Metastasis. This solitary lesion had no features specific to a metastasis and could have been a primary carcinoma; histology showed it to be a secondary from a previously resected carcinoma of the bowel.

Clinical context

The presence of changes elsewhere in the body, such as hypertrophic pulmonary osteoarthropathy (Fig. 2.25), may be of help in the diagnosis of pulmonary masses. This is most commonly seen in carcinoma of the bronchus, usually squamous cell, and occasionally in adenocarcinoma, but not in oat cell carcinoma. It is also seen in benign fibroma of the lung or pleura. A history of treatment for a primary malignant neoplasm elsewhere in the body suggests that the thoracic mass may be a metastatic tumour (Fig. 2.26), but the possibility of a second primary tumour should not be forgotten, especially if the patient is a smoker. The pulmonary lesion should be fully investigated until its nature is proved.

The solitary round nodule in the lung

Frequently a circumscribed opacity in the lung is a chance finding on a routine radiograph and poses a diagnostic problem. The approach to diagnosis should begin with establishing, if possible, how long the lesion has been present. If calcification is present within the lesion it is almost certainly benign, except for the occasional carcinoma developing in association with an old tuberculous focus or other calcified granuloma. It may be necessary to perform tomography to demonstrate calcification or to show abnormal feeding vessels in arteriovenous fistula but, in most instances, with good-quality, high-kilovoltage radiographs, tomography nowadays adds little or no useful additional information. Rather, an attempt at obtaining a histological or cytological diagnosis should be made. Sputum should be examined; if negative, fibreoptic bronchoscopy, with washing and brushings, and transbronchial biopsy may be undertaken. Recourse to direct percutaneous aspiration needle biopsy under fluoroscopic or CT control (Fig. 2.27) may be necessary if results so far have been unrewarding. Finally, it may be necessary to perform a thoracotomy and open biopsy to establish a diagnosis. The general clinical picture, including the age of the patient and the smoking history, will obviously influence the degree to which investigation is pursued.

The use of CT in the diagnosis of the solitary pulmonary nodule has in recent years received impetus following reports from a few centres that the density of the lesion indicates whether it is benign or malignant. Many benign lesions are more dense, with a higher CT number, than malignant lesions; this is probably because of microscopic amounts of calcification present within them.

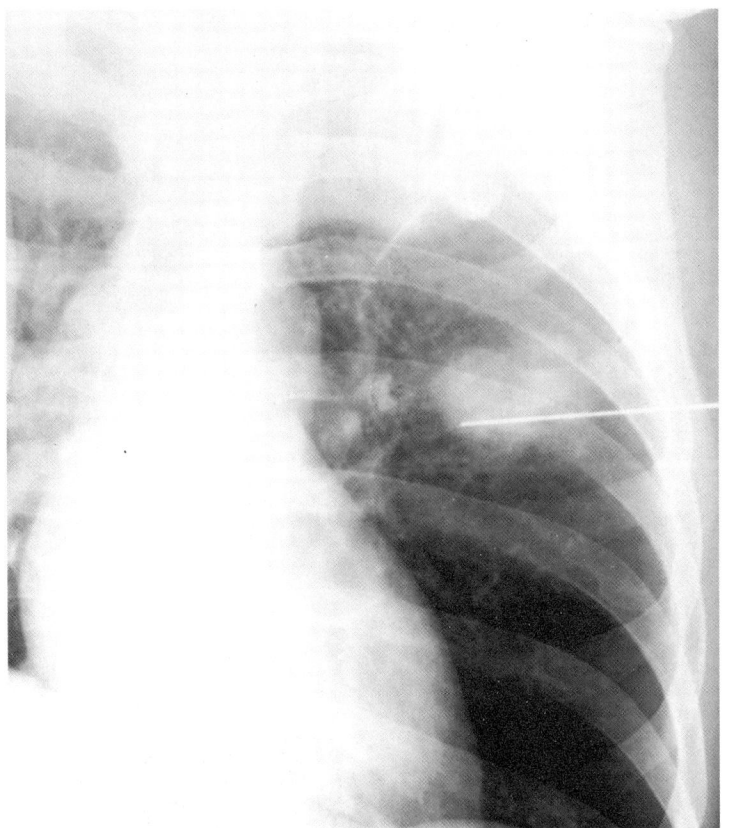

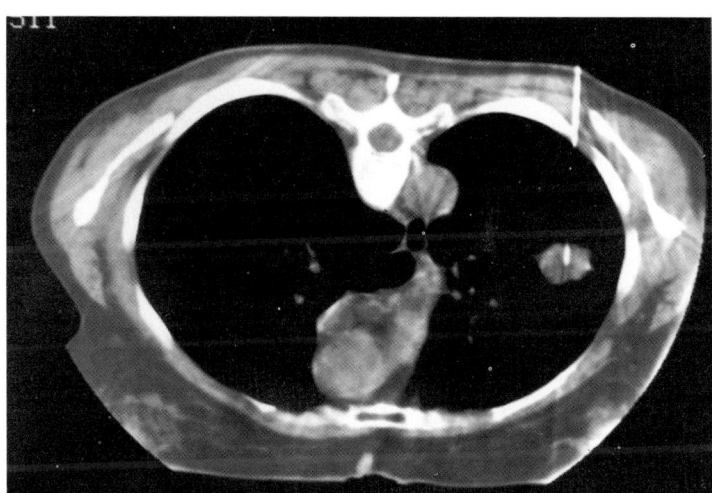

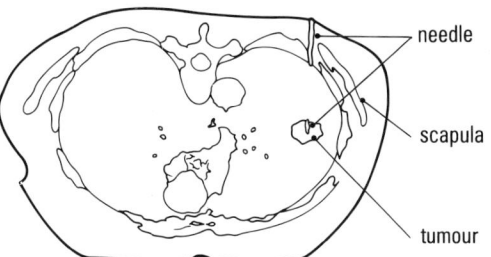

Fig. 2.27 Carcinoma. The radiograph was taken during aspiration needle biopsy under fluoroscopic control and shows the tip of the needle in a nodule in the lung. Histology revealed a squamous cell carcinoma. The CT scan shows a needle in a carcinoma of the left lung during biopsy under CT control. The needle can be seen in the soft tissues, with its tip in the lesion; the portion between is not visible on this window setting.

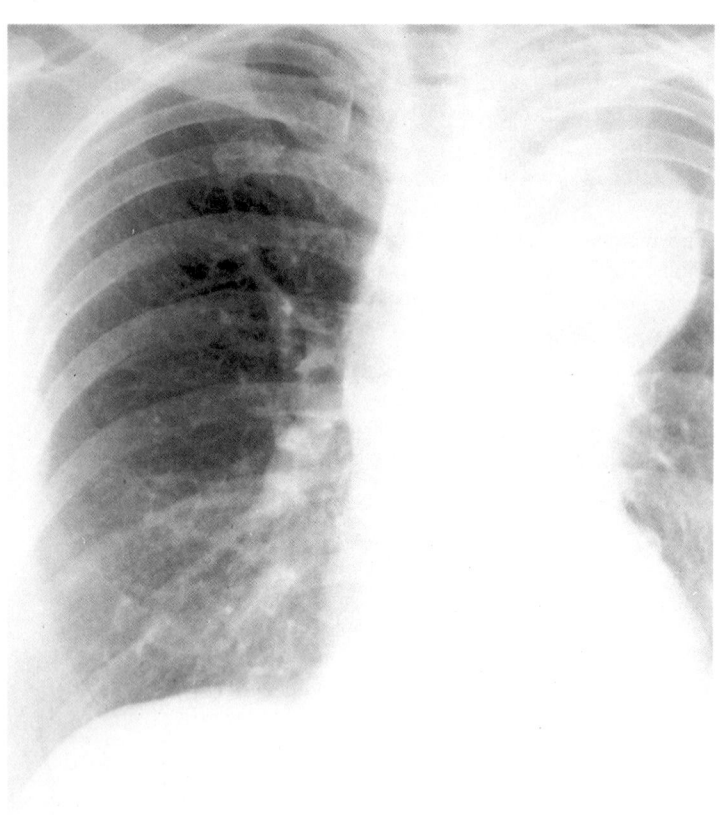

Masses at the Hilum

Masses at the hilum that have irregular margins are usually carcinomas (Fig. 2.28), though occasionally inflammatory masses occur in the perihilar region to mimic central carcinomas. Actinomycosis is one such inflammatory mass (Fig. 2.22) but is rare. Hilar nodes, when enlarged by inflammatory or neoplastic disease, are usually well defined. Bilateral and symmetrical hilar node enlargement is most commonly seen in sarcoidosis (Fig. 2.29). Hilar node enlargement is also seen in lymphoma (Fig. 2.30) but asymmetrical involvement is more common here. Asymmetrical hilar nodes are also seen in tuberculosis, usually in children (Fig. 2.31).

Fig. 2.28 Carcinoma of the left hilum with collapse of the left upper lobe. Note the metastasis in the right sixth rib in the axilla.

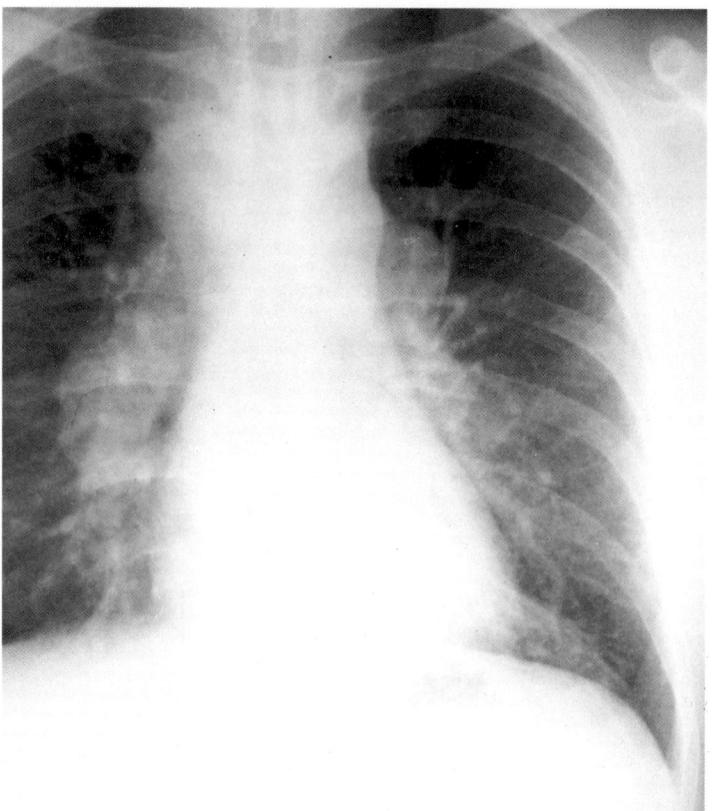

Fig. 2.29 Sarcoidosis. There is bilateral hilar node enlargement. A large paratracheal node is seen on the right side of the superior mediastinum. A few small pulmonary nodules can be identified.

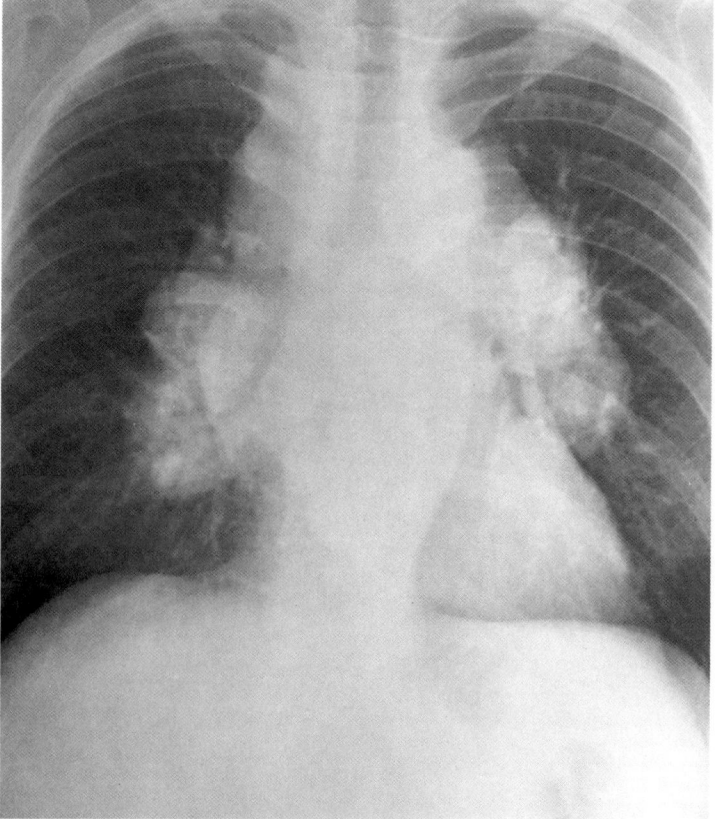

Fig. 2.30 Hodgkin's disease. Hilar and mediastinal lymphadenopathy is present. The nodes in this case are unusually symmetrical and difficult to distinguish from the nodes of sarcoidosis; more commonly the nodes are asymmetrical.

Mediastinal Masses

Some of the largest masses in the chest arise from mediastinal organs. It may be difficult, on plain radiographs or conventional tomography, to distinguish a mediastinal mass from a mass in the lung adjacent to the mediastinum. Computed tomography (CT) is of immense help in mediastinal lesions. A much more accurate assessment of the origin of various tumours can be made and, with contrast enhancement, vascular lesions such as aneurysms can readily be diagnosed without recourse to arteriography. Arteriography, however, still provides useful information regarding the extent of lesions of the aorta and great vessels, and should be used in hospitals in which CT is not yet available.

The position in the mediastinum of a mass may give a clue to its nature (see Chapter 8). Cystic lesions have clearly defined rounded smooth margins. A retrosternal thyroid (Fig. 2.32) is usually in the superior mediastinum and displaces the trachea to the right or to the left, and either forwards or backwards. The trachea is often compressed by a retrosternal thyroid and this may be so severe as to embarrass respiration. Thymic cysts and tumours (Fig. 2.33) are anterior mediastinal tumours occurring from a level of the upper part of the heart to the level of the arch of the aorta. Some tumours of the thymus are associated with myasthenia gravis and others with severe anaemia. Calcification is often seen in thymic tumours. Thymic lesions frequently bulge to both sides of the mediastinum on a frontal radiograph of the chest, whereas dermoid cysts (Fig. 2.34), which also occur in the anterior

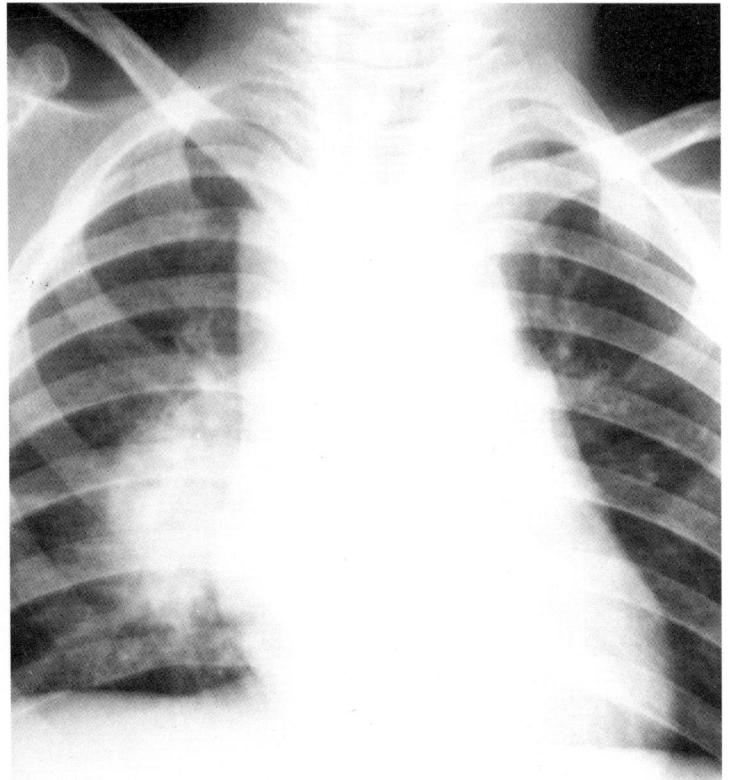

Fig. 2.31 Primary tuberculosis. Enlarged nodes at the right hilum in this three- year-old child are producing a mass. Some patchy shadowing is also seen in the right lower zone and the superior mediastinum is wider than normal.

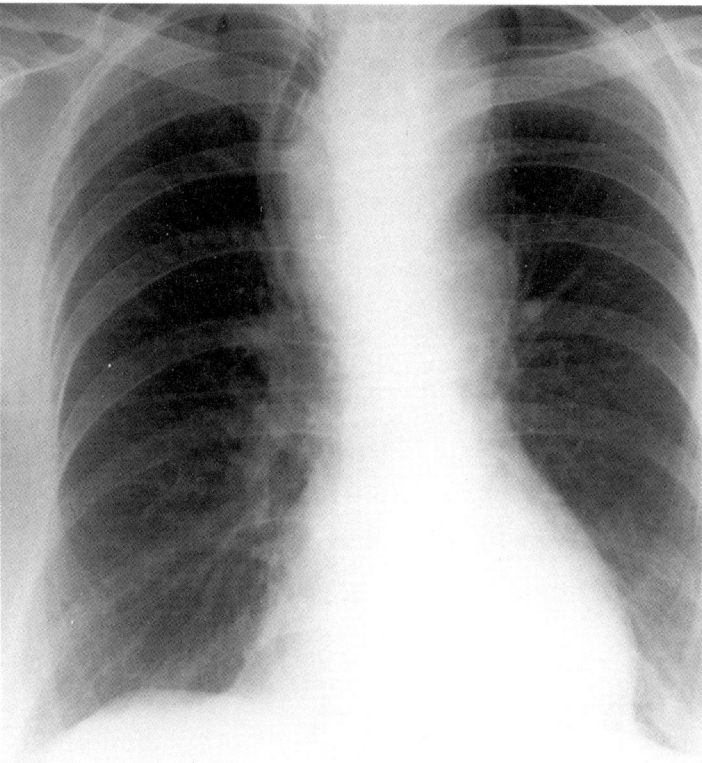

Fig. 2.32 Retrosternal thyroid. The trachea is deviated to the right and forwards, and also compressed by this retrosternal goitre.

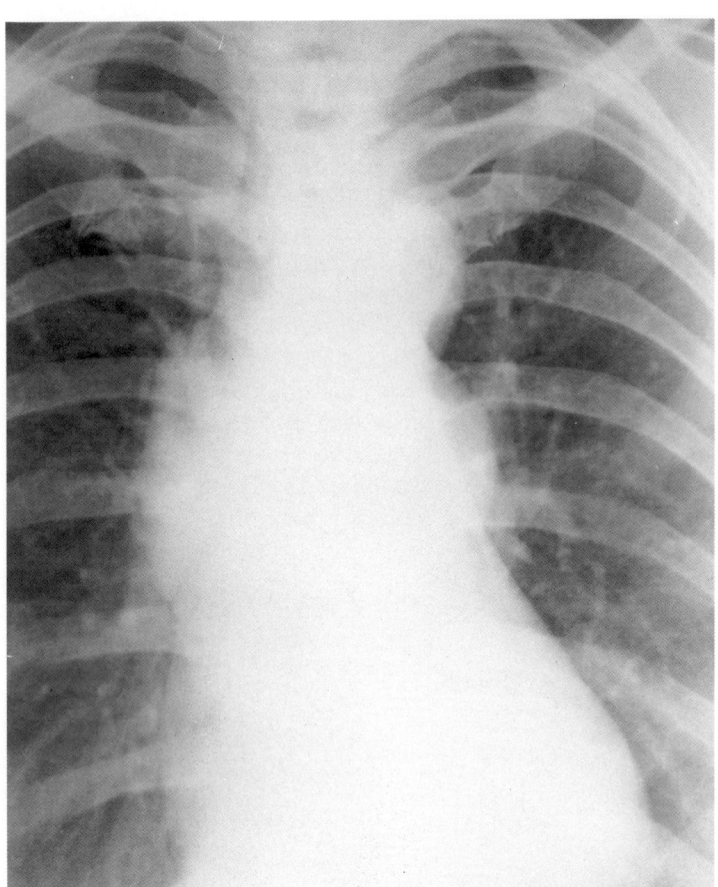

mediastinum, frequently bulge only to one side. Dermoid cysts and teratodermoid tumours may contain calcification, sometimes in the form of a recognizable tooth, and may contain sufficient low-density fat or cholesterol to be detected by CT. Dermoid cysts may become infected and then they increase in size, become less sharply defined on the chest radiograph and give rise to a severe mediastinitis. Other tumours causing masses in the mediastinum include germ cell tumours (seminomas) (Fig. 2.35) and lipomas (Fig. 2.36). Pleuropericardial cysts (Fig. 2.37) arise from the pericardium and are seen as clearly defined rounded opacities on the chest radiograph, attached to the heart border on either the left or right side. They do not usually become infected and, though they may increase slowly in size, are extremely benign. They may communicate with the pericardial sac.

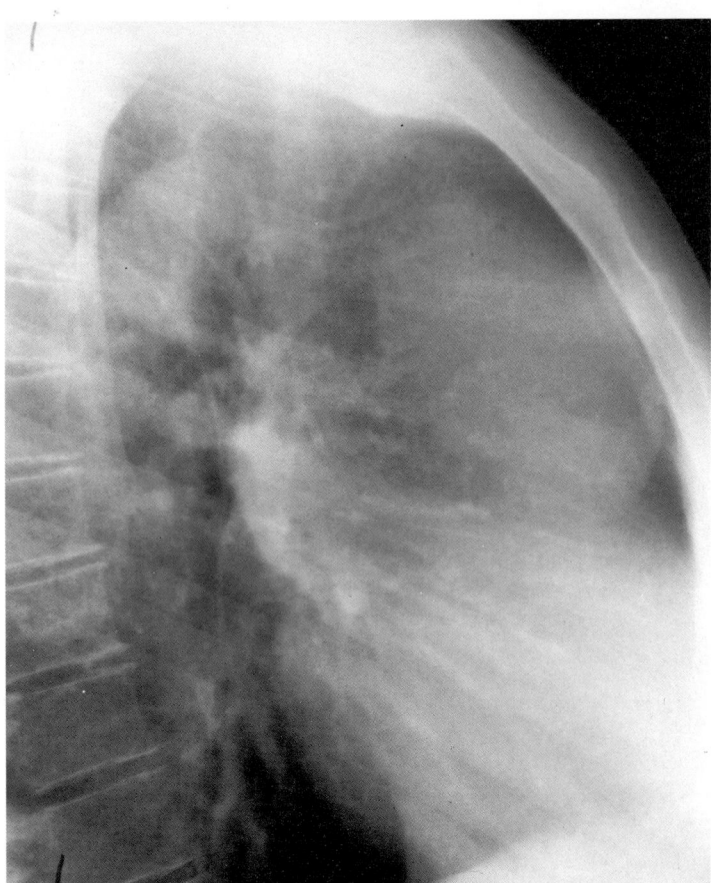

Fig. 2.33 Thymic tumour. A clearly defined oval mass bulging to both sides of the mediastinum is seen to lie behind the sternum on the lateral radiograph.

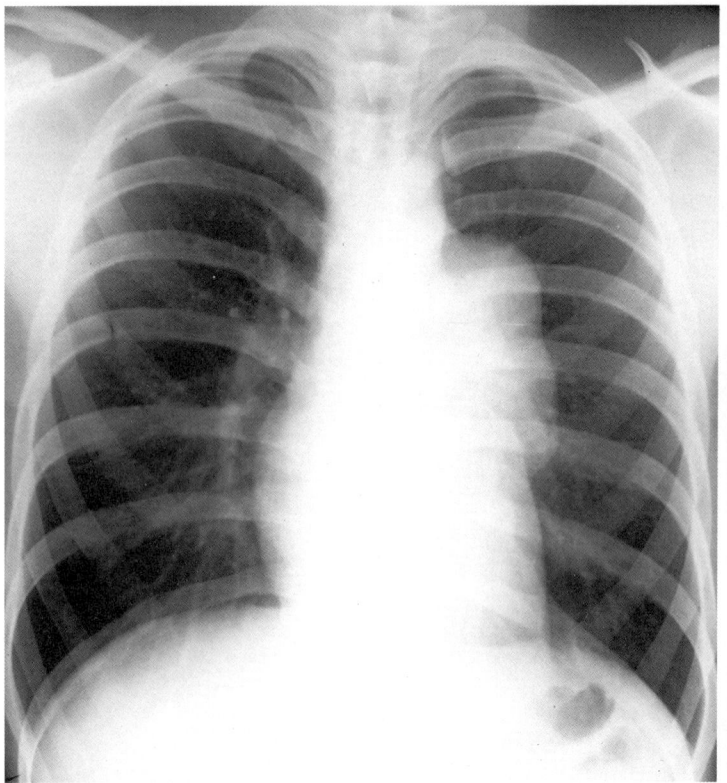

Fig. 2.34 Dermoid cyst. A lobulated, smooth, clearly defined opacity in the anterior mediastinum is bulging towards the left in front of the left hilum, which is seen through it.

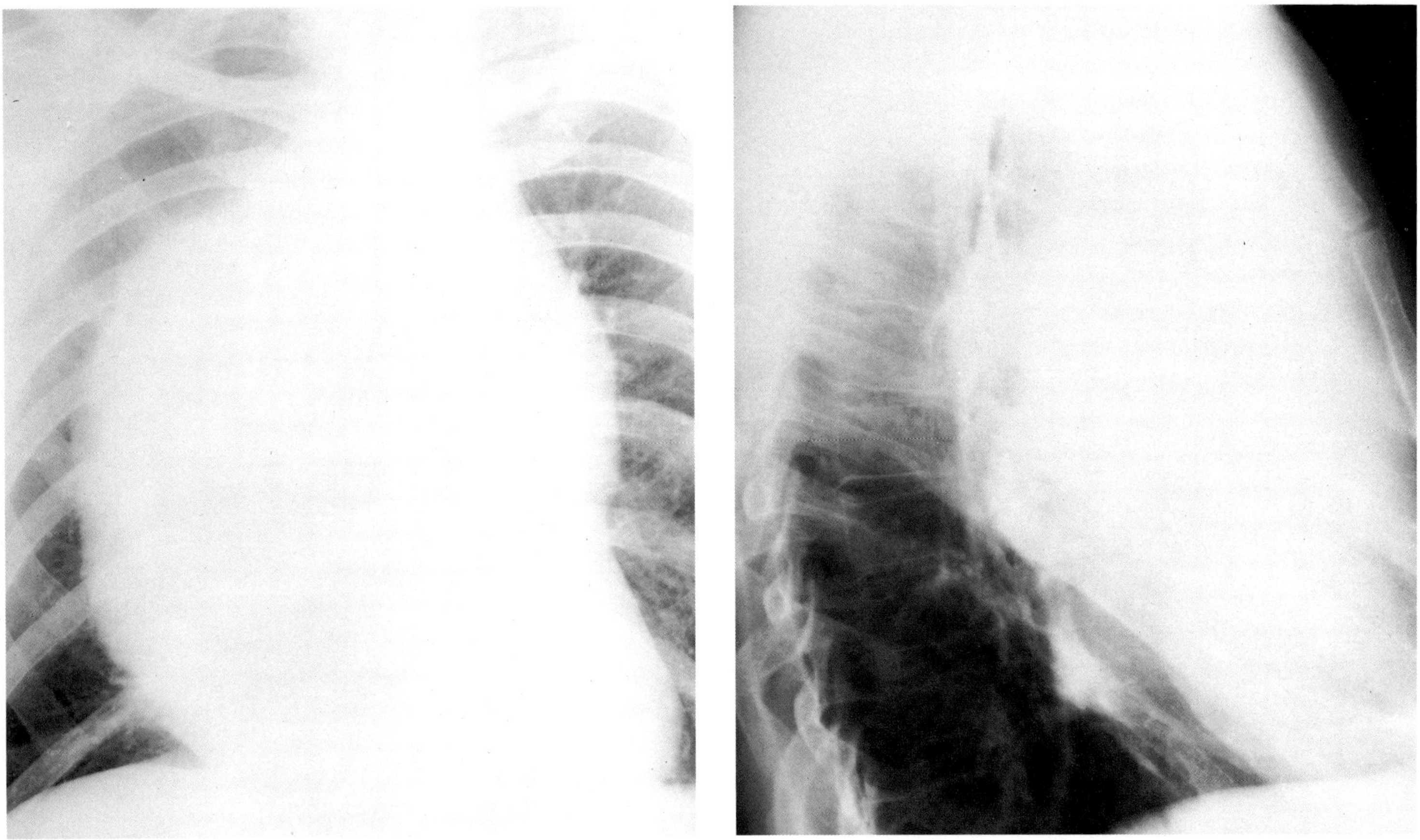

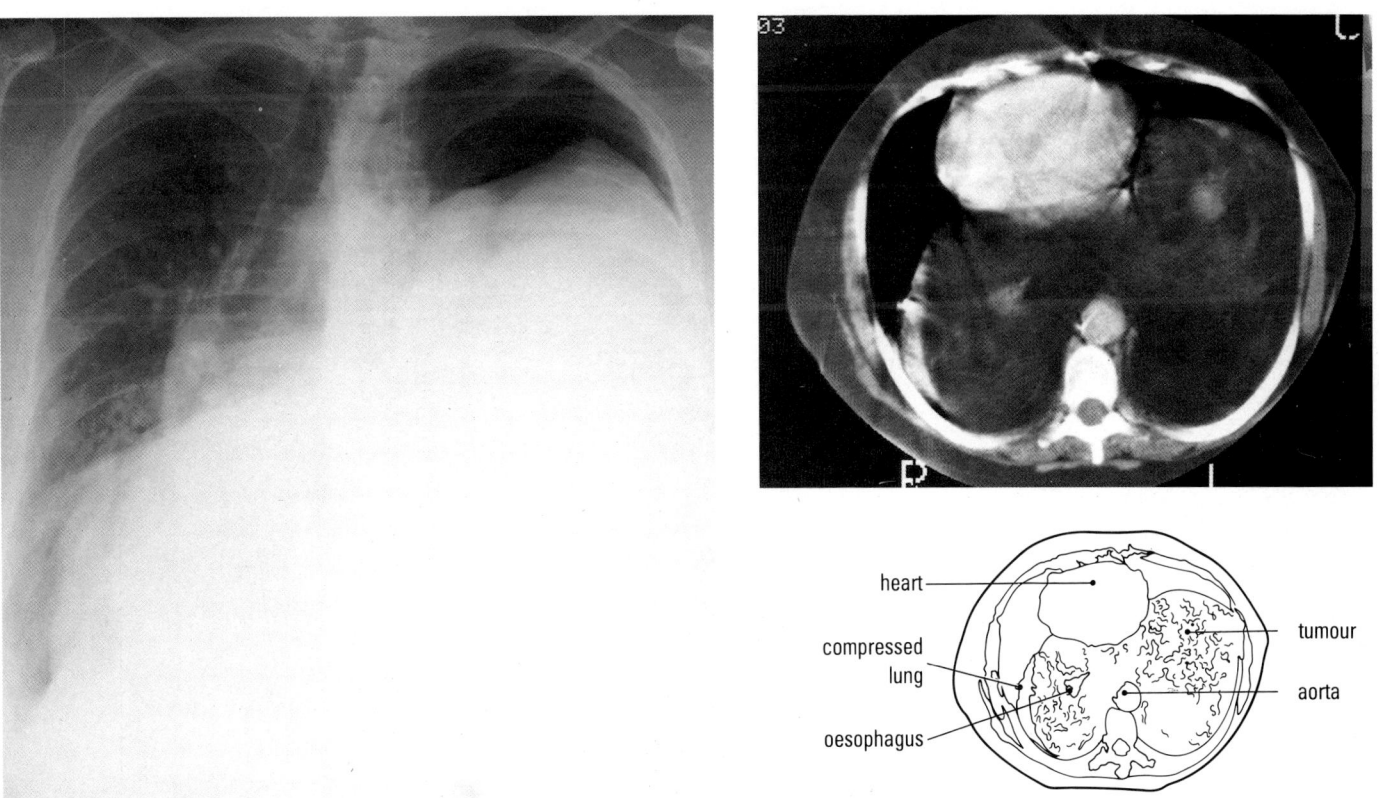

Fig. 2.35 Seminoma. This large retrosternal mass, due to a primary germ cell tumour in the mediastinum, responded dramatically to radiotherapy.

heart

compressed
lung

oesophagus

tumour

aorta

Fig. 2.36 Lipofibrosarcoma. A very large mass obscures the cardiac outline and bulges to both sides of the mediastinum. A left pneumothorax is present following a needle biopsy. The low density of the mass, due to fat, is demonstrated by CT.

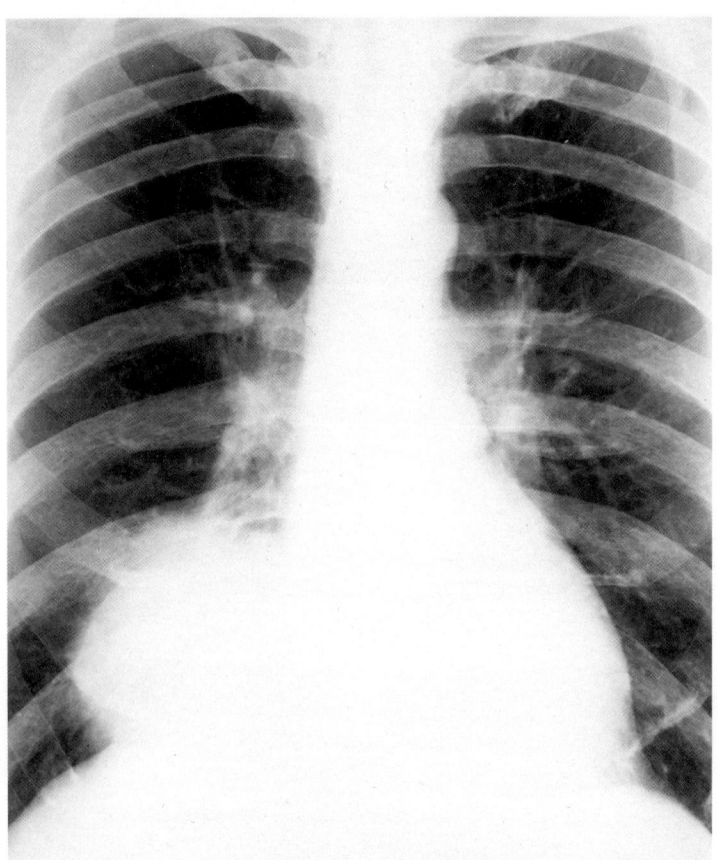

Aneurysms of the aorta may be saccular or fusiform (Figs 2.38 and 2.39). They are seen to be continuous with the aortic shadow at some point, though with saccular aneurysms it may occasionally be difficult to identify this connection. The aneurysm is often filled with layers of thrombus (Fig. 2.40) and fluoroscopy to observe pulsation is therefore useless. Most lesions in the mediastinum will transmit pulsation from the great vessels and it is not possible to distinguish transmitted pulsation from expansile pulsation on fluoroscopy. Aneurysms should be diag-

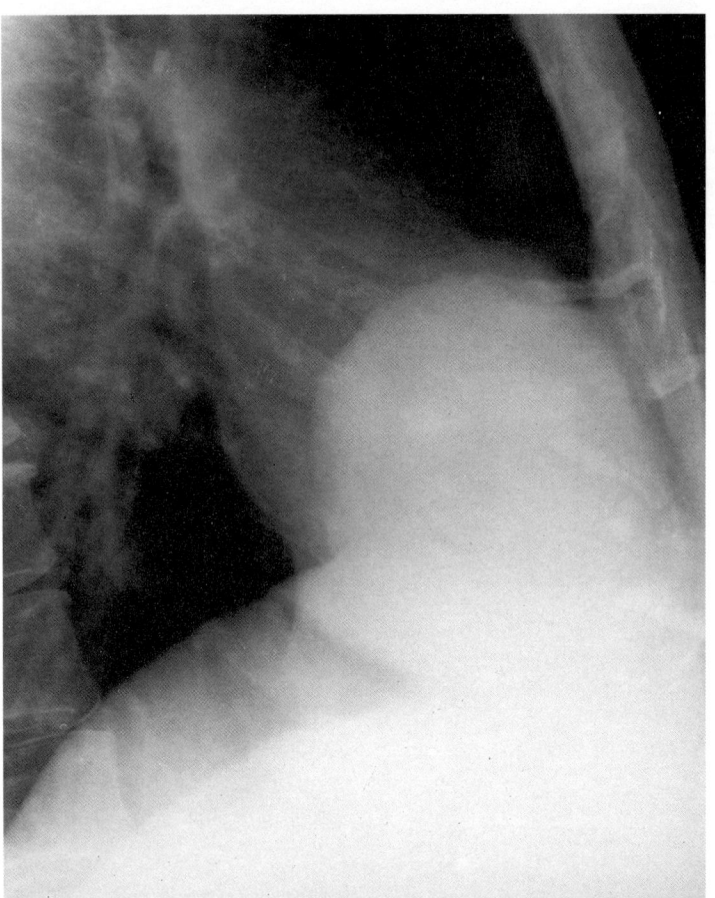

Fig. 2.37 Pleuropericardial cyst. This cyst lies in the right cardiophrenic angle. The slightly hazy outline is probably due to some compression and collapse of adjacent lung. Differential diagnosis includes a Morgagni hernia (see Fig. 2.41).

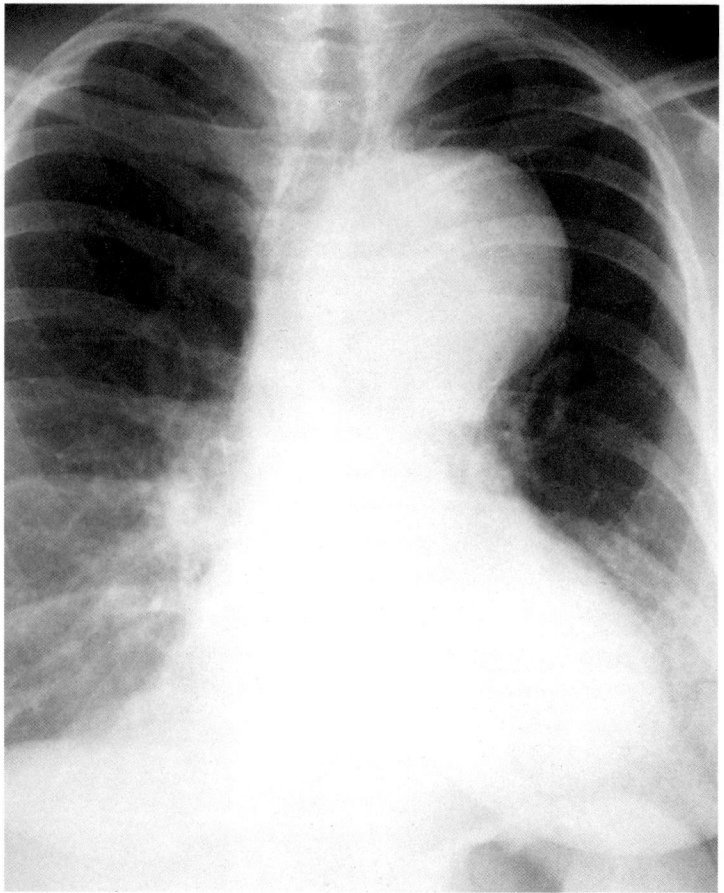

Fig. 2.38 Aneurysm of the arch of the aorta. The aneurysm is causing some compression and displacement of the trachea and left main bronchus. The mass is obscuring the normal aortic arch 'knuckle'.

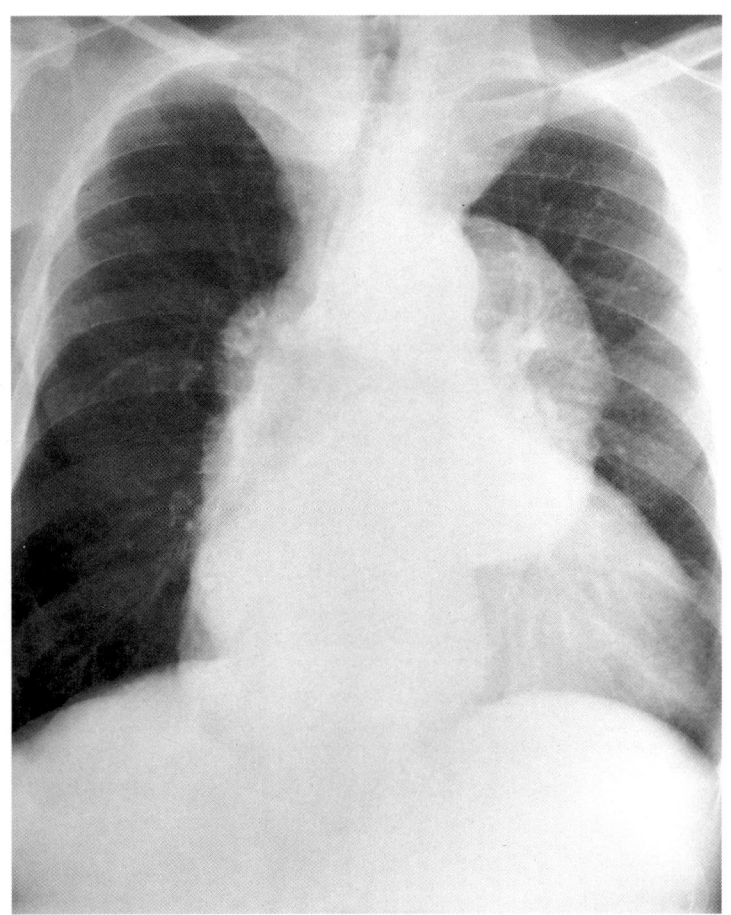

nosed by CT, radioisotope studies or arteriography and it may be important to do these before other procedures, such as biopsy or thoracotomy, are performed. The possibility that a mediastinal mass is an aneurysm should always be borne in mind. Sometimes an aneurysm will expand into the lung, and bleeding from it can be a cause of haemoptysis. The edge of the aneurysm may in these circumstances become indistinct and the appearances can be confused with a carcinoma of the lung.

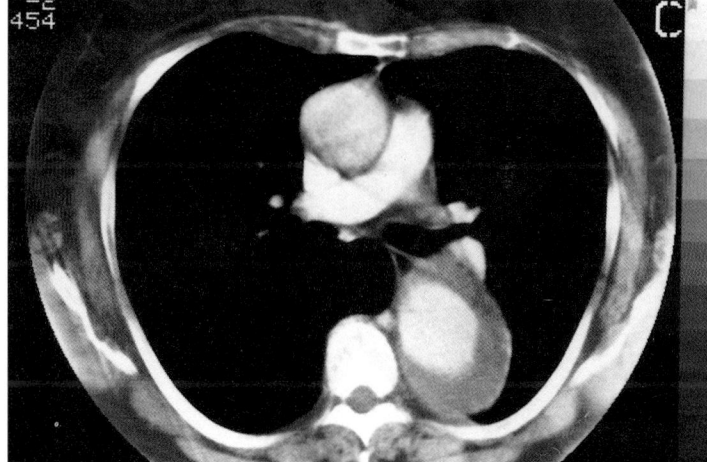

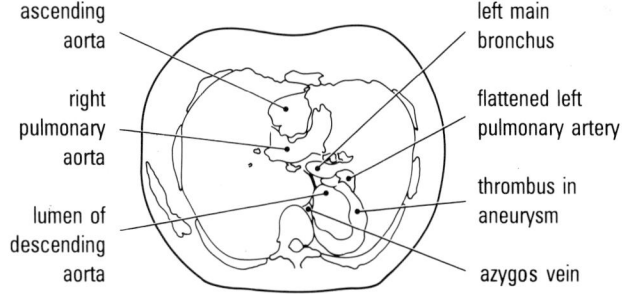

ascending aorta

right pulmonary aorta

lumen of descending aorta

left main bronchus

flattened left pulmonary artery

thrombus in aneurysm

azygos vein

Fig. 2.40 Aneurysm of the descending aorta. This CT scan shows clot within the dilated aorta. Contrast medium enhances the lumen, where there is free blood flow. The left pulmonary artery is adjacent to the anterolateral margin of the aneurysm; the left main bronchus is just in front.

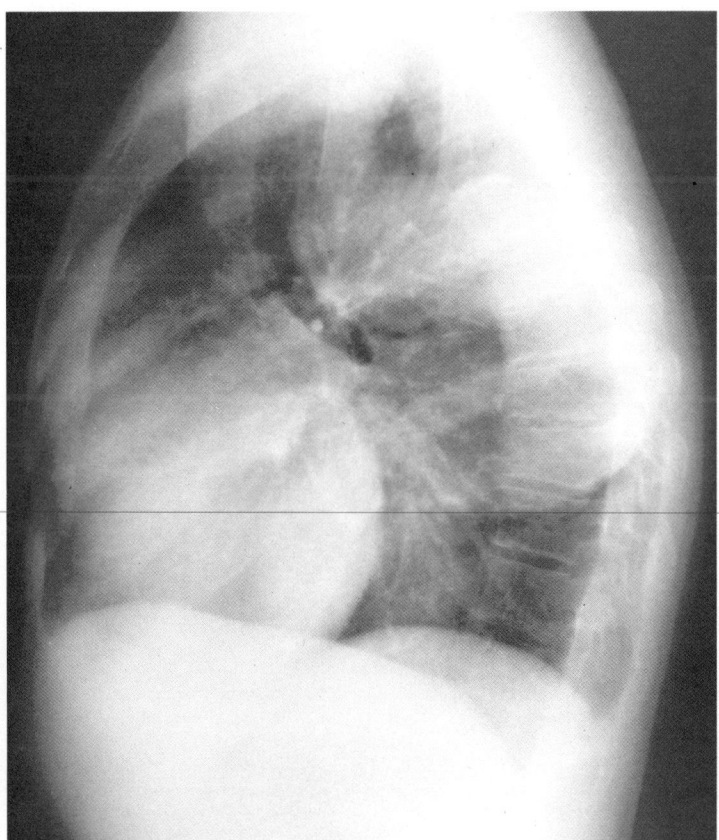

Fig. 2.39 Aneurysm of the descending aorta. In this case the aortic 'knuckle' is visible in front of the mass, but the mass cannot be separated from the shadow of the descending aorta from which it arises.

Hernia of the diaphragm

Hernia of the diaphragm may give rise to a large mass-like lesion in the chest. Bowel may be present in the hernia, but frequently most of the hernia contains omentum, which has a high fat content, and liver. Hernias of the foramen of Morgagni occur anteriorly, usually in the right cardiophrenic angle, and produce a round swelling arising from the anterior part of the diaphragm (Fig. 2.41). Hernias of the foramen of Bochdalek occur posteriorly and contain kidney, bowel, liver or spleen (Fig. 2.42); they are nearly always seen on the left side. Hiatus hernias are the commonest and produce a mass, nearly always with an air/fluid level, behind the heart, due to the herniated stomach. A barium study will demonstrate a hiatus hernia and late films may show bowel in Bochdalek or Morgagni hernias (Fig. 2.43). Congenital hernias of the diaphragm cause respiratory distress in the neonatal period and may be very large. Rupture of the diaphragm and herniation may occur after trauma.

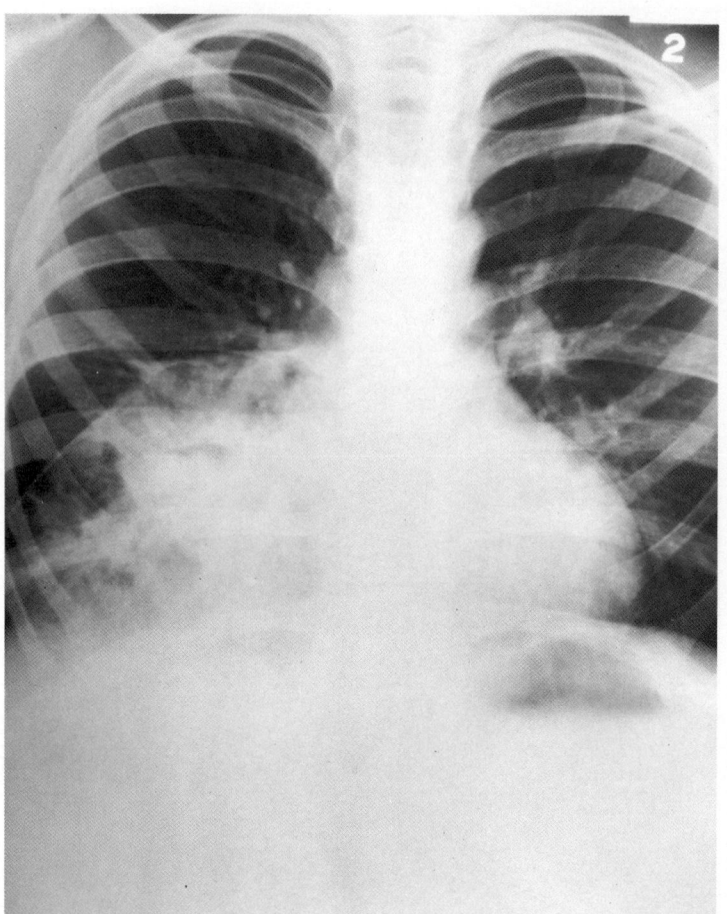

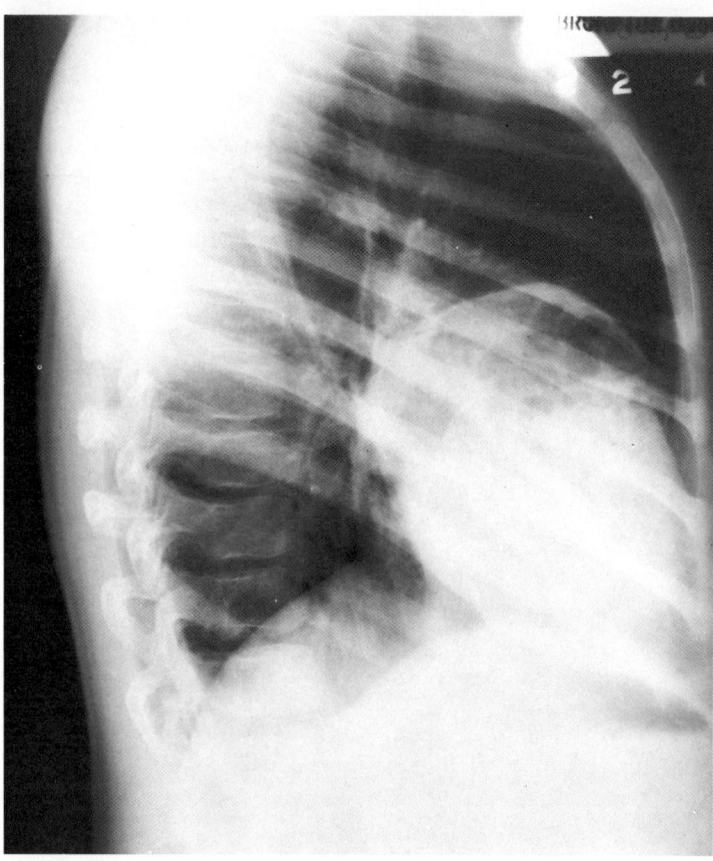

Fig. 2.41 Morgagni hernia. This hernia is filled with bowel which contains gas and faeces. Often only omentum is present.

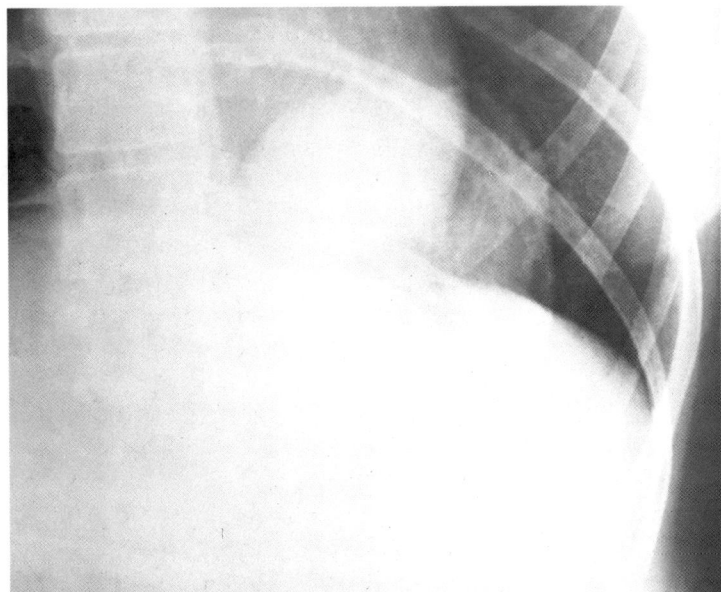

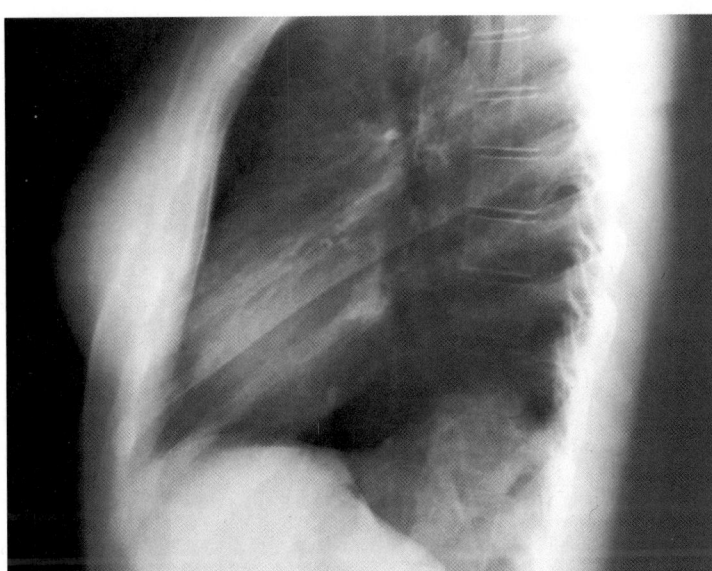

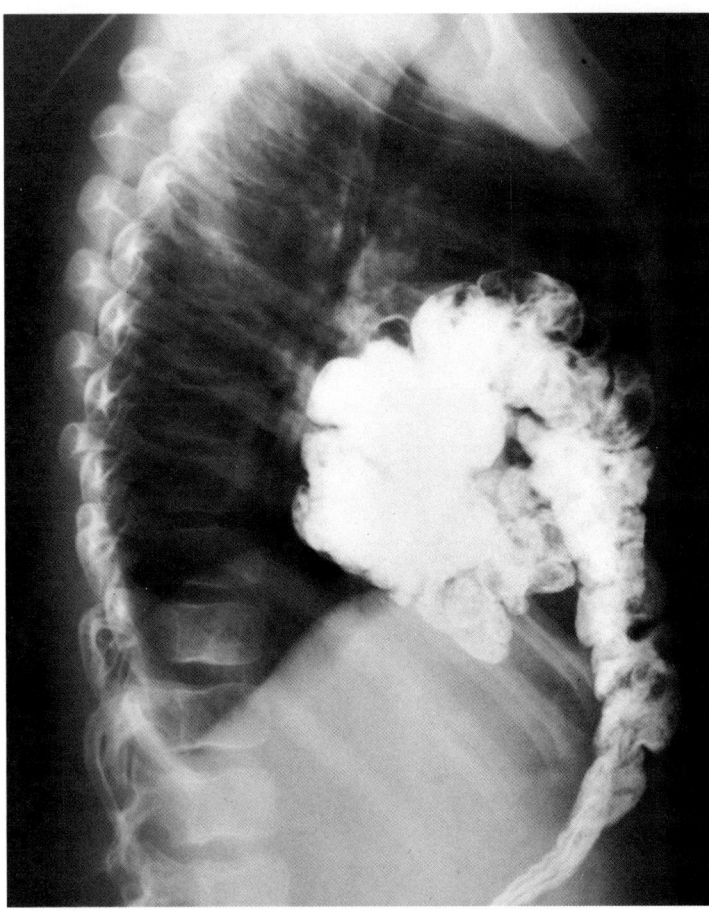

Fig. 2.43 Morgagni hernia. Barium-filled loops of bowel lie in the hernia.

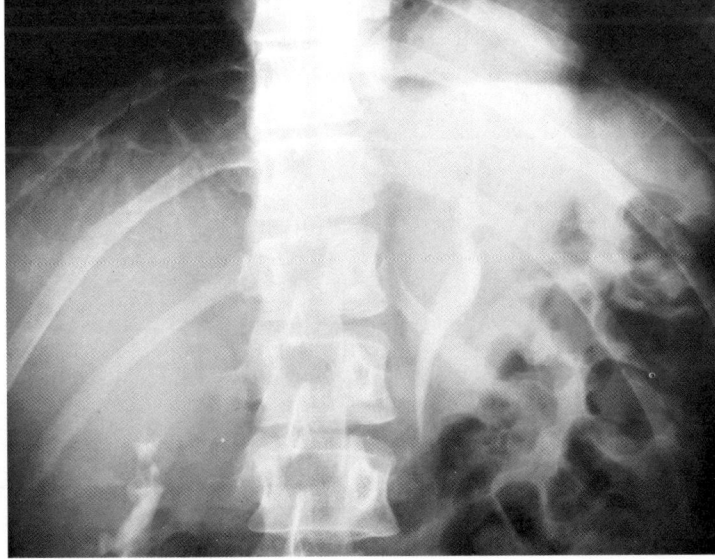

Fig. 2.42 Bochdalek hernia. A bulge is seen arising from the posterior part of the diaphragm behind the heart. The intravenous urogram (bottom) shows that the left kidney lies within this hernia, which also contains perirenal fat.

3

Tumours

Carcinoma of the Bronchus

Chest radiograph

The chest radiograph may initially be normal or show no definite mass (Fig. 3.1) but any of the following may occur:

A solitary nodule or 'coin' lesion of any size may be present. An opacity with an irregular margin adjacent to the hilum is a very common radiological appearance (Fig. 3.2) — this can be caused by the tumour itself or by metastases to the hilar lymph nodes. Cavitating lesions

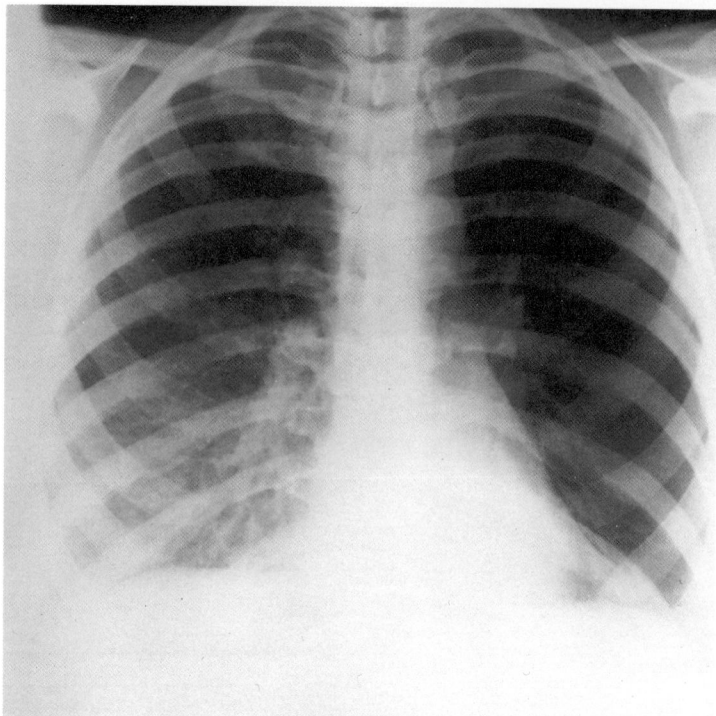

Fig. 3.1 Carcinoma of the bronchus showing obstructive overinflation (obstructive emphysema). The left lung shows decreased vascularity but no definite mass can be identified. There is a carcinoma of the left main bronchus. On expiratory film there was air trapping in the left lung.

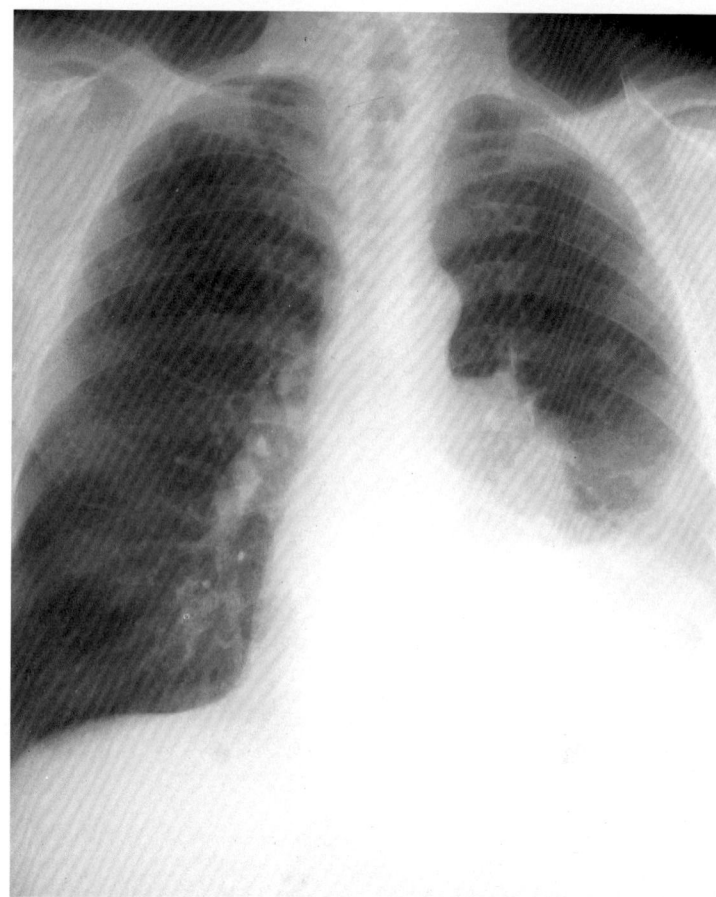

Fig. 3.2 Oat cell carcinoma mass at the left hilum with a left pleural effusion.

may be present (Fig. 3.3). The collapse of a lobe or a whole lung (Fig. 3.4) may be present with the signs of mediastinal displacement. The appearance may be of pneumonia distal to a still relatively small carcinoma. Lymphangitis carcinomatosa causes linear shadows which may be unilateral or bilateral (Fig. 3.5). Pleural effusion can be present. Bony metastases involving the rib cage can occur. The mediastinum may be widened due to lymph node metastases. Elevation of the hemidiaphragm due to a phrenic nerve palsy (Fig. 3.6) is possible and multiple pulmonary metastases can occur.

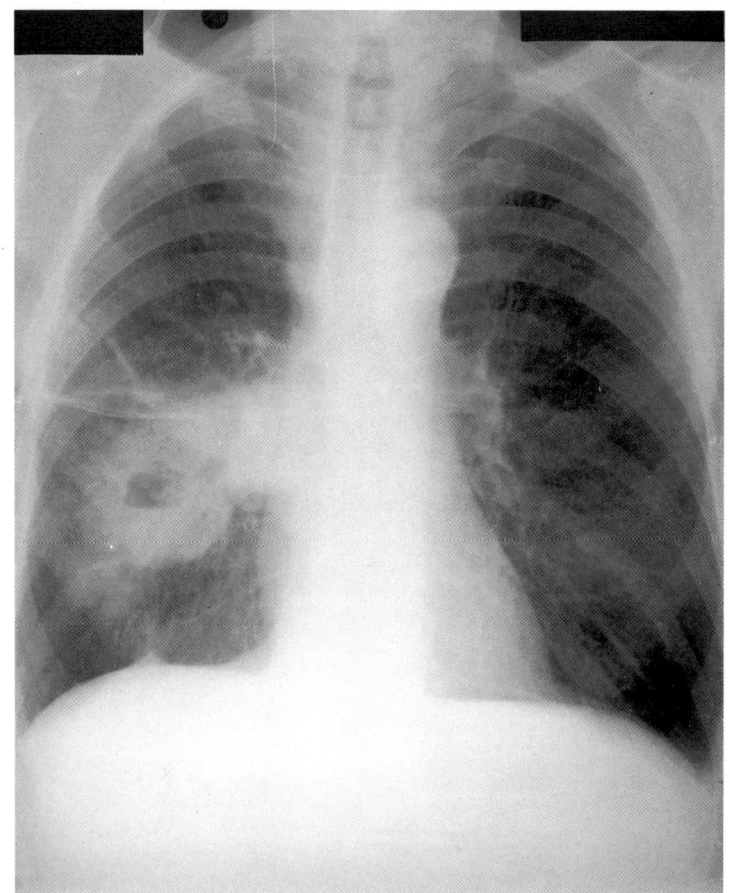

Fig. 3.3 Cavitating carcinoma of the bronchus in a patient with coal miners' pneumoconiosis. There is lymph node involvement at the right hilum.

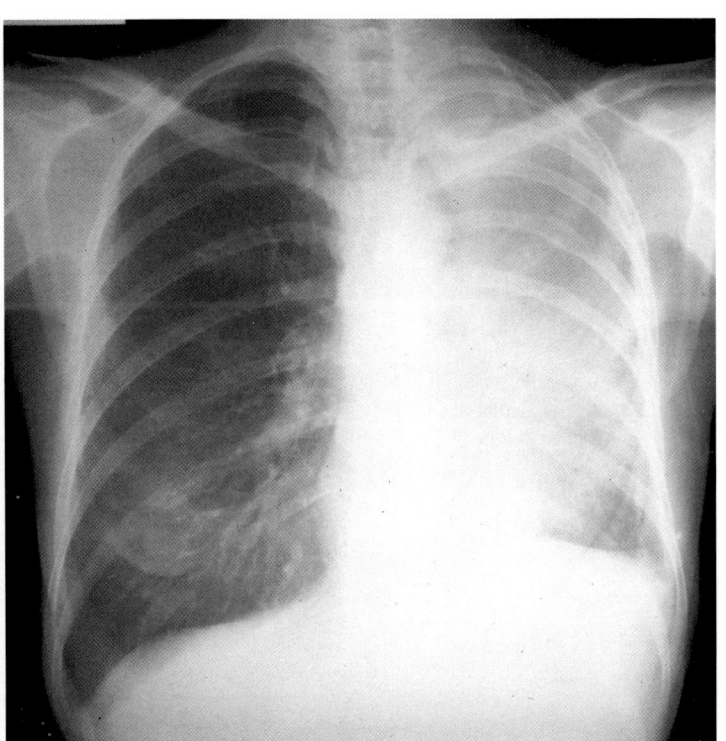

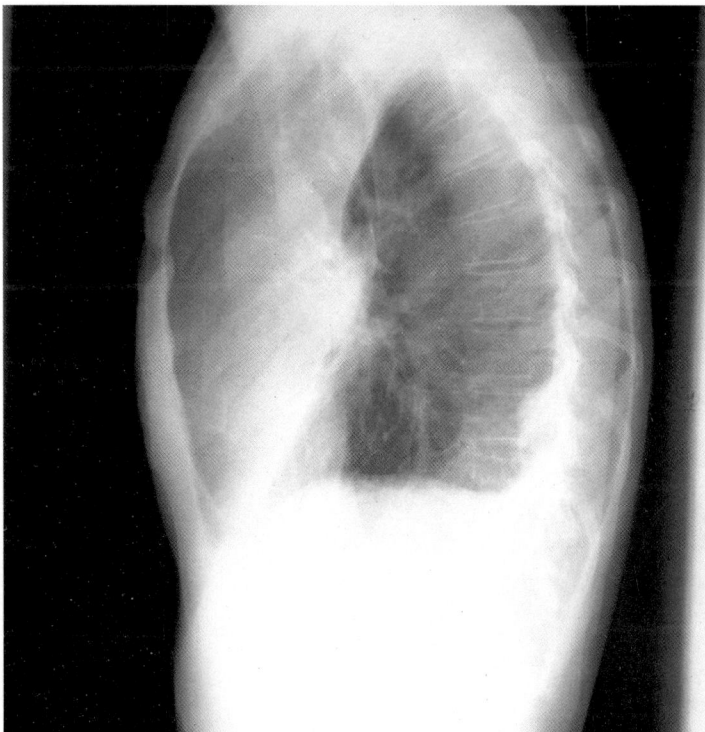

Fig. 3.4 Frontal view shows collapse of the left upper lobe. Posterior part of the left sixth rib shows an area of destruction. The lateral view shows a pleural nodule posteriorly above the diaphragm.

Percutaneous needle biopsy

This is carried out under fluoroscopic control. It is particularly useful for peripheral tumours not accessible to the fibreoptic bronchoscope (Fig. 3.7).

Barium swallow

If a patient has dysphagia a barium swallow is indicated to see if there is enlargement of mediastinal nodes pressing on the oesophagus (Fig. 3.8).

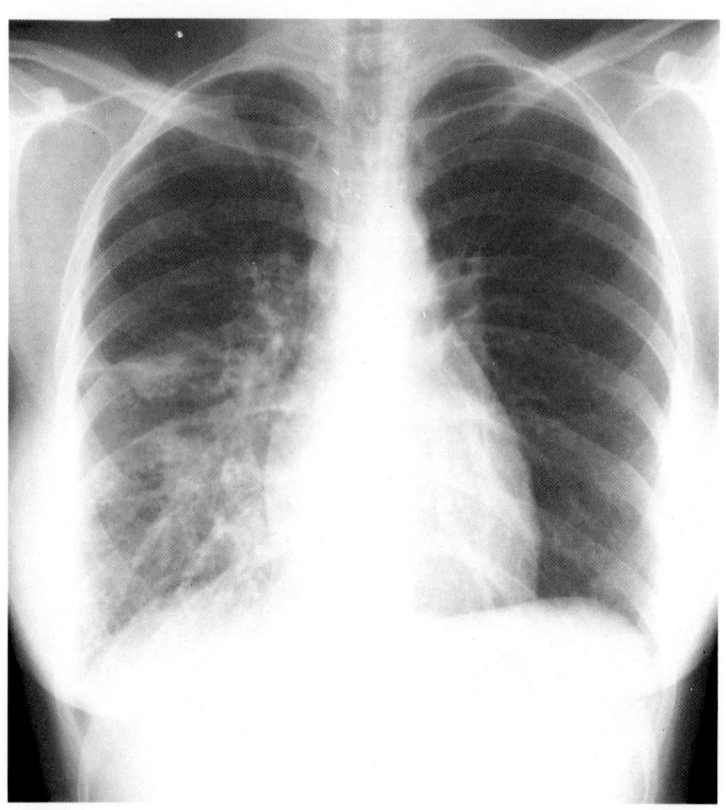

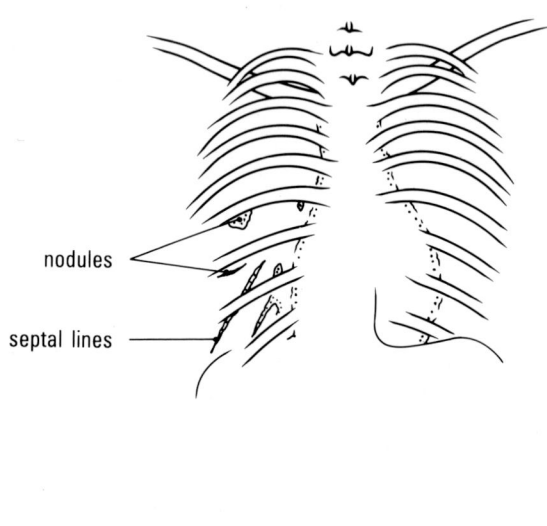

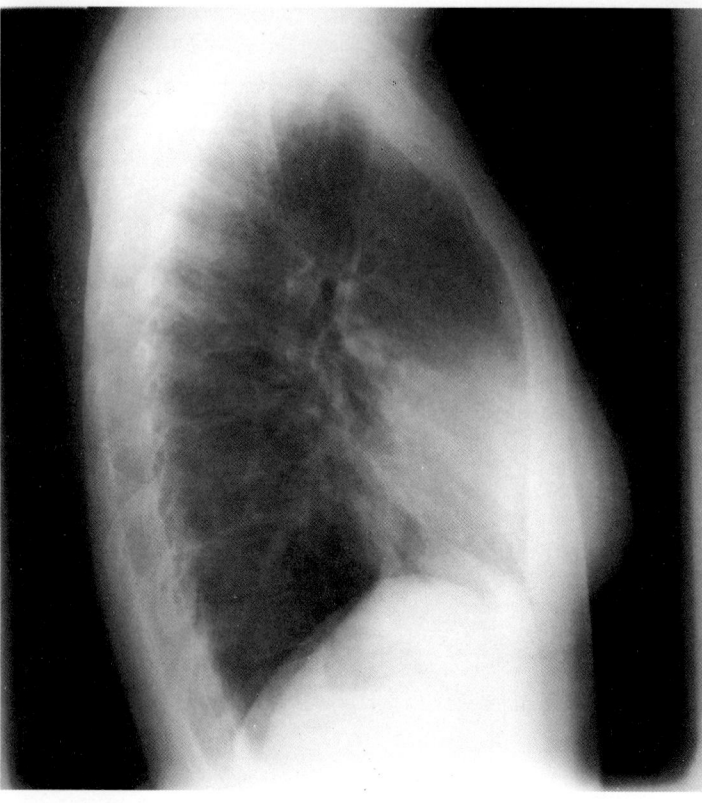

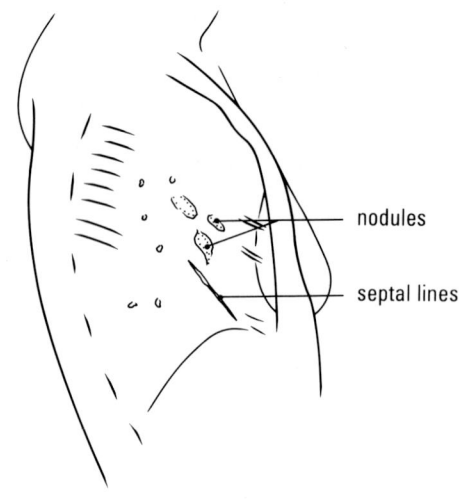

Fig. 3.5 Right unilateral lymphangitis carcinomatosa, primary unknown. Extensive shadowing, predominantly linear, is seen in the right lung. Prominent septal lines are present and a few nodules of varying sizes are also present in the right lower zone. The left lung is clear.

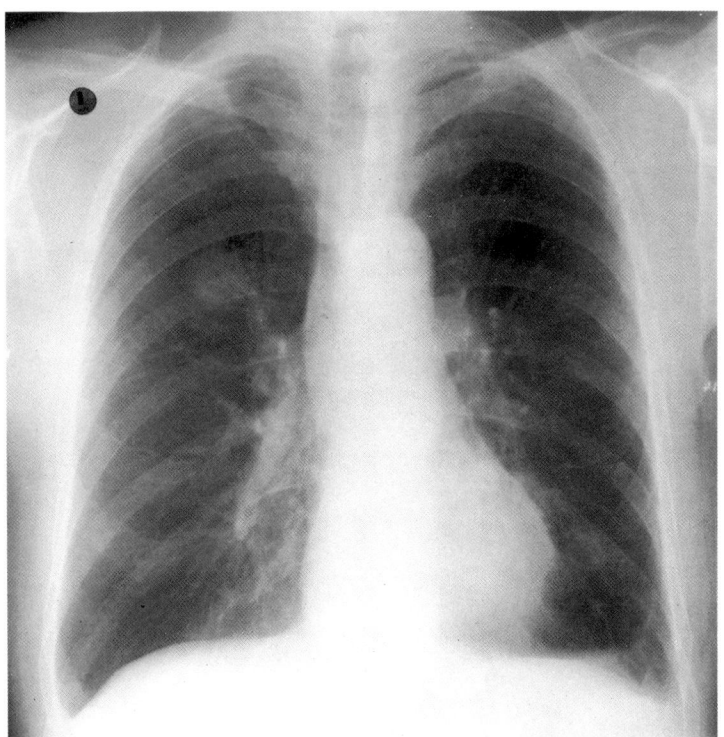

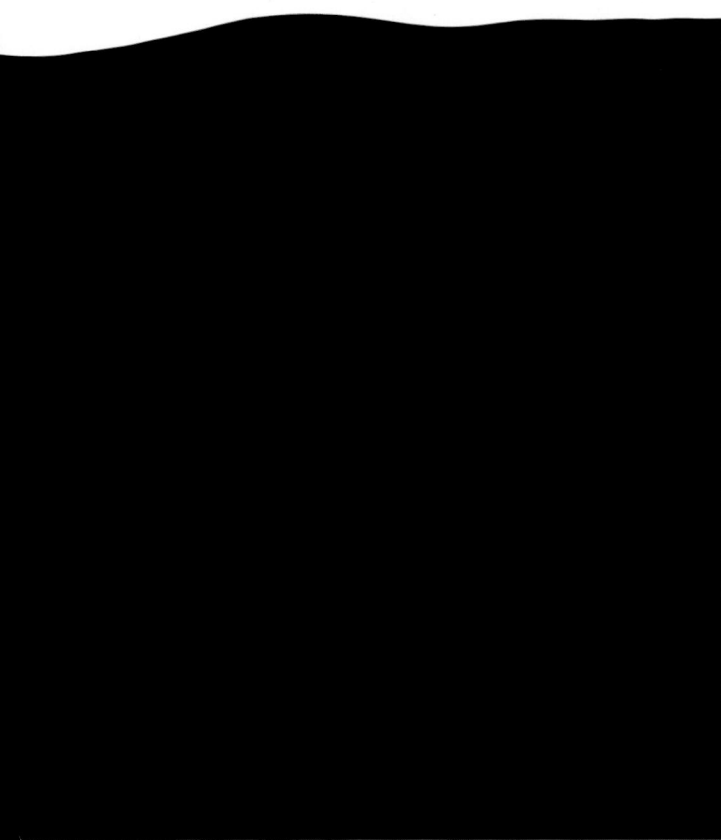

Fig. 3.6 Carcinoma of the bronchus with right phrenic nerve paralysis. A mass is present at the right hilum and there is elevation of the right dome of the diaphragm.

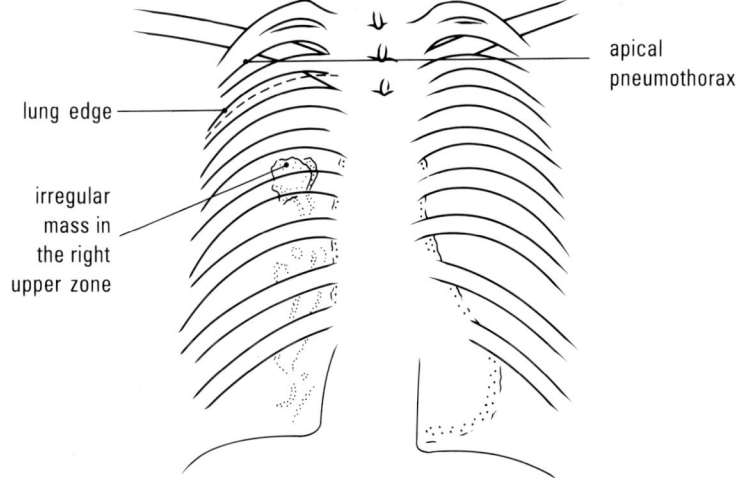

Fig. 3.7 A slightly irregular opacity in the right upper lobe with no specific radiological features. A small pneumothorax is present following needle aspiration and biopsy.

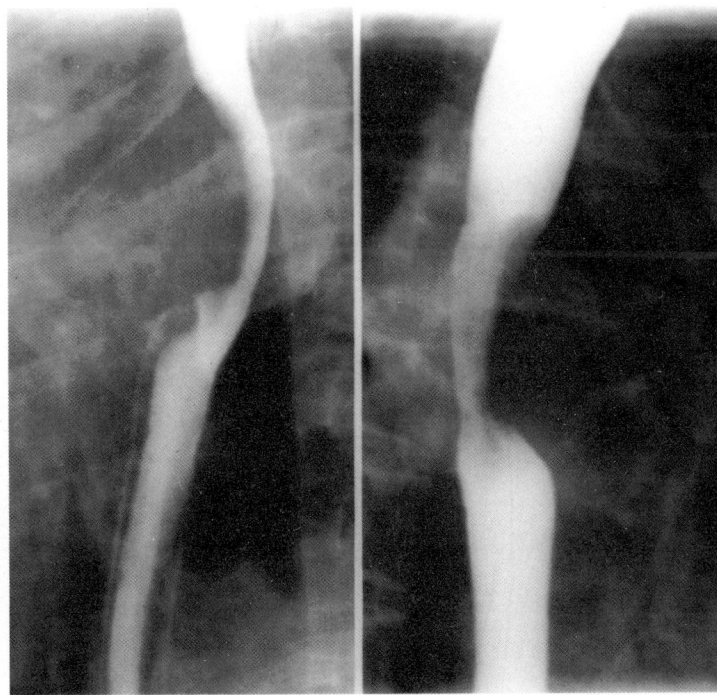

Fig. 3.8 Small cell carcinoma of the bronchus. The patient presented with dysphagia. Barium swallow shows compression and marked narrowing of the oesophagus by enlarged lymph nodes.

Screening of the diaphragm

Involvement of the phrenic nerve by tumour can cause paralysis of the diaphragm which can be confirmed by screening (Fig. 3.9).

Computerized tomography (CT)

CT scan of the thorax will help to determine the extent of the tumour, identifying lymphadenopathy or the presence of metastases in the chest (Figs 3.10–3.13). It should be noted that enlargement of the lymph nodes does not necessarily indicate that they are invaded by tumour.

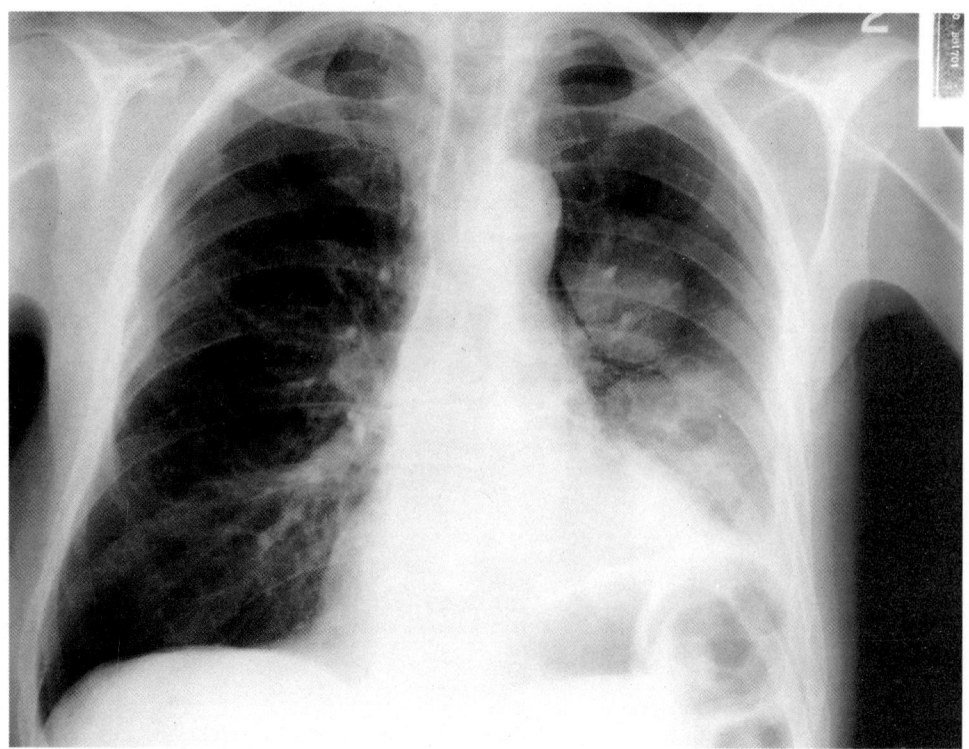

Fig. 3.9 Small cell carcinoma: a cavitating mass in the left lower lobe. A small left pleural effusion is present and the left dome of the diaphragm is elevated due to phrenic nerve involvement. An oval opacity above the carcinoma has well defined inferior margins and poorly defined upper margins. This is due to a loculated effusion in the oblique fissure. There are pathological fractures of several ribs on the right due to metastases.

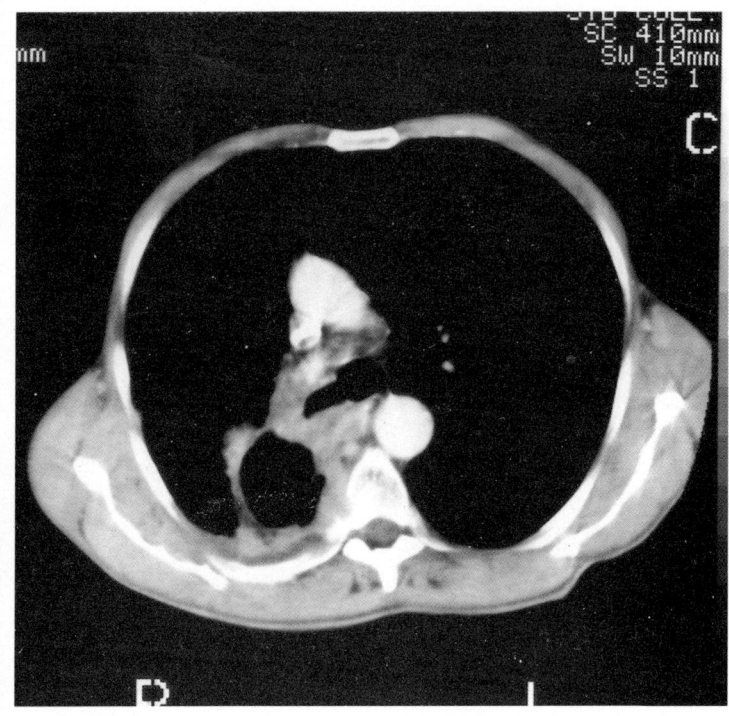

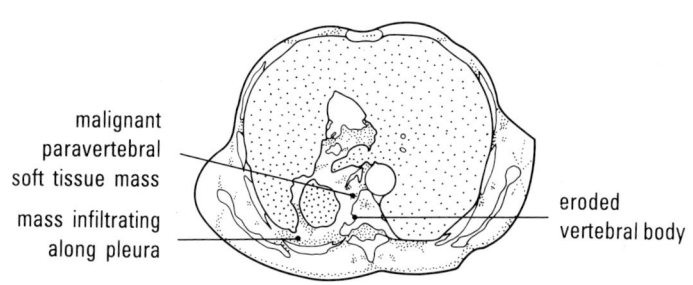

Fig. 3.10 CT scan showing carcinoma involving vertebrae. Malignant infiltrates are seen in the right paravertebral gutter with destruction of the right posterior parts of the vertebrae.

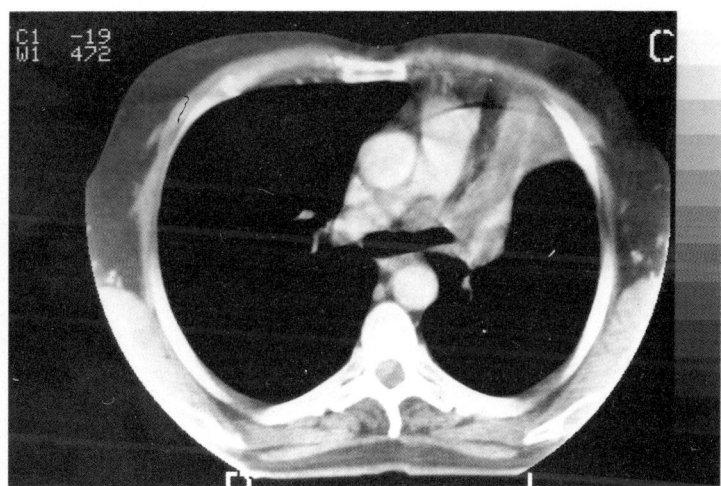

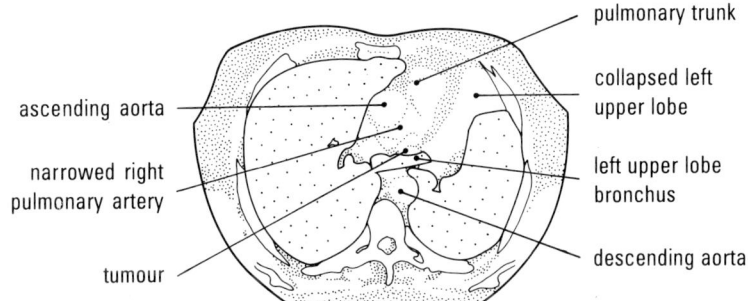

Fig. 3.11 CT scan showing collapse of the left upper lobe. Tumour is seen extending into the mediastinum in front of the bronchus and causing compression of the right pulmonary artery at its origin from the pulmonary trunk. The tumour has occluded the upper left lobe bronchus.

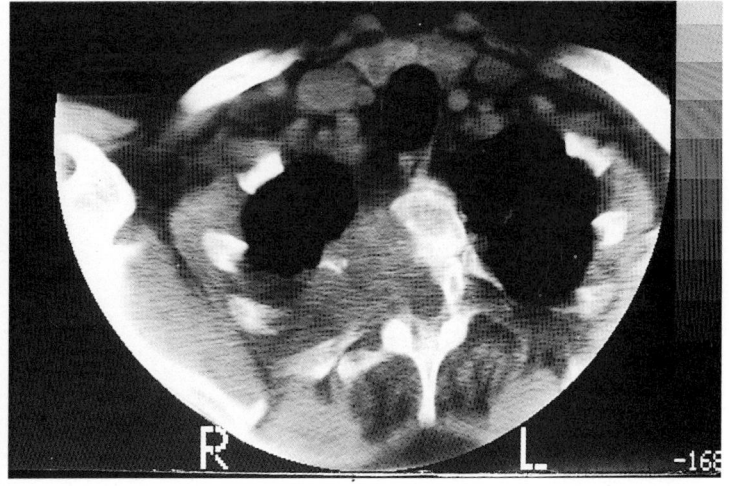

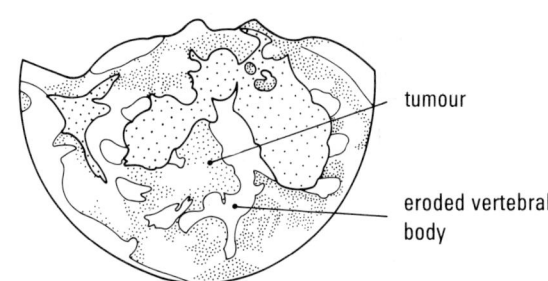

Fig. 3.12 CT scan of chest: Pancoast's tumour destroying part of the right side of the vertebrae and posterior ends of adjacent ribs.

Pulmonary lymphomas

These arise from lymphoid tissue within the lung and typically remain localized for considerable periods of time. They may be Hodgkin's or non-Hodgkin's lymphomas and presentation may be similar to other types of pulmonary tumour (Fig. 3.15). The radiological appearance includes glandular enlargement, pulmonary infiltrates, disseminated nodules, coin lesions, or unilateral hilar masses

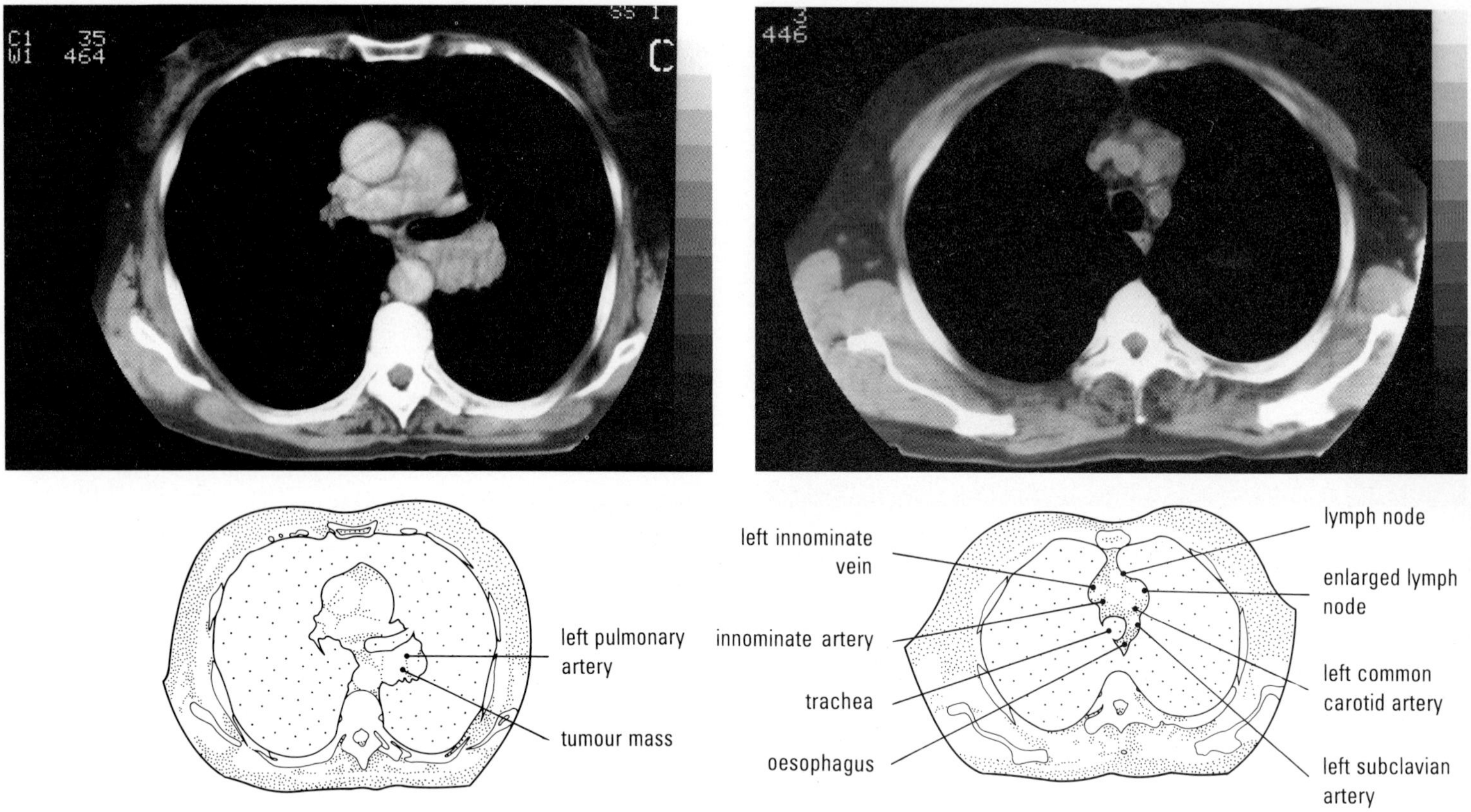

left pulmonary artery

tumour mass

left innominate vein

innominate artery

trachea

oesophagus

lymph node

enlarged lymph node

left common carotid artery

left subclavian artery

Fig. 3.13 Carcinoma of the bronchus. CT scans showing: (a) Following contrast enhancement the left pulmonary artery is seen to be considerably compressed by the mass. (b) Enlargement of nodes in the left superior mediastinum in front of the left common carotid artery.

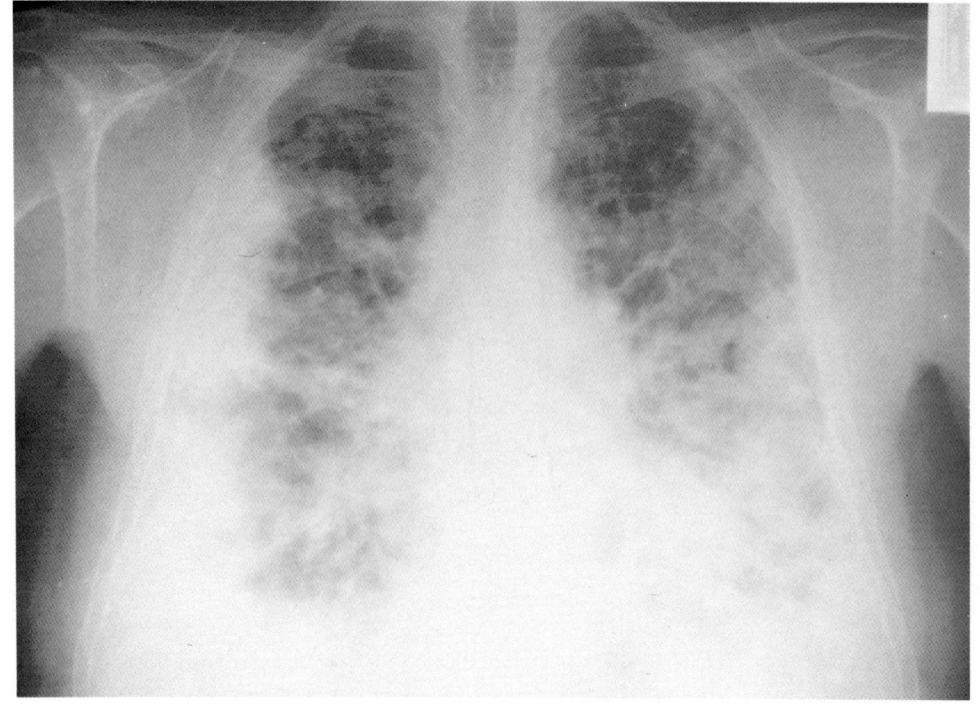

Fig. 3.14 Bronchiolo-alveolar cell carcinoma: widespread poorly defined nodular shadowing which is confluent over a large area in both lungs, particularly peripherally.

resembling carcinoma of the bronchus. Pleural effusions may also be present. Treatment is by chemotherapy and/or radiotherapy, as for other lymphomas. The pulmonary lesion has however usually to be removed to make the diagnosis.

Pulmonary blastoma

This is derived from undifferentiated embryonic connective tissue (Fig. 3.16) and is another very rare tumour which sometimes has a benign course but may metastasize.

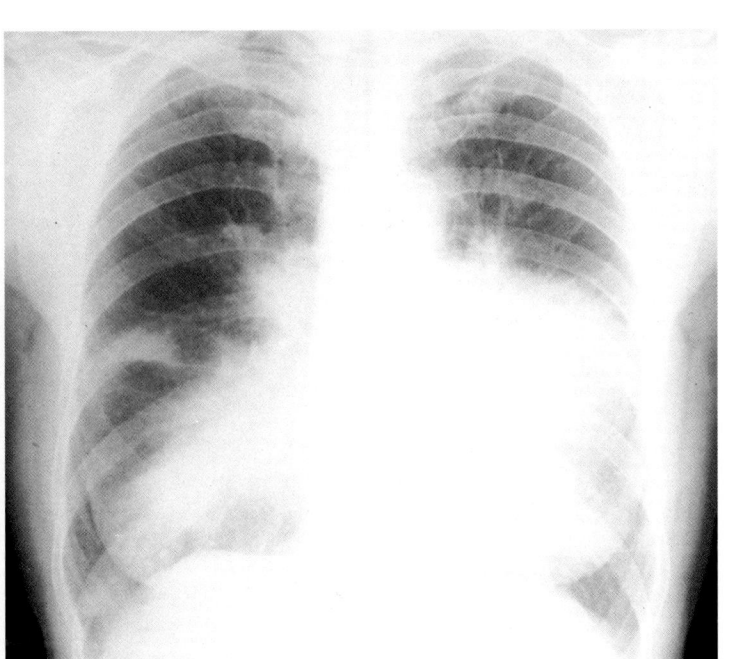

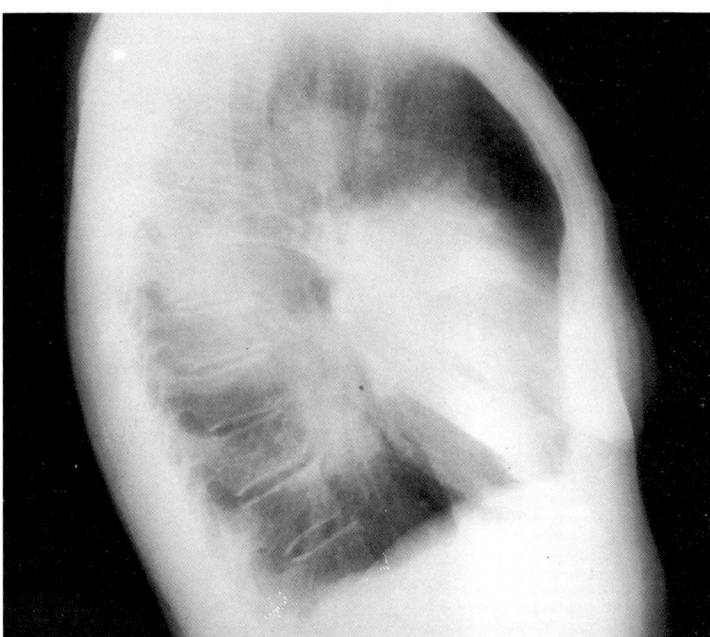

Fig. 3.15 Lymphocytic lymphoma of the lung. Ill-defined areas of dense opacification are present in both lungs; similarly areas of consolidation. These developed slowly over several years.

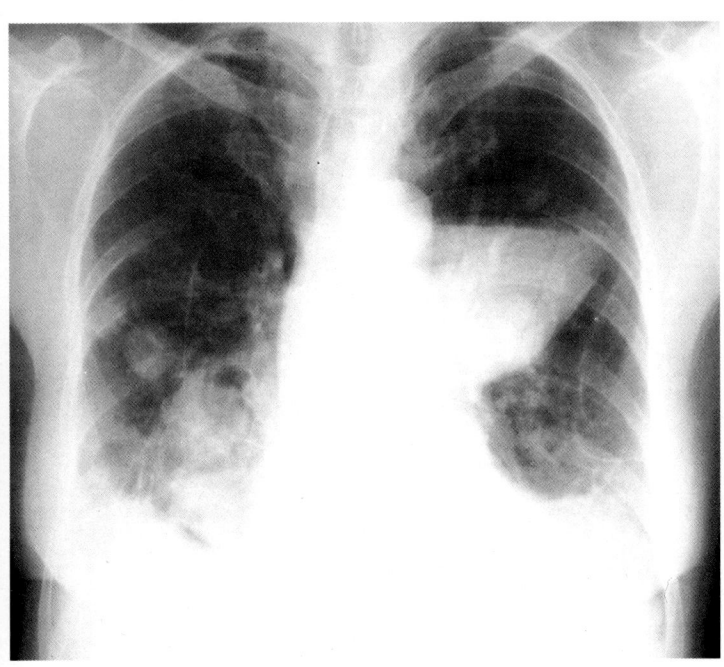

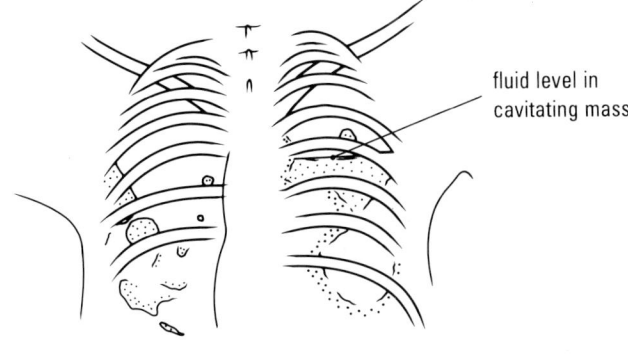

Fig. 3.16 Pulmonary blastoma: multiple round opacities some of which have cavitated (an air fluid level is seen opposite the aortic knuckle in one large lesion.

Carcinoids

This is the commonest of the bronchial adenomas and may present as a polyp (Fig. 3.17) in the bronchus. A bronchial carcinoid tumour (see Fig. 2.17) may give rise to the carcinoid syndrome which consists of intermittent cyanotic flushes, abdominal cramps, diarrhoea, wheezing and dyspnoea. These symptoms are thought to be due to the production of serotonin and kinins. Breakdown products of serotonin can be identified in the urine. Most patients with carcinoid symptoms have metastases, usually in the liver, in which case valvular disease affecting the right heart may develop. The chest radiograph may be abnormal, but it is often normal and diagnosis is made following bronchoscopy and biopsy.

Bronchial gland tumours

Adenocystic carcinoma (cylindroma) (Fig. 3.18), muco-epidermoid carcinoma and mixed tumours all arise from the bronchial mucous glands, often in the large bronchi, whose wall they infiltrate. They may present with recurrent haemoptysis, cough, unilateral wheezing, pulmonary collapse and infection. These tumours may metastasize but many of the tumours grow slowly.

Hamartoma

This tumour is composed of different tissues which normally appear in the lung but they are abnormally organized to form a tumour (see Fig. 2.9). The lesion usually arises in the periphery of the lung and may be found on a routine chest X-ray, and usually occurs after the age of fifty years. Hamartoma should be considered in the differential diagnosis of any solitary pulmonary nodule. Treatment is by surgical resection.

Leiomyoma

Leiomyoma are rare and arise from the smooth muscle found in airways and alveolar ducts (Fig. 3.19).

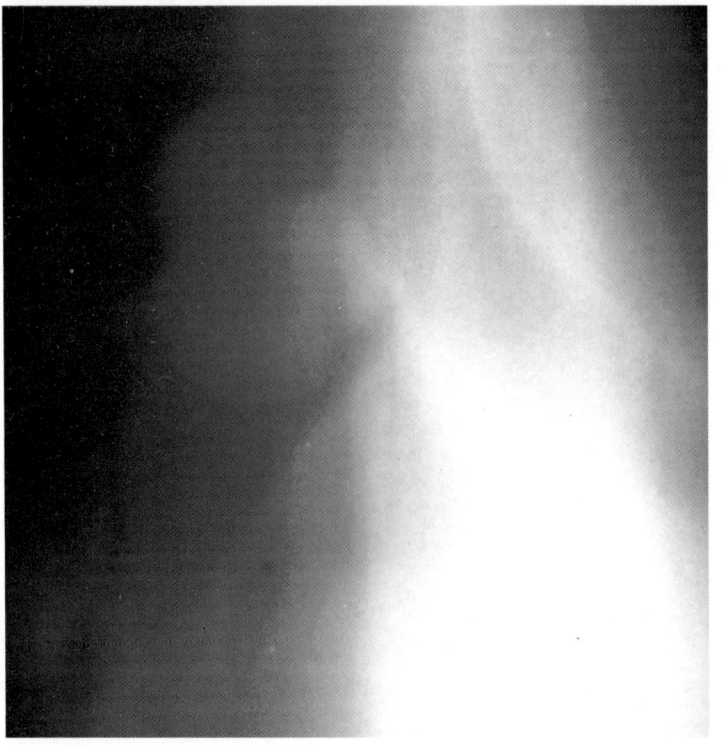

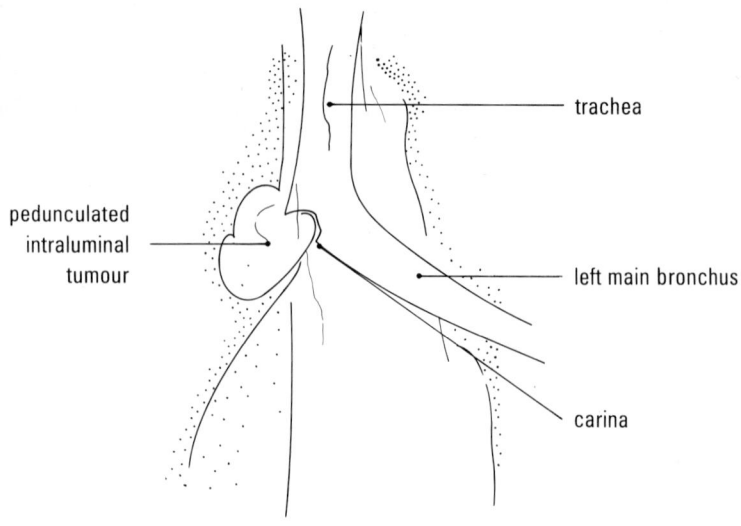

Fig. 3.17 Bronchial carcinoid tumour. The tomogram shows a pedunculated intraluminal tumour at the origin of the right main bronchus.

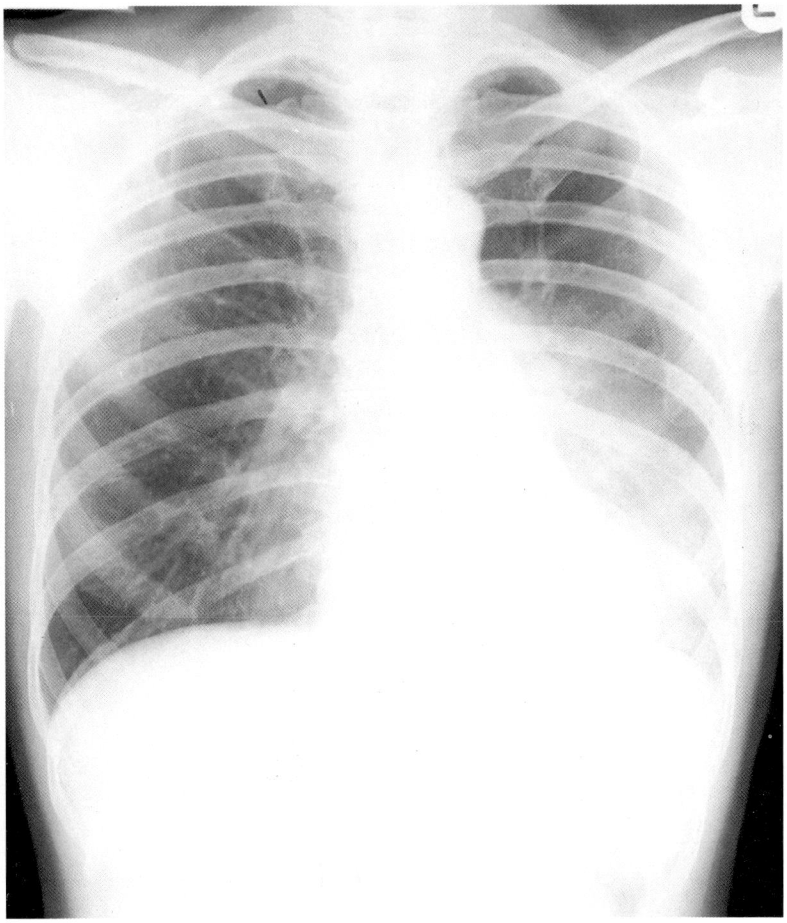

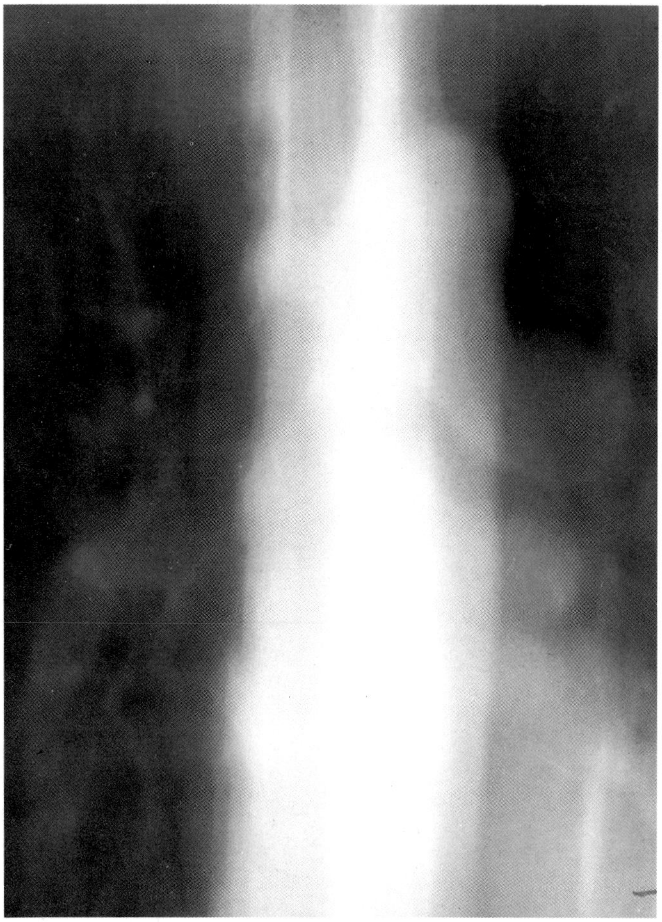

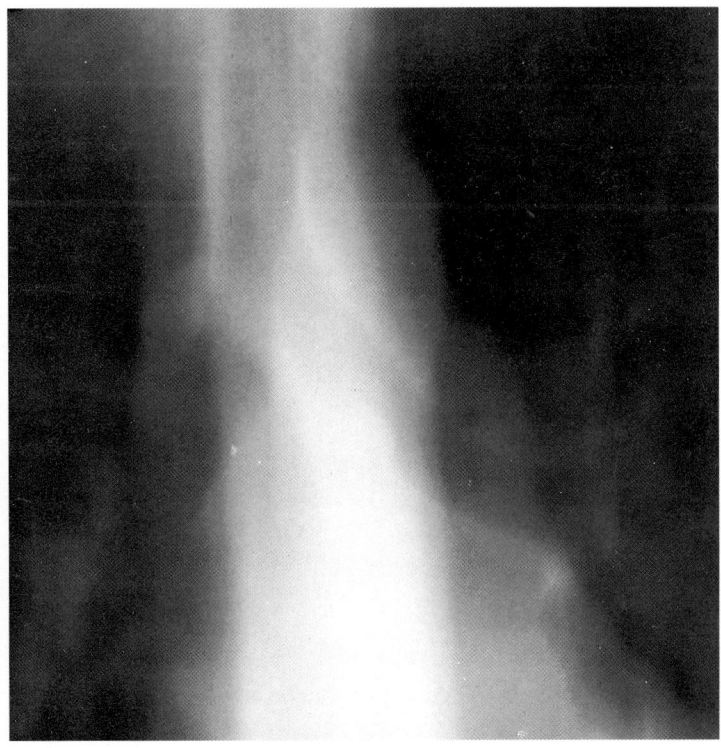

Fig. 3.18 Adenoid cystic carcinoma (cylindroma). The mass at the left hilum is due to nodal involvement. There is some consolidation of the left lower lobe. Tomogram shows a tumour almost totally occluding the left main bronchus at its origin.

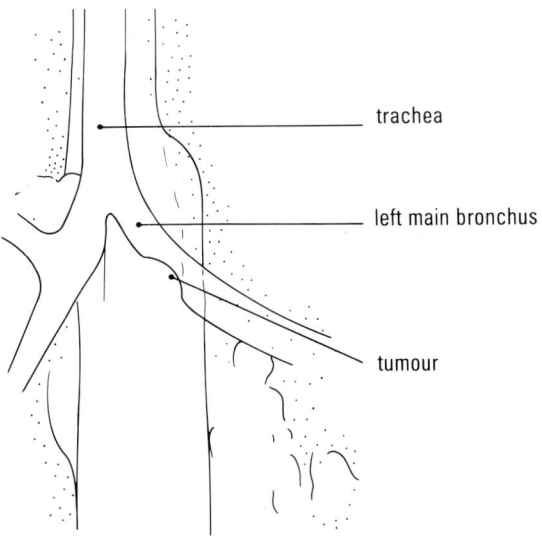

trachea

left main bronchus

tumour

Fig. 3.19 Leiomyoma of the left main bronchus. This patient presented with stridor and haemoptysis. The frontal view was normal on inspiration but the tomogram shows the tumour arising from the inferior wall of the left main bronchus.

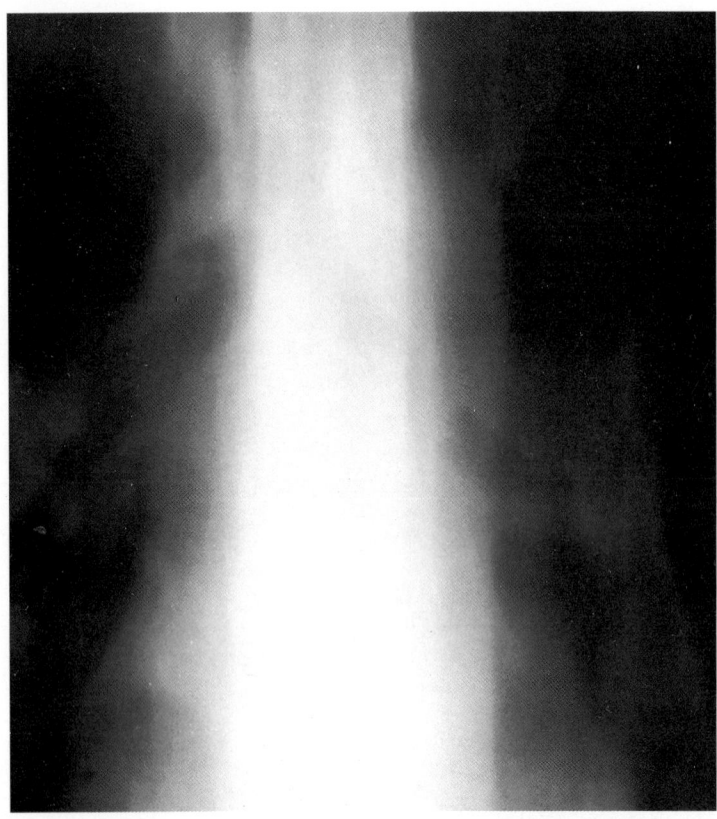

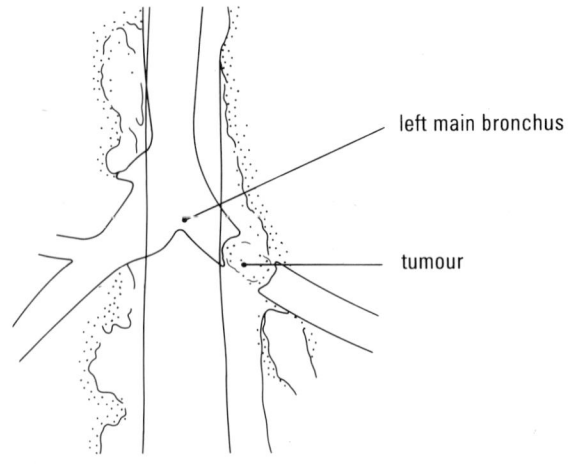

Fig. 3.20 Papilloma of the left main bronchus. The tomogram shows tumour of the left main bronchus (an anomalous bronchus rises from the right main bronchus).

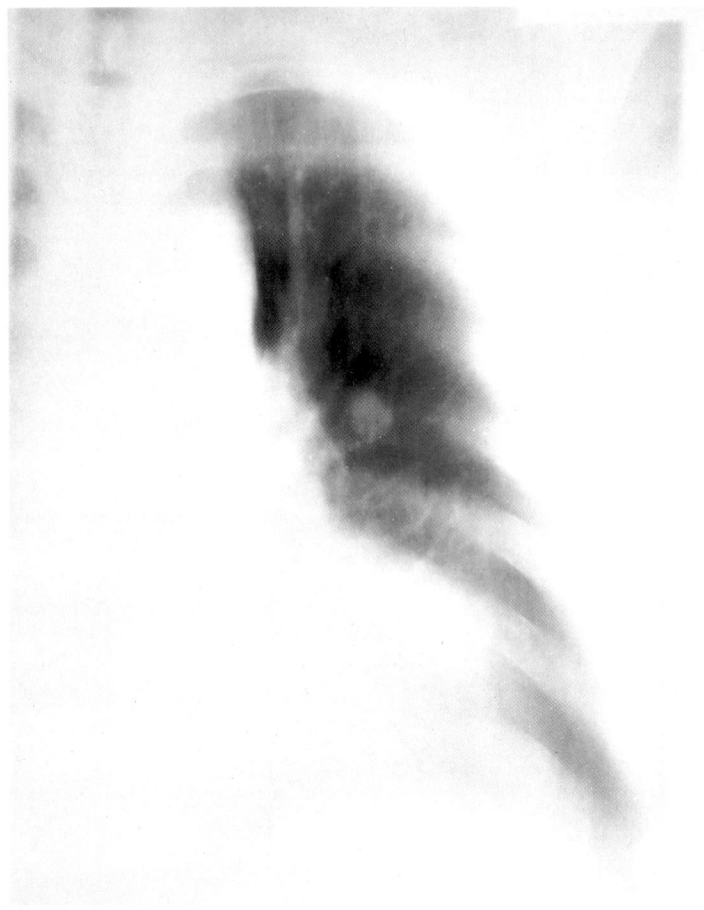

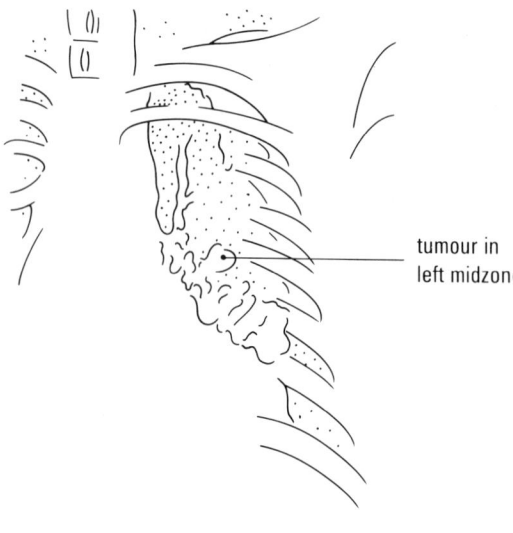

Fig. 3.21 Plasma cell granuloma. The tomogram shows the clearly defined tumour in the left middle zone. There are no specific radiological features.

Papilloma

Papillomata of trachea or bronchus are rare and usually occur in young people (Fig. 3.20). This tumour consists of a connective tissue core covered by squamous epithelium.

Plasma cell granuloma

This lesion consists of plasma cells, spindle cells, lymphocytes and blood vessels. Haemoptysis is a frequent presenting symptom. The lesion is usually within the lung substance and may involve the bronchus (Fig. 3.21).

Pulmonary metastases

The common sites of a primary tumour which metastasizes to the lungs are breast, pancreas, stomach, skin, kidney, ovary, prostate, uterus, thyroid (Fig. 3.22) and testes. Pulmonary metastasis may cause the following radiographic appearances: extensive lesions (Fig. 3.23), solitary pulmonary nodules, multiple nodules or lymphangitis carcinomatosa. Many pulmonary metastases do not cause any symptoms but breathlessness may occur with the development of lymphangitis carcinomatosa. Pleural effusions may form due to secondary malignant deposits in the pleura.

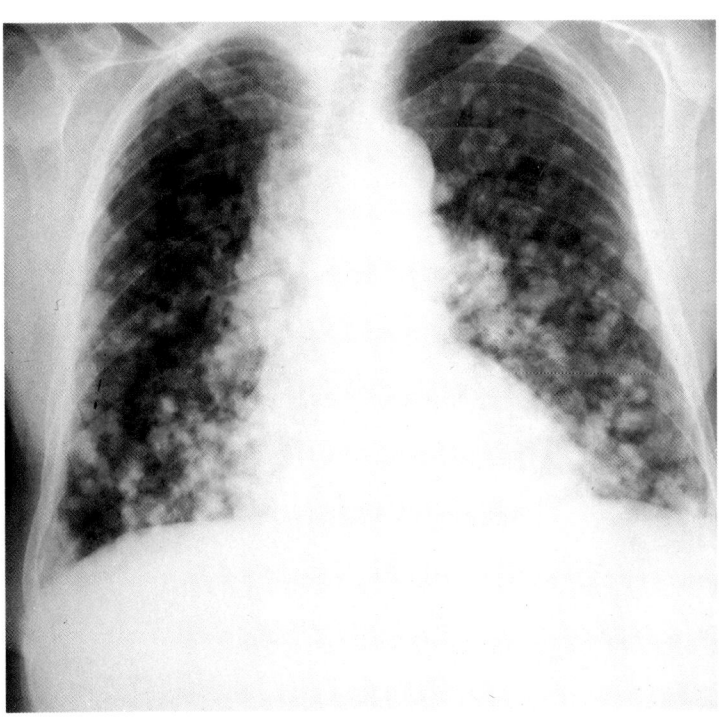

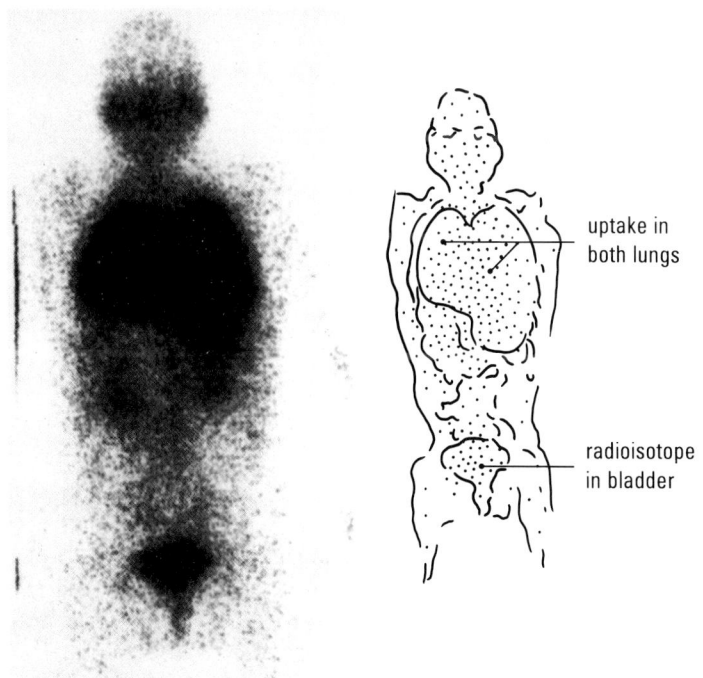

uptake in both lungs

radioisotope in bladder

Fig. 3.22 Metastases from a follicular cell carcinoma of the thyroid. Frontal view shows multiple round opacities in both lungs with lymphadenopathy at the right hilum and right paratracheal region. Radioiodine scan of the lungs shows uptake in both lungs.

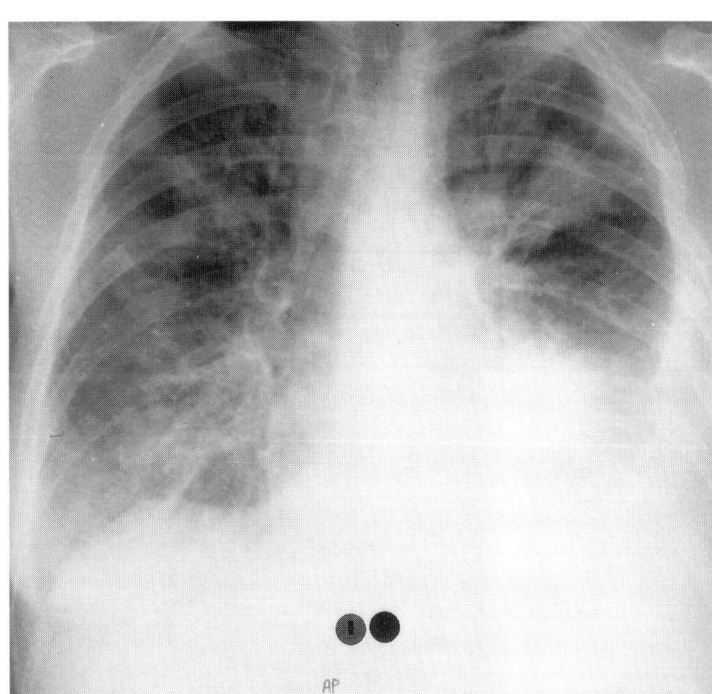

Fig. 3.23 Carcinoma of the breast with extensive pulmonary and bone metastases. Frontal view shows that a left mastectomy has been performed. There is a left pleural effusion and diffuse nodular shadowing confluent in places. Linear shadowing is present in both lungs due to extensive intrapulmonary spread. The left 4th rib is destroyed in the axilla by metastases.

4

Diseases of the Airways

Chronic Bronchitis

The chest radiograph is usually normal. During an exacerbation, hyperinflation secondary to gas trapping may cause a low diaphragm (Fig. 4.1).

Thus, a low flat diaphragm during an exacerbation does not necessarily indicate a co-existent emphysema. Other abnormalities, when present, are due to complications. Pneumonic shadowing may be seen during an acute exacerbation; cardiomegaly usually indicates the development of cor pulmonale, and cough fractures are frequently seen (Fig. 4.2). Bronchography reveals irregular, narrowed or distorted bronchi, with lack of side-branching and peripheral pruning. Diverticula in the larger bronchi may be demonstrated by contrast medium entering dilated ducts of the mucous glands. Bronchography may also demonstrate associated centriacinar emphysema (Fig. 4.3), but this investigation is not indicated routinely in chronic bronchitis. Lung function testing is helpful in defining the functional impairment, in assessing the degree of reversibility and also in monitoring progression of the disease.

Emphysema

Emphysema can only be diagnosed with absolute certainty at postmortem or at operation. It is defined as an increase in size of the air spaces distal to the terminal bronchioles with destruction of their walls. Since emphysema is mainly induced by smoking, most patients also have a clinical history of chronic cough and sputum (i.e. chronic bronchitis). However, some patients deny cough and sputum and

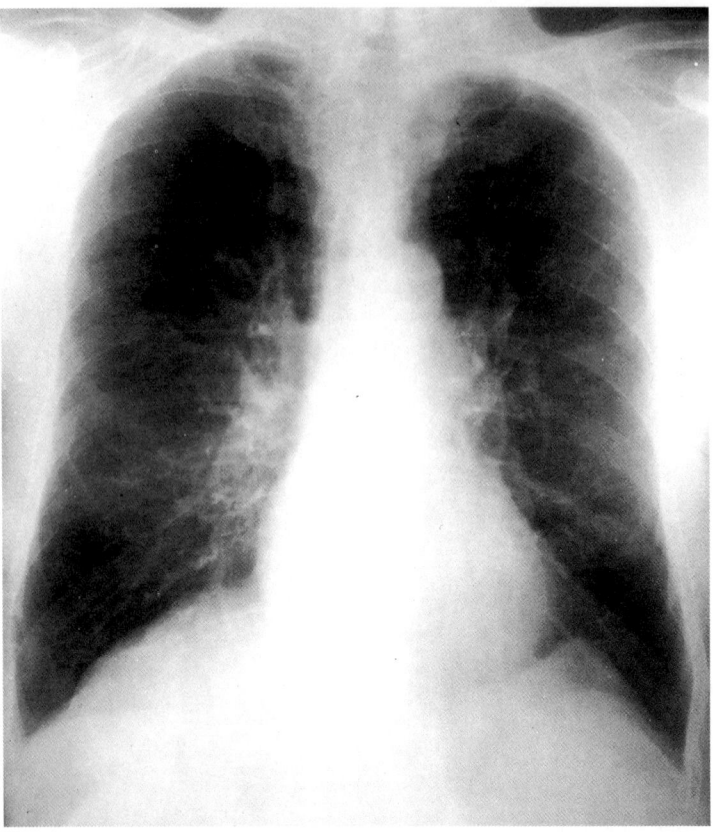

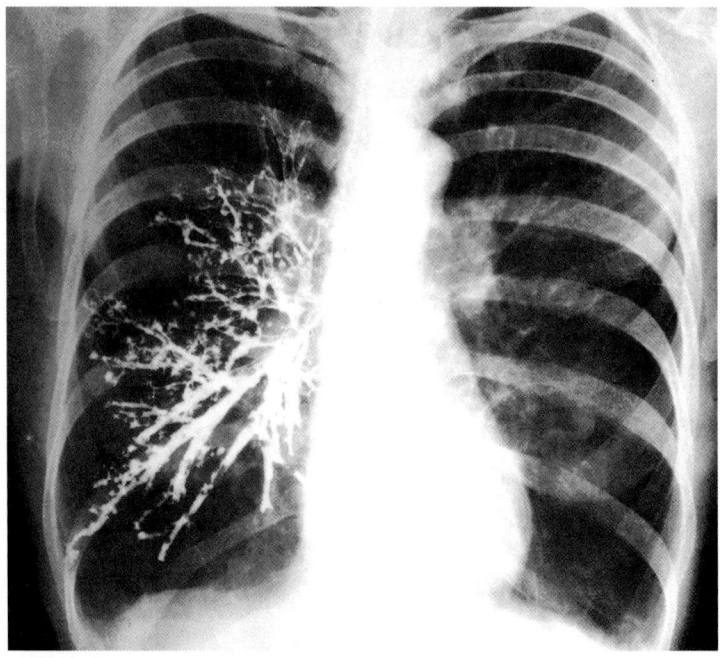

Fig. 4.1 Chronic bronchitis. A low diaphragm indicates over-inflation of the lungs, but otherwise the chest radiograph is normal.

Fig. 4.2 Chronic bronchitis. The chest radiograph shows multiple deformities of the left ribs with callus formation due to cough fractures; the diaphragm is slightly flattened.

Fig. 4.3 Chronic bronchitis. The bronchogram shows lack of side branching and peripheral pruning. Where the bronchi have filled a 'mimosa blossom' pattern due to centriacinar emphysema is evident.

have relatively pure emphysema. Two forms of emphysema are commonly described: centriacinar emphysema and panacinar emphysema. The latter can be secondary to alpha-1-antitrypsin deficiency, when its distribution is predominantly basal.

Essential radiographical features are overinflation with diminished vascular markings. Overinflation is judged on a low flat diaphragm with a thin vertical heart and enlarged retrosternal space on the lateral chest film. The pattern of vascular deficiency is usually generalized, although one or more lobes may be spared (Fig. 4.4) and in alpha-1-antitrypsin deficiency the distribution is mainly basal (Fig. 4.5).

Bullous Lung Disease

Air-containing cysts which occur in the lung are usually associated with chronic, emphysematous lung disease, in which case they are known as bullae. Similar cysts may occasionally be congenital, or acquired after staphylococcal or tuberculous infection.

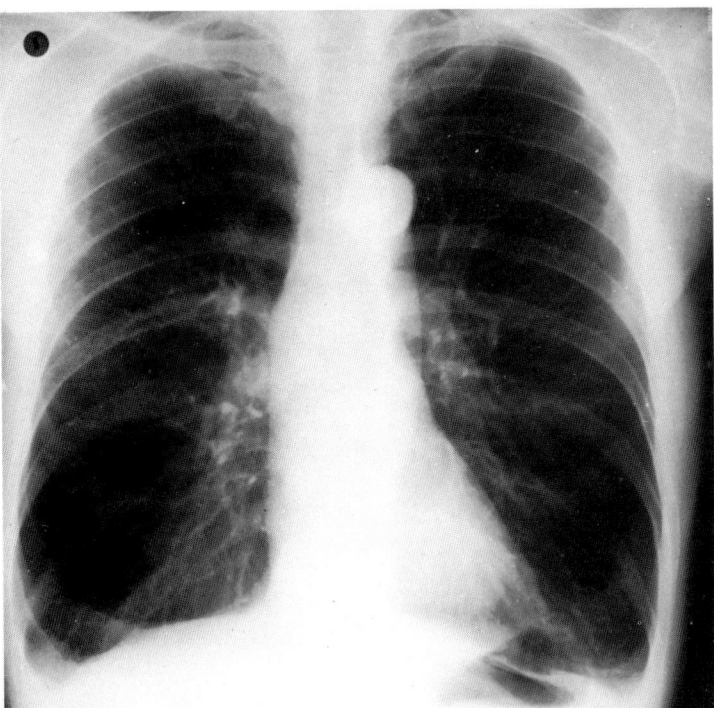

Fig. 4.4 Emphysema. Chest radiograph showing low, flat diaphragm. The vessels are severely reduced in middle and peripheral lung fields in all zones. The left upper zone is least affected.

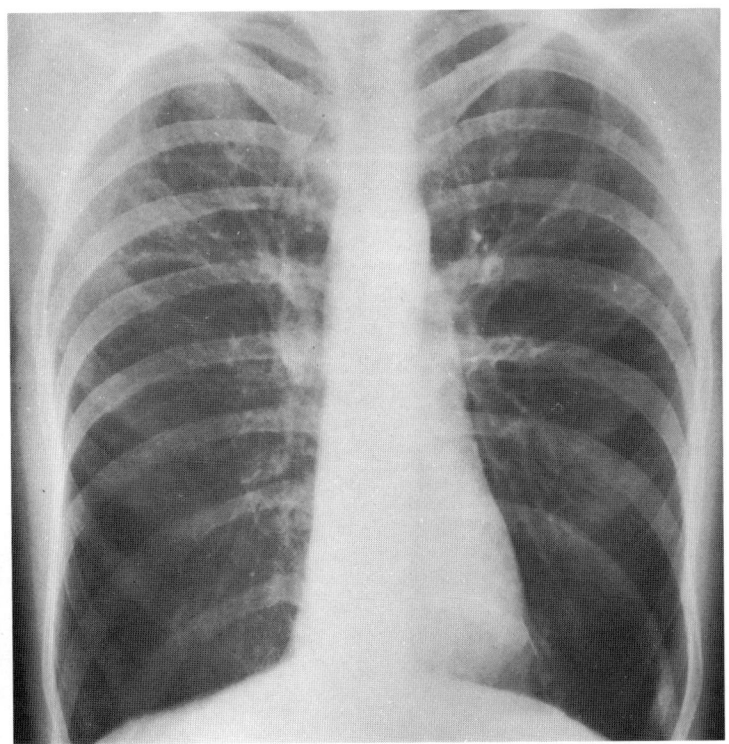

Fig. 4.5 Emphysema due to alpha-1-antitrypsin deficiency. Chest radiograph showing low, flat diaphragm and greatly reduced lung vessels in the middle and lower zones. The upper zones are relatively spared and upper zone vessels are prominent since they carry most of the cardiac output.

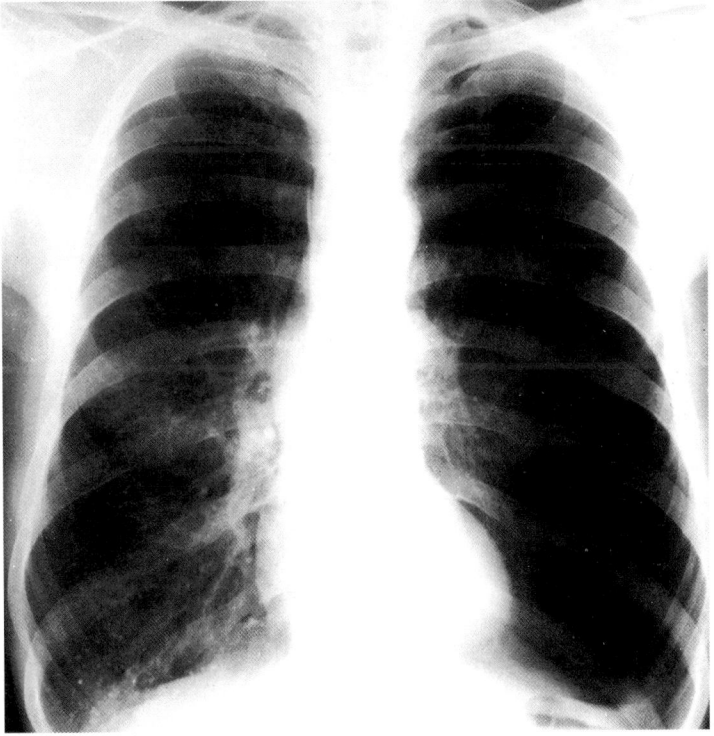

Fig. 4.6 The plain radiograph shows a large bulla in the left lung and evidence of old chickenpox pneumonia in the right.

Plain chest radiograph

In many cases bullae can be clearly demonstrated by standard plain films (Fig. 4.6), or in whole lung tomography, where they appear as avascular areas with curvilinear boundary shadows. Extrapolation of the shape and size of a single bulla is usually possible from these landmarks on the PA and lateral views. It may also be possible to obtain simple functional information about the ventilation of a solitary cyst or cluster of bullae from inspiratory and expiratory films.

However, in the majority of cases bullae are not solitary and the edges are ill defined, so that it is not always possible to describe the three-dimensional configuration from the confusion of curvilinear shadows that usually compose a bullous system.

Computed tomography

This should now be the radiological investigation of choice. In addition to identifying the position and number of bullae, it can also give functional information about the change of volume of a bulla with a breath and some indication of the condition of the surrounding lung. Bullae are easily seen on CT and can be clearly identified even in those areas which tend to be hidden in conventional radiography, such as the apices, costophrenic sinuses and the paramediastinal areas. They can also be distinguished when they are associated with other conditions which may make the plain film difficult to interpret, for example in pulmonary fibrosis or scoliosis. Since a large bulla can be clearly outlined, its volume can be measured by summing the area of the bulla in consecutive slices, and if the scans are taken in inspiration and expiration then the ventilation can be measured. It is, however, important to measure the whole volume and not rely upon the area change of a single slice to assess ventilation, since there can be considerable distortion without a change in volume. Finally, CT allows some assessment of the non-bullous lung. It may identify unsuspected bullae or the lung may be of generally poor quality with areas of low attenuation and disrupted vasculature indicating emphysema. It must be remembered, however, that CT is relatively insensitive in identifying emphysema that is not gross, other functional measurements being more sensitive for this (Fig. 4.7).

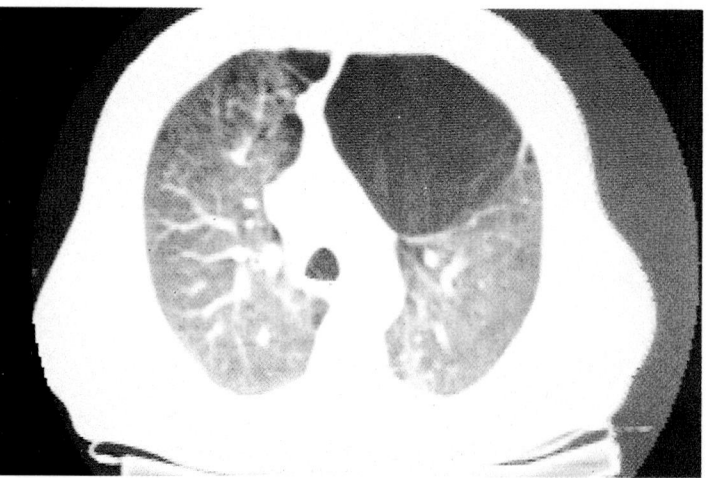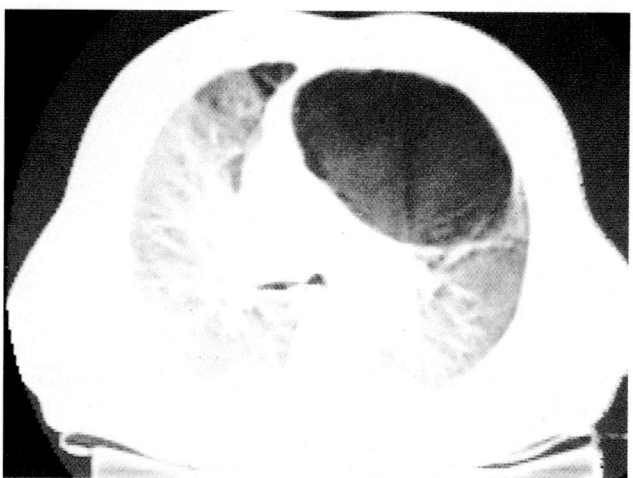

Fig. 4.7 CT scans at the same level in inspiration (left) and expiration (right) in the same patient. The left anterior bulla is well defined and does not diminish in area during expiration. The surrounding lung is of good quality and ventilates normally. The mediastinum is displaced to the opposite side by the bulla in expiration. Lastly it is a good example of the motion of the lungs with the thorax during expiration when the carina comes into view as the bronchial tree moves cephalad.

Bronchiectasis

Bronchiectasis is defined as a permanent dilatation of the bronchi. In recent years the incidence of bronchiectasis in developed countries has declined as a result of the improved treatment of childhood respiratory infections and the partial control of whooping cough and measles by vaccination.

Bronchiectasis may be saccular or cylindrical and is usually acquired during childhood following pneumonia, measles, whooping cough or inhalation of a foreign body. Primary tuberculosis can also cause bronchiectasis through pressure of an enlarged lymph node on a bronchus, lead-ing to distal dilatation and bronchiectasis. In adult life, bronchiectasis can be acquired following a suppurative pneumonia, tuberculosis, bronchial adenoma, allergic bronchopulmonary aspergillosis or chronic sinusitis. It occasionally occurs in conjunction with gross pulmonary fibrosis, although usually only when secondary infection is present. Congenital causes of bronchiectasis include Kartagener's syndrome, unilateral emphysema and sequestration. Cystic fibrosis and hypogammaglobulin-aemia are inherited defects which also predispose to bronchiectasis.

The characteristic symptoms of bronchiectasis are cough and sputum and haemoptysis is common. A patient with extensive disease may also complain of dyspnoea. On examination the patient may have finger clubbing and there may be coarse crepitations over the part of the lung affected by bronchiectasis. The plain radiograph may be normal but bronchial wall thickening is often visible. The diagnosis can be confirmed by a bronchogram or CT (Figs 4.8 and 4.9).

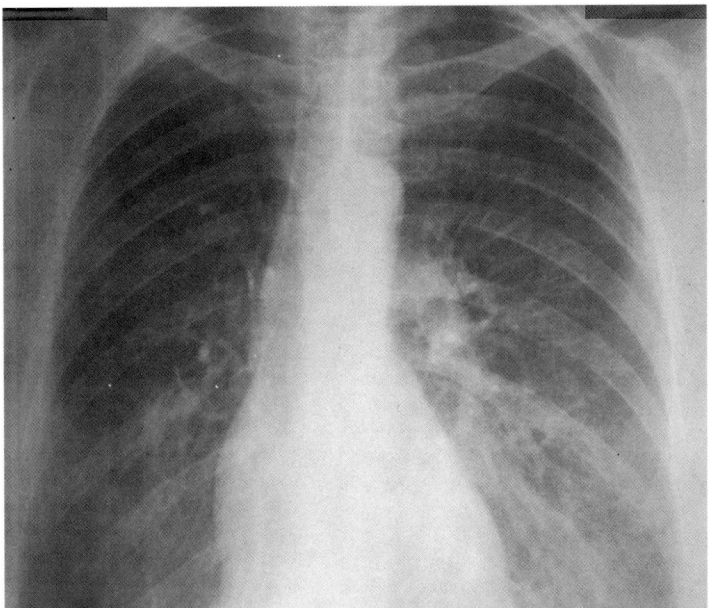

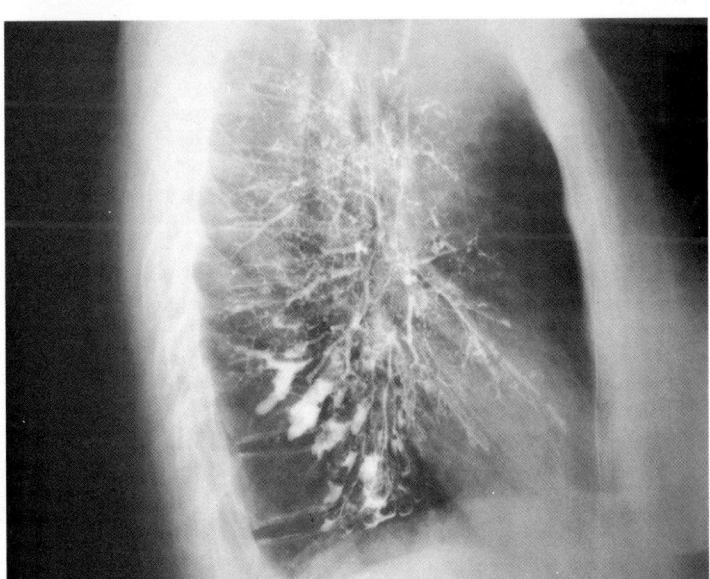

Fig. 4.8 Bronchiectasis. Collapsed right lower lobe with parallel line shadows on a plain film (upper) suggests bronchiectasis which is confirmed on the bronchogram (lower).

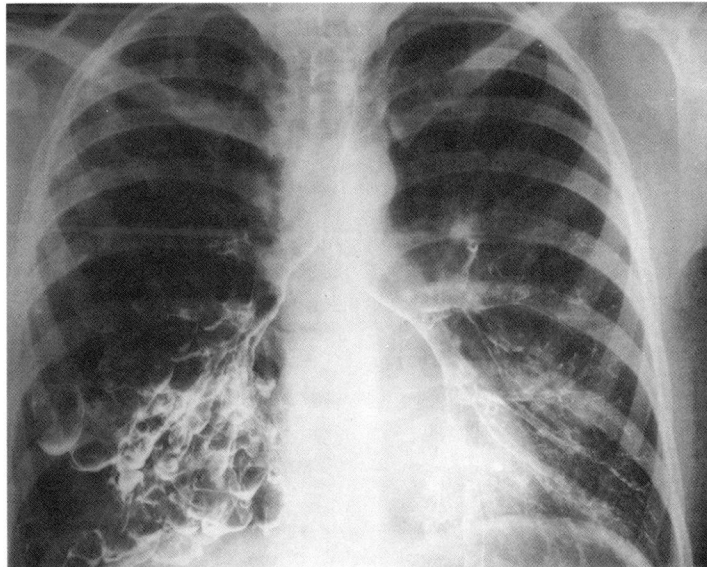

Fig. 4.9 Bronchogram showing cystic bronchiectasis of the right lung in an adult.

Cystic Fibrosis

Cystic fibrosis is characterized by chronic bronchopulmonary infection, malabsorption and a high sweat sodium concentration. It is assuming importance as a cause of bronchiectasis especially in developed countries where bronchiectasis following childhood infections is now less common.

The chest radiograph is usually normal at birth. In children the earliest change is bronchial wall thickening (Fig. 4.10). Some patients, however, retain a normal radiograph into adult life. As the disease progresses, overinflation of the lungs may occur with depression of the diaphragm. Ill-defined nodular shadows 2–5mm in size appear and may be transient or persistent. Parallel line shadows occur due to bronchial wall thickening and bronchiectasis (Fig. 4.11).

The pulmonary complications of cystic fibrosis include progressive respiratory failure, cor pulmonale, atelectasis, allergic bronchopulmonary aspergillosis, pneumothorax and haemoptysis (Fig. 4.12).

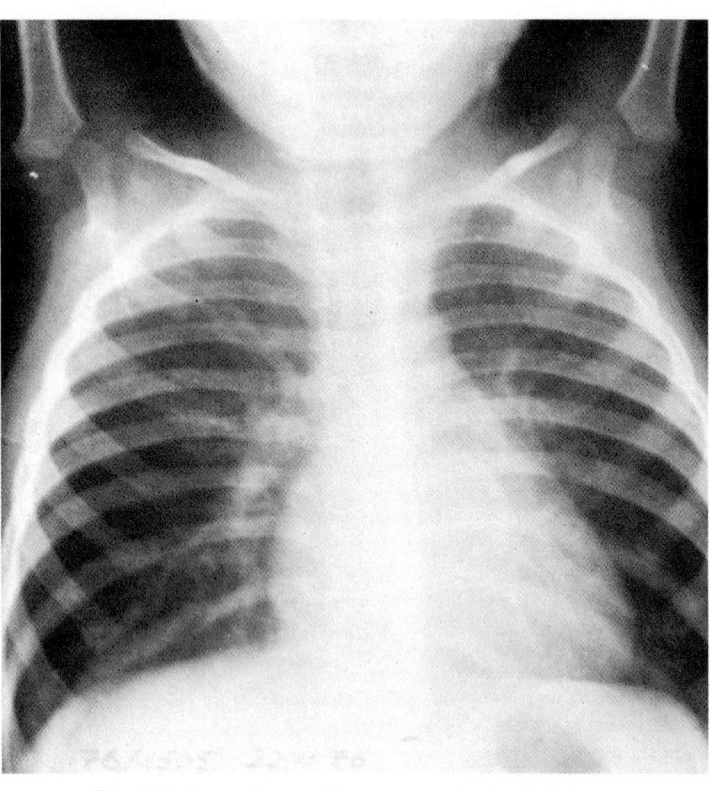

Fig. 4.10 Cystic fibrosis. Chest radiograph of a child showing large volume lungs with some bronchial wall thickening, mainly in the middle and upper zones.

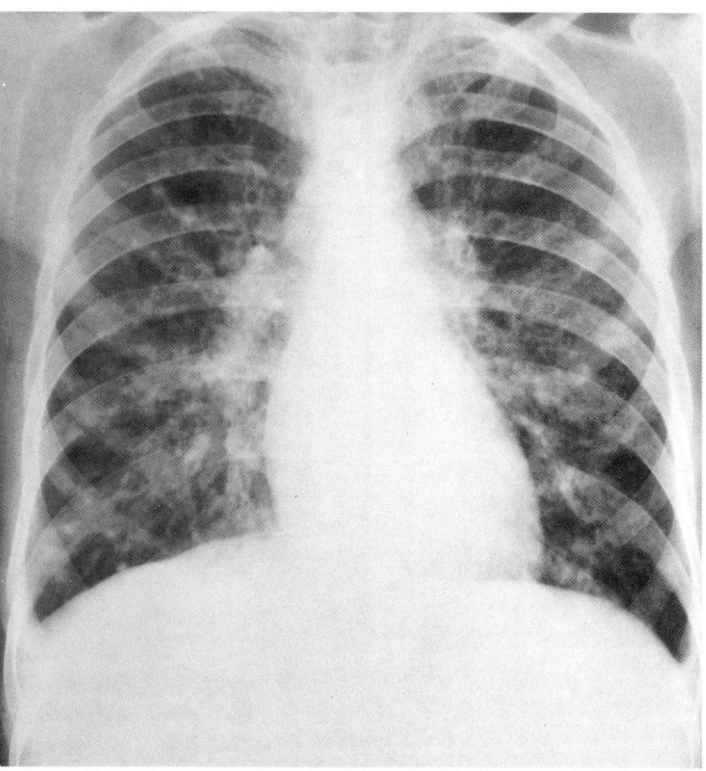

Fig. 4.11 Cystic fibrosis. Chest radiograph of an adult: widespread irregular and patchy shadowing throughout all lobes, several ring shadows and parallel line shadows are present due to bronchial wall thickening and bronchiectasis and the hila are prominent.

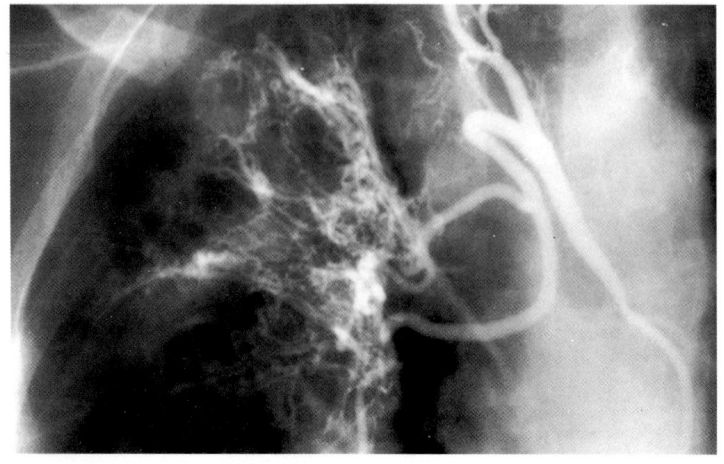

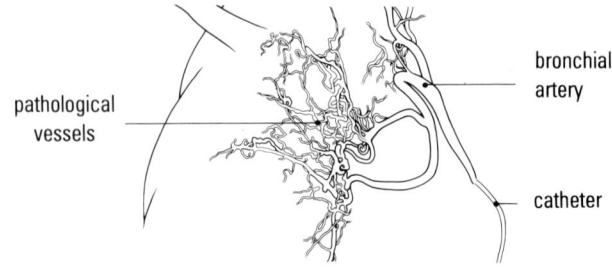

Fig. 4.12 A bronchial arteriogram showing a large bronchial artery supplying the right upper lobe. There are multiple pathological vessels within this diseased lobe.

5

Infections and Allergic Disorders

Pneumonia

Bacterial pneumonias

Streptococcus pneumoniae (also called pneumococcus) is the commonest cause of acute bacterial pneumonia in previously healthy young adults. Chest radiographs show lobar consolidation (Fig. 5.1).

Pneumonia due to *Staphylococcus pyogenes* may be found among patients who are debilitated, immunosuppressed or have some other focus of staphylococcal infection. Cases also occur following influenza epidemics (Fig. 5.2). Pneu-monia is often severe and cavities may form. Infection with *Haemophilus influenzae* is usually found in patients with pre-existing lung disease as is infection with *Klebsiella pneumoniae*, which can cause extensive consolidation.

Other causes of bacterial pneumonia are *Streptococcus pyogenes*, *Escherichia coli*, *Pseudomonas aeruginosa* and *Bacteroides*. Infection with Gram-negative organisms, particularly *Pseudomonas aeruginosa*, is often found among patients with pre-existing lung disease, such as bronchiectasis or cystic fibrosis. Other groups particularly at risk are those with diabetes mellitus, alcoholism or impaired immune defences and those receiving mechanical ventilation.

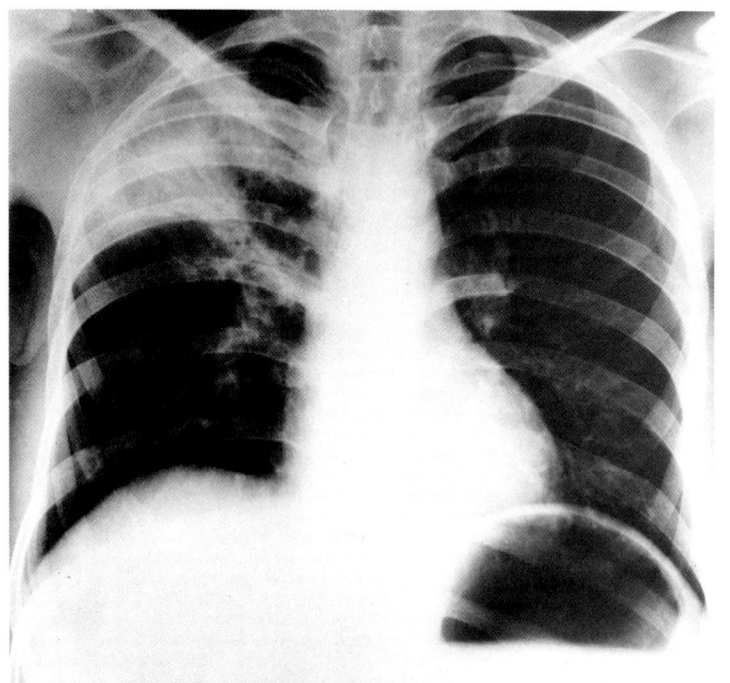
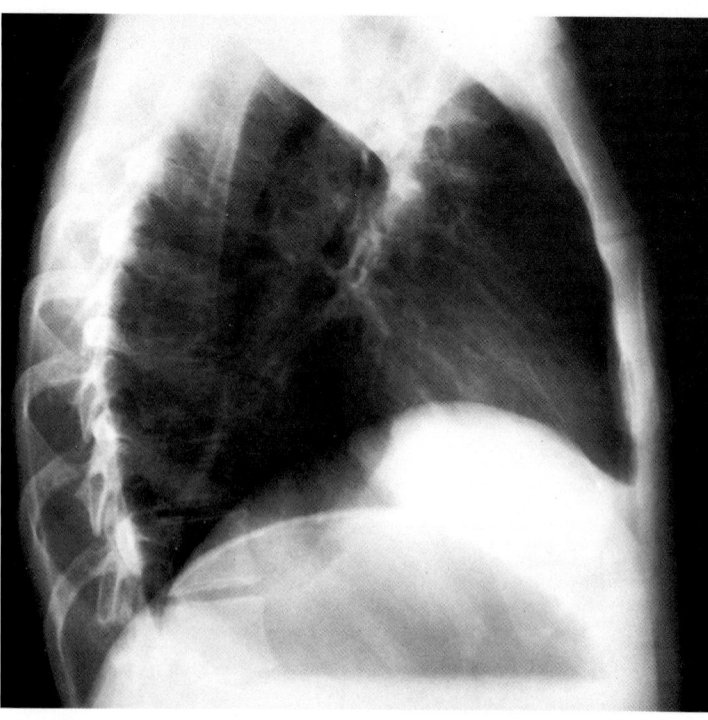

Fig. 5.1 Pneumococcal pneumonia. There is dense homogenous opacification of the right upper lobe, mainly the posterior segment. Note the air bronchogram indicating solid lung with patent airways. The patient developed sudden onset of cough and pleuritic chest pain; he had herpes simplex on his lips, a temperature of **39.9°C** and a WBC of **20 × 10⁹/l**. *Streptococcus pneumoniae* was isolated from sputum and blood culture.

Legionella pneumophilia was first described in 1976 after an outbreak among American legionnaires in Philadelphia. It is now realized that this type of pneumonia can occur in a mild form, but some outbreaks have shown a high mortality. Many systemic features such as headache, confusion, abdominal pain and diarrhoea occur, in addition to pulmonary symptoms such as cough and pleuritic chest pain. There is often leucopenia, associated hyponatraemia and albuminuria.

Bacterial pneumonia may also accompany a systemic bacterial disease such as pertussis, typhoid, brucellosis, or plague (Fig. 5.3).

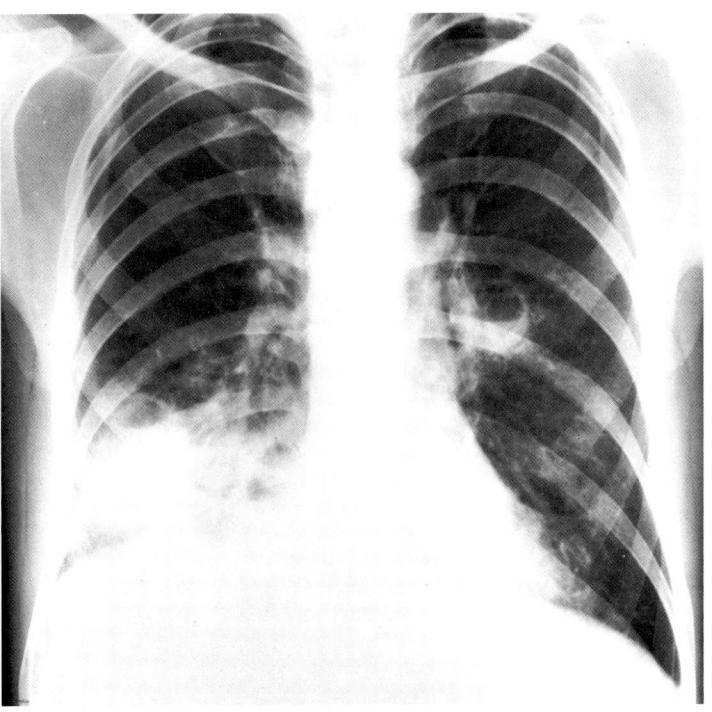
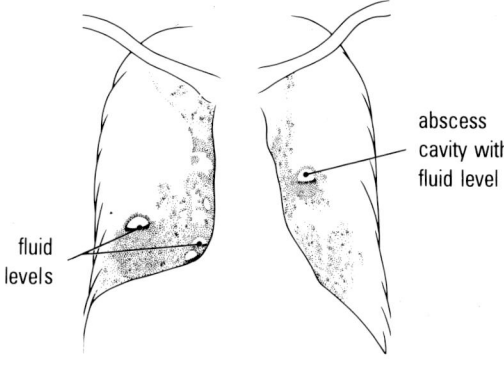

Fig. 5.2 Staphylococcal pneumonia. There is consolidation at the right base and thin-walled cavities with fluid levels at the right base and left mid-zone.

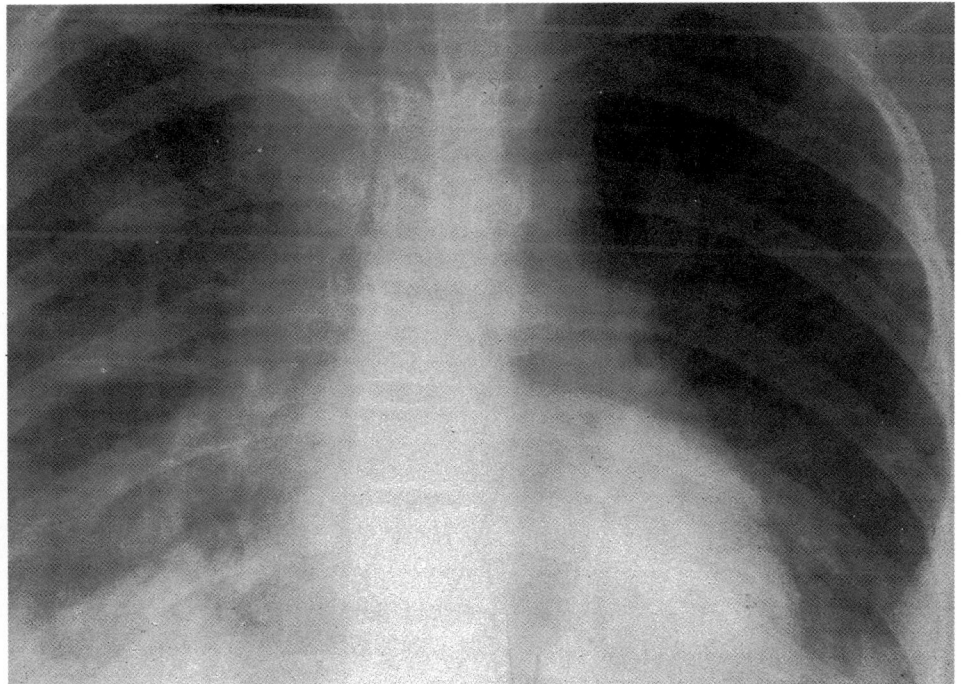
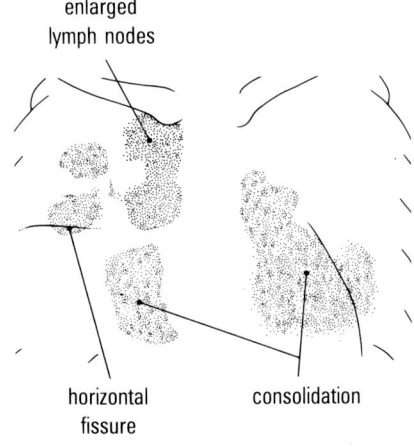

Fig. 5.3 Pulmonary involvement in bubonic plague. Infection of the lungs is via the blood. There are enlarged hilar and paratracheal lymph nodes with patchy consolidation in both lungs.

Viral, chlamydial, rickettsial and mycoplasmal pneumonias

Viruses which may cause pneumonia include influenza virus (Fig. 5.4), measles virus, cytomegalovirus, adenoviruses, parainfluenza viruses, rhinoviruses, varicella virus, herpes viruses and respiratory syncytial virus.

Varicella pneumonia can be florid (Fig. 5.5), or fine residual calcified opacities may be found in the lungs many years later.

Pneumonia due to *Chlamydia psittaci* is usually found where there is a history of contact with birds, and rickettsial pneumonias where there is contact with animals. Mycoplasmal pneumonia (Fig. 5.6) is commonly the cause of outbreaks in schools, military camps and other institutions.

Pneumonia due to viruses, rickettsia, mycoplasma and chlamydia is less dramatic in onset than bacterial pneumonia. Some patients have few abnormal physical signs in the chest and the radiograph often shows less extensive consolidation than in bacterial pneumonia. Occasional cases may, however, be fulminating.

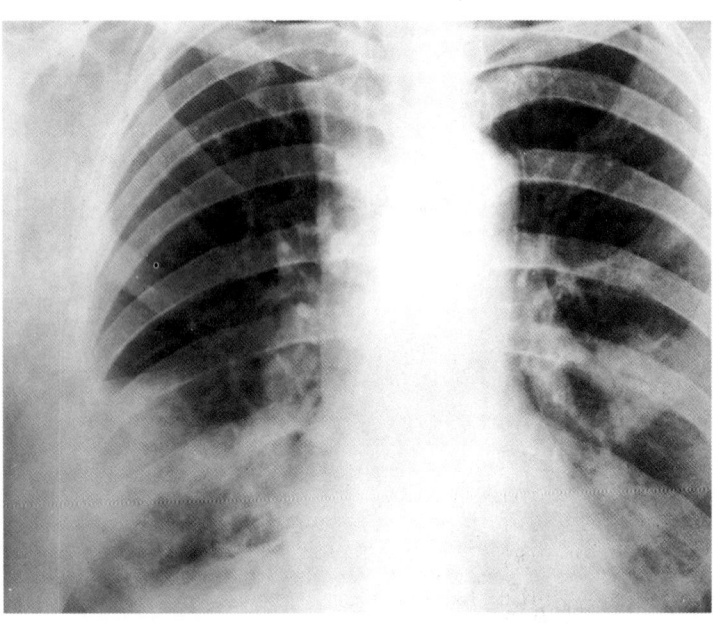

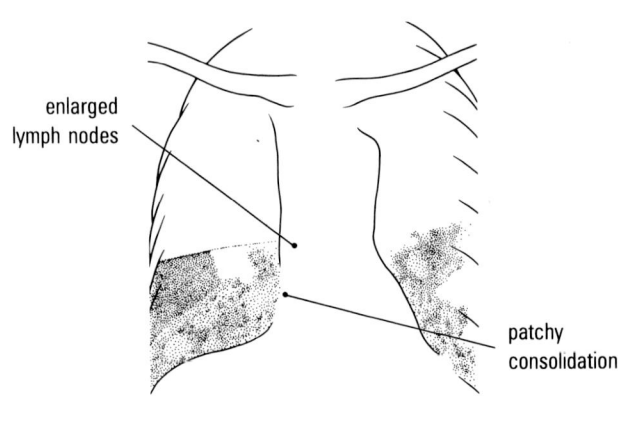

enlarged lymph nodes

patchy consolidation

Fig. 5.4 Influenza virus pneumonia. Non-segmental, poorly defined areas of opacification are present predominantly in the middle lobe and lingula. The patient had a temperature of 39.9°C, a WBC of 12 × 10⁹/l and no response to antibiotics. A complement fixation text revealed a four-fold rising titre to influenza A.

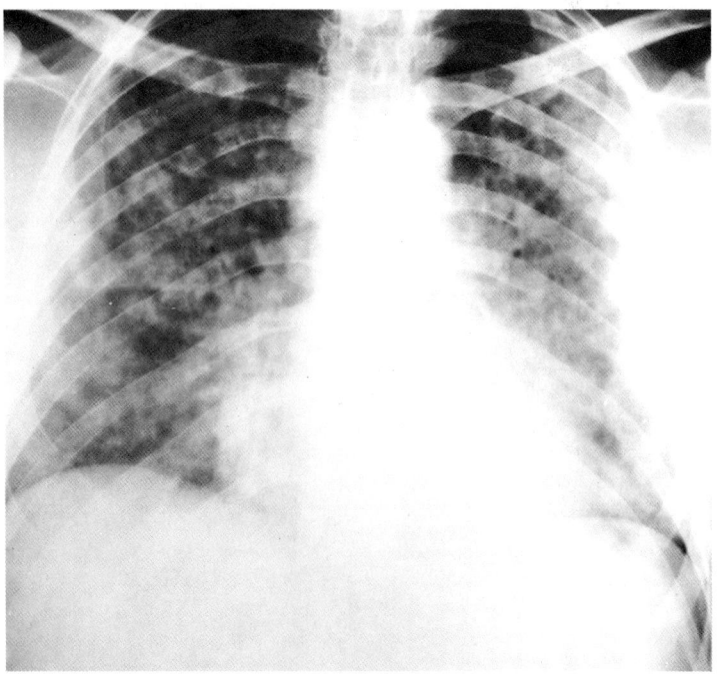

Fig. 5.5 Chickenpox pneumonia. In the acute florid form widespread poorly defined opacities are confluent in places and, where confluent, an air bronchogram is seen. The lung apices are less affected than other areas. The patient is extremely ill and is unable to maintain a satisfactory position, hence part of the lung is obscured by the scapulae.

Actinomycetes, fungi, yeasts and protozoa

Pneumonia due to *Histoplasma capsulatum* (Fig. 5.7) or *Coccidioides immitis* (see later) must be considered in patients who have travelled in endemic areas. Infection with *H. capsulatum* may be asymptomatic, may take the form of an acute fulminating disease, or may simulate chronic tuberculosis. Similarly, infection with *C. immitis* may be asymptomatic but it also has acute and chronic

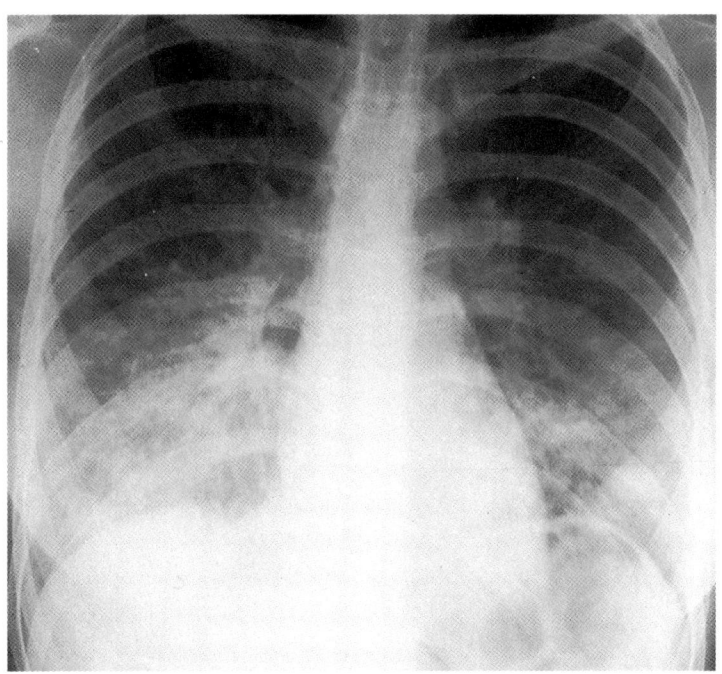

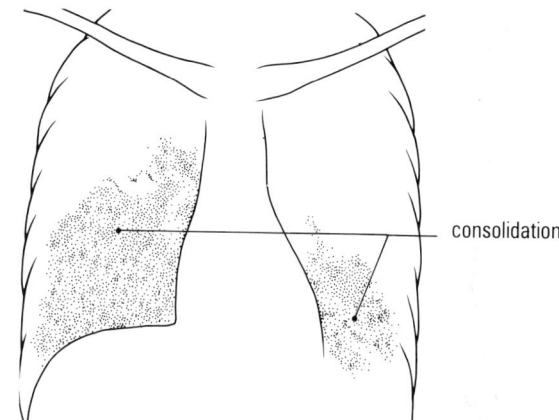

Fig. 5.6 Mycoplasma pneumonia. This patient presented with eight days of fever, malaise, cough and sputum. The temperature was 39°C and WBC 7.5 × 10⁹/l. Cold agglutinin and the complement fixation test were positive for *Mycoplasma pneumoniae*.

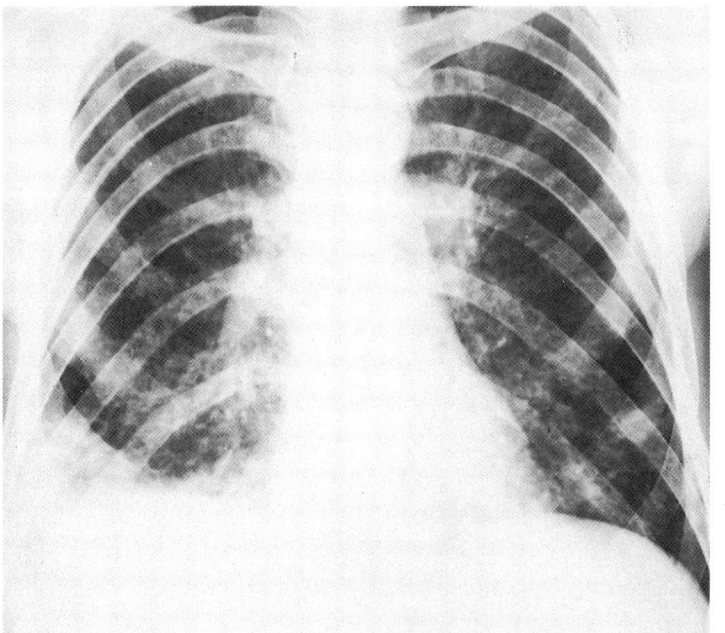

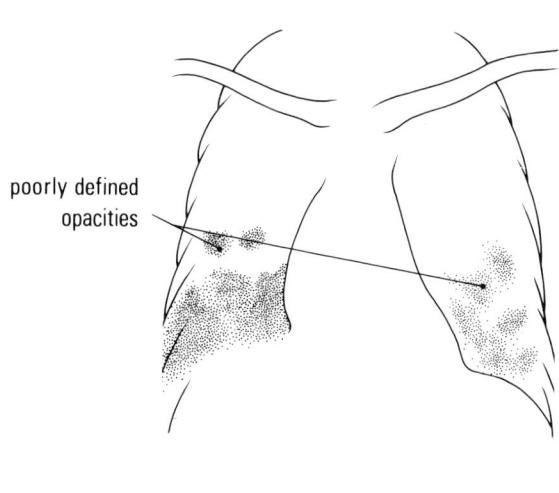

Fig. 5.7 Pneumonia due to *Histoplasma capsulatum*. There are widespread poorly defined mottled opacities which have become confluent at the right base. This patient had travelled widely in the USA and Middle East.

forms. *Actinomyces israelii* (see Fig. 2.22), *Nocardia asteroides* (Fig. 5.8), cryptococci, *Aspergillus fumigatus* and the protozoans *Pneumocystis carinii* and *Toxoplasma gondii* must be considered in cases of unusual pneumonia occurring in immunosuppressed patients. *P. carinii* presents in a susceptible patient with increasing breathlessness, and a chest radiograph shows widespread pulmonary infiltrates (see Fig. 5.20). This organism is the commonest cause of pneumonia in patients with AIDS.

Allergic, chemical and physical causes of pneumonitis
An allergic reaction to *A. fumigatus* can cause 'flitting' pulmonary shadows. Lipoid pneumonia may result from the aspiration of oils, taken in nasal drops or as an aperient. Aspiration pneumonia may also be due to oesophageal disease (Fig. 5.9). Inhalation of vomit, which usually occurs when consciousness is impaired, may cause widespread pneumonia. This is due to gastric acid being inhaled into the lungs, and may be associated with infection by a mixed population of bacteria including anaerobes. Irradiation and inhalation of a variety of irritant gases may also cause pneumonitis.

Carcinoma presenting as pneumonia
In patients who have been smokers it must always be remembered that pneumonia may be distal to a carcinoma

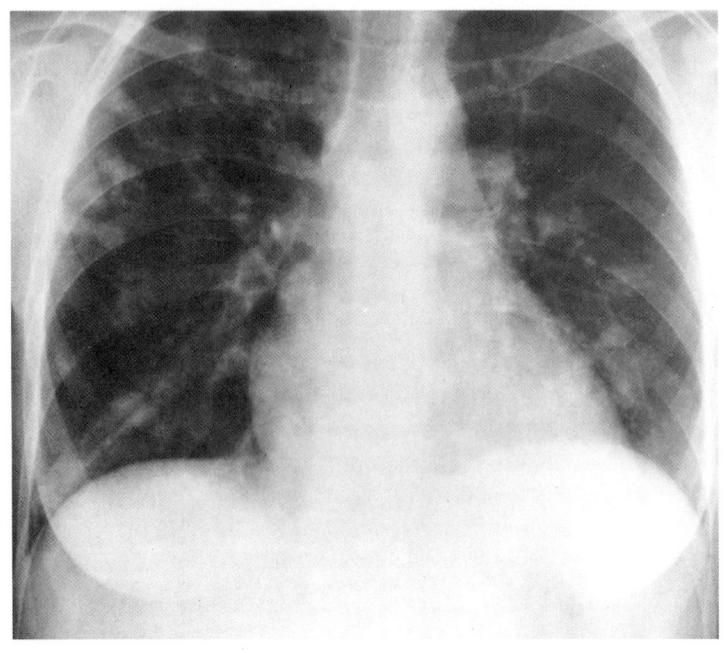

Fig. 5.8 Pneumonia due to *Nocardia asteroides*. This patient had had a successful renal transplant. Moderately well-defined opacities, 1–2cm in diameter, occur in both lungs. Some of the lesions have cavitated and appear as ring shadows.

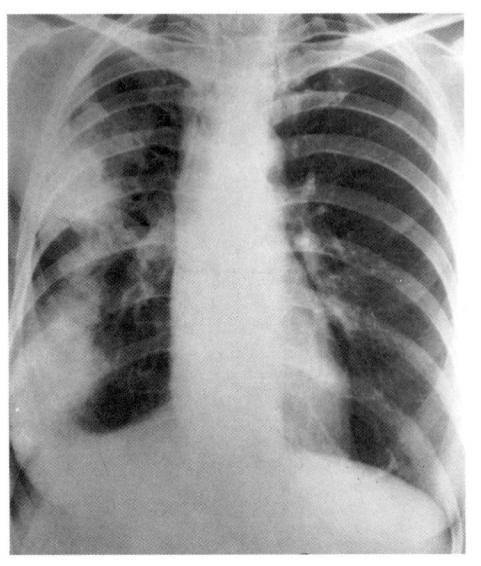
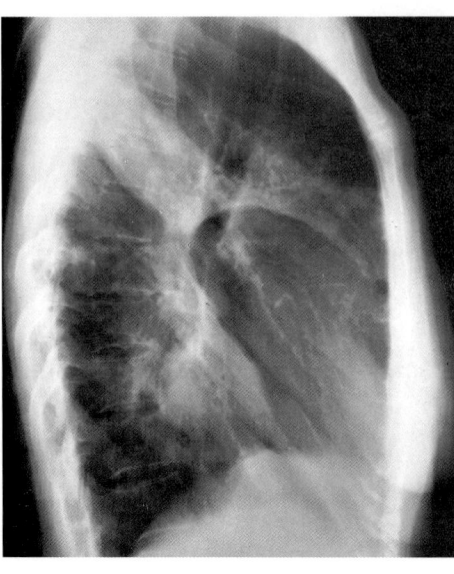

Fig. 5.9 Aspiration pneumonia due to achalasia. Ill-defined areas of opacification are present in the anterior and posterior segments of the right upper lobe and right lower lobe. The gastric air bubble is absent and the mediastinum has a straight right border due to a dilated oesophagus.

causing obstruction in the bronchial tree (Fig. 5.10). All patients recovering from pneumonia should have a chest radiograph six weeks after all symptoms have disappeared to make sure that there is no underlying pathology, such as carcinoma.

Radiological appearance

Radiological appearances in patients with pneumonia are very varied. Lobar consolidation without shrinkage may be seen, as may widespread bilateral foci of consolidation. Local areas of consolidation are more common in bacterial pneumonia than in those of other aetiology. Abscesses are more commonly seen in pneumonia due to *Staphylococcus pyogenes*, *Klebsiella pneumoniae* and anaerobes, whilst *Mycobacterium tuberculosis* pneumonia typically cavitates. In some cases, miliary shadows, atelectasis and pleural effusion will be found. In all cases of pneumonia, a chest radiograph should be taken when the patient has recovered clinically to make sure that there is no residual pathology.

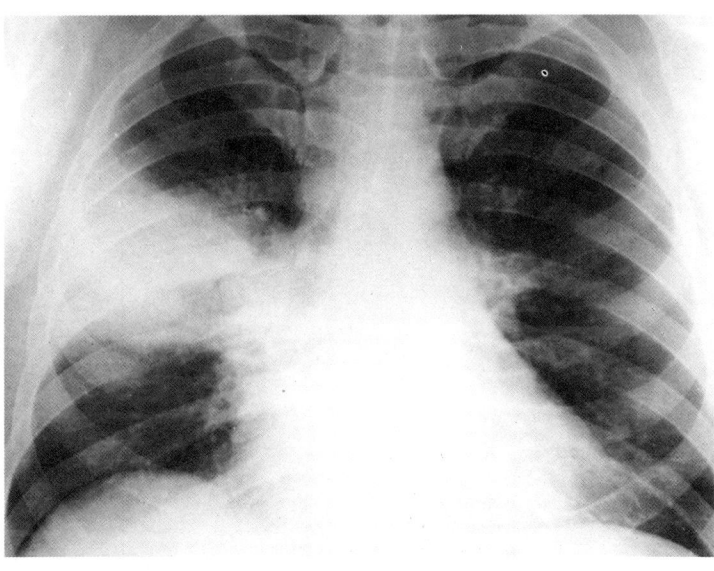

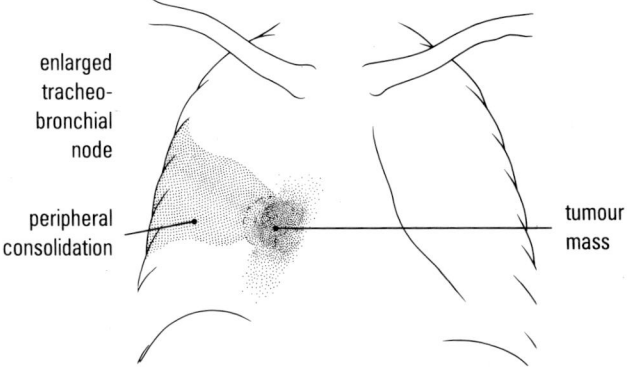

enlarged tracheo-bronchial node

peripheral consolidation

tumour mass

Fig. 5.10 Pneumonia distal to carcinoma. There is a segmental area of opacification in the right middle zone with a density at the right hilum. No air bronchogram is present.

Opportunistic and Fungal Infections

The pathogenicity of microorganisms varies greatly. Some highly pathogenic organisms cause disease whenever they are present in sufficient numbers, for example chickenpox virus or *Streptococcus pneumoniae*. Other organisms, for example *Mycobacterium tuberculosis*, cause disease in individuals whose natural resistance to infection is lowered by factors such as malnutrition or alcoholism, as well as in a proportion of normal individuals. A third group of organisms causes disease only in subjects who are severely debilitated or who have a deficiency in their immune defence mechanisms caused by disease, for example the acquired immune deficiency syndrome or leukaemia, or by therapeutic intervention, for example cytotoxic agents or corticosteroids. These organisms include *Pneumocystis carinii* or *Aspergillus* species. In addition, normally mild infections, such as measles or chickenpox, may be rapidly fatal if the patient is immunosuppressed.

Actinomycetaceae

This family includes two genera of organisms that may cause disease in man: *Actinomyces* (see Fig. 2.22) and *Nocardia*. In the lungs, actinomycosis is often initially unilateral, taking the form of pneumonia, lung abscess or sinus.

Nocardia infection characteristically produces multiple nodular opacities on the chest radiograph (see Fig. 5.8), and medium-sized and large nodules tend to cavitate. A pleural effusion may occur, and there may also be a periosteal reaction with new bone formation at the surface of a rib or vertebra adjacent to a peripheral pulmonary lesion. In immunosuppressed patients, the infection may spread to involve a lobe or a whole lung.

Zygomycetes

The Zygomycetes (formerly known as Phycomycetes) include several orders of fungi of which the order Mucorales includes the genera *Mucor*, *Rhizopus* and *Absidia*. These are normally saprophytic organisms but may become pathogenic in immunocompromised individuals (Fig. 5.11). Among cases of fungal pneumonia in such individuals, zygomycetes are found infrequently; they may be identified to some degree by their morphology.

Deuteromycetes
Aspergillus species

Allergic bronchopulmonary aspergillosis is discussed in a later section (see p. 81).

When cavitation or extensive fibrous scarring occurs in a lung the site may become colonized by *Aspergillus* species. The resulting fungus ball is termed an aspergilloma (Figs 5.12 and 2.16). The fungus ball may be expectorated piecemeal, leaving an apparently empty cavity, but active fungal growth in the wall of the cavity will cause the

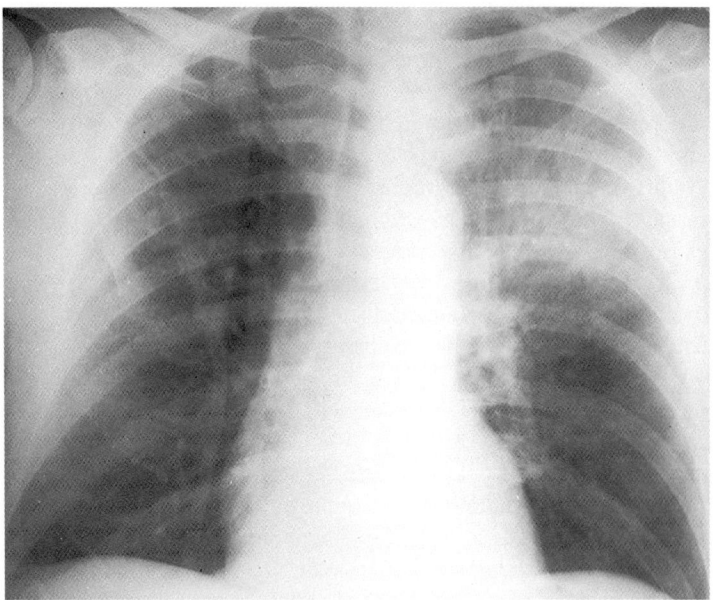

Fig. 5.11 *Mucor* pneumonia. This 54-year-old man had received intensive chemotherapy for acute myeloid leukaemia. He complained of cough, breathlessness and pleuritic pain in the left upper chest. The radiograph shows extensive consolidation of the left upper lobe. He was treated for a bacterial pneumonia and the correct diagnosis was only made at postmortem.

aspergilloma to re-form. Continued increase in the size of the cavity leads to progressive deterioration of lung function. Haemoptysis is frequent and may be massive or even fatal, and high titres of precipitating antibodies are found in the serum.

Pneumonia and disseminated aspergillosis may occur in immunocompromised individuals in whom *Aspergillus* species may not remain confined within a bronchus or cavity, but may rapidly progress into the lung parenchyma. *Aspergillus* pneumonia may produce a variety of appearances on the chest radiograph, including multiple nodules which may cavitate (Fig. 5.13) and widespread reticular shadowing.

Candida species

Patients who are seriously ill, debilitated or immunosuppressed may experience increased colonization of the mouth and pharynx by *Candida* species, most commonly *C. albicans*. This organism is a normal commensal of mucous membranes but frequently becomes locally invasive, causing oral candidosis.

Severe oral candidosis is frequently accompanied by candida oesophagitis (Fig. 5.14) which causes retrosternal discomfort or pain, aggravated by swallowing. When candida oesophagitis develops it is frequently followed by deep invasion and systemic spread of the organism via the

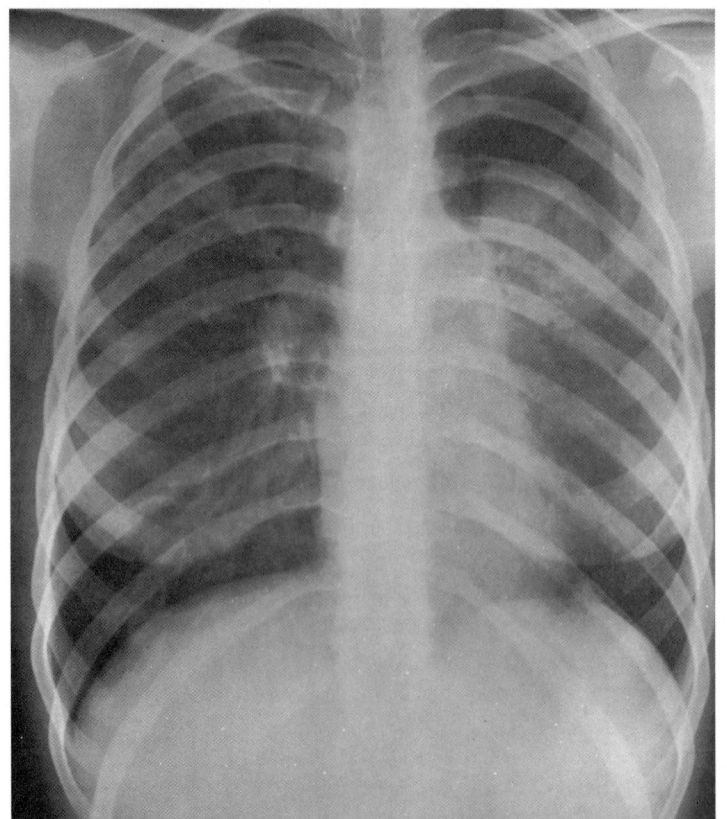

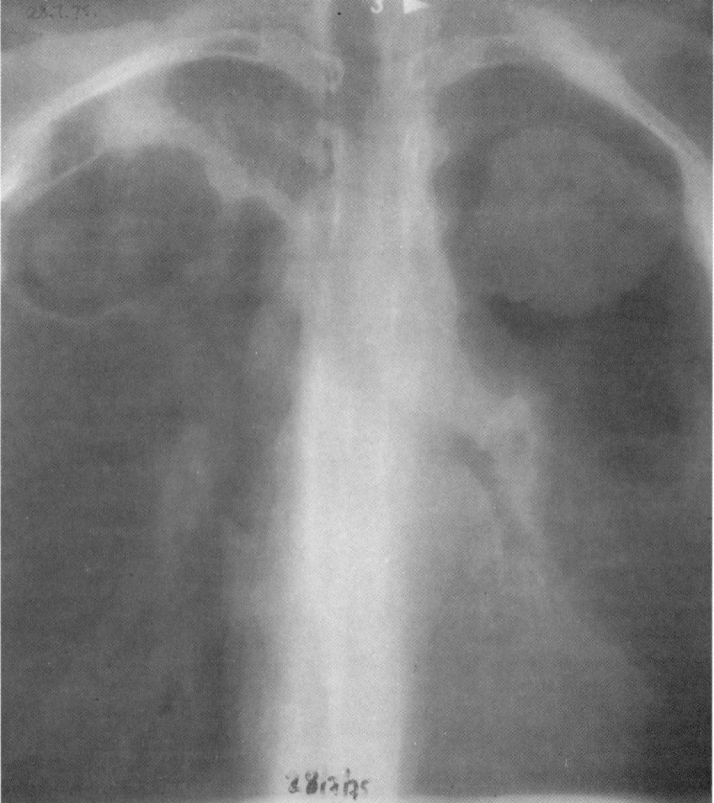

Fig. 5.12 Aspergilloma. The chest radiograph shows a well-defined cavity containing a fungus ball in the left upper lobe and the same features, less clearly defined, in the right upper lobe. Both aspergillomata are confirmed by the tomogram.

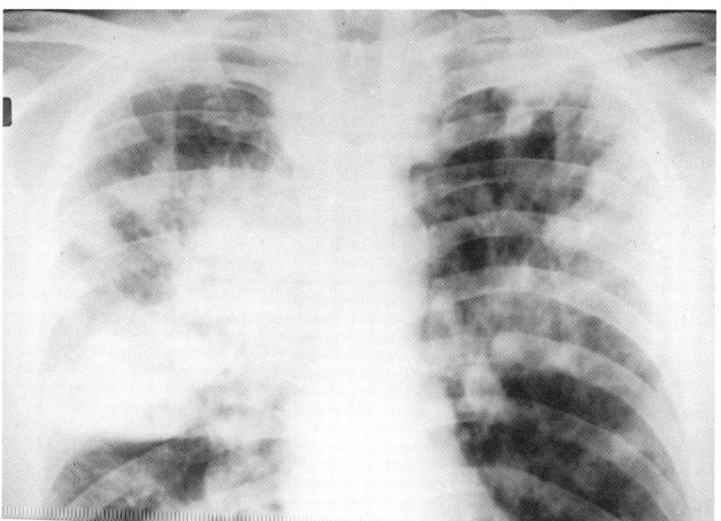

Fig. 5.13 Aspergillus pneumonia. This patient had very severe asthma, only controlled by prednisolone 120mg daily; on this regimen he developed increasing breathlessness and bilateral widespread shadows. His sputum contained *A. fumigatus* and no other pathogen. There was rapid extension of shadowing despite intravenous amphotericin B and attempted lowering of prednisolone dosage. Autopsy showed extensive invasive aspergillosis.

bloodstream. Candida pneumonia usually develops late in the course of disseminated (systemic) candidosis (compare aspergillus pneumonia).

Cryptococcus neoformans

Pulmonary infection with *C. neoformans* may be clinically silent, particularly when it occurs in an immunologically competent individual. It may then be discovered on a routine chest radiograph as a cryptococcoma (Fig. 5.15). Cryptococcus pneumonia occurs more frequently in immunocompromised individuals, and there is a particular association with Hodgkin's disease, the precise reason for which is unclear.

Histoplasma capsulatum

Histoplasma capsulatum is a small yeast that is endemic in   central USA. The infection may be asymptomatic, leading only to a positive reaction to the histoplasmin intradermal skin test (delayed hypersensitivity, Type IV, reaction). Patients presenting with mild respiratory symptoms may be discovered to have a peripheral infiltrate together with hilar lymphadenopathy, for which treatment is unlikely to be required. Healed lesions may result in a single dense small peripheral shadow on the chest radiograph.

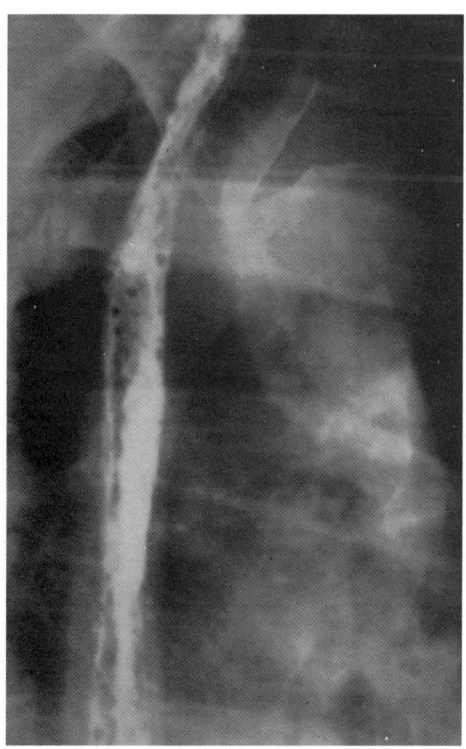

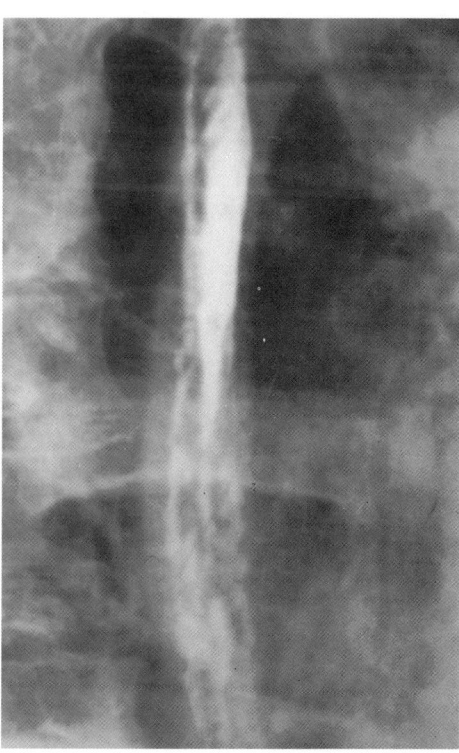

Fig. 5.14 Oesophageal candidosis: barium swallow. The mucosal outline is irregular and there are many 'filling defects' due to mucosal plaques of candida.

More severe infections may follow heavy exposure to the organism, when an acute bronchopneumonia may develop (see Fig. 5.7). Healing is followed by widespread fibrosis and calcification ('buckshot calcification'), the size and number of the calcified lesions corresponding to the size and number of the original infiltrates. Typical lesions on the chest radiograph are composed of a central calcified core and a surrounding, less dense halo.

Inhalation exposure most commonly gives rise to very widespread, medium-sized to small nodular lesions (Fig. 5.16), but may also produce very fine nodular lesions in the granulomatous form of the disease.

Coccidioides immitis

Coccidioides immitis is a soil-dwelling fungus that is found in the south-western USA and in central parts of South America. Primary infections may cause hilar lymphadenopathy (Fig 5 17), patchy opacities in the lung fields or pleural effusions. An inactive lesion may appear as a dense rounded opacity on the chest radiograph and is termed a coccidioidoma (Fig. 5.18).

Progressive coccidioidomycosis follows the primary infection in about one percent of cases. Progressive disease may take a number of forms, of which the commonest is bronchopneumonia; the healing of such a lesion may result in the formation of a thin-walled or 'eggshell' cavity, which may contain a fluid level. Other forms of progressive coccidioidomycosis include miliary dissemination, which is usually rapidly fatal, and a chronic granulomatous reaction in the lungs, skin, joints, meninges and brain.

Blastomyces dermatitidis

Blastomyces dermatitidis is a soil fungus found in the south-eastern USA. Pulmonary involvement is usually part of a systemic disease, which may involve the genito-urinary and central nervous systems, and there may be miliary shadowing on the chest radiograph Massive opacities in the lungs may cavitate, the cavities frequently persisting after treatment (Fig. 5.19).

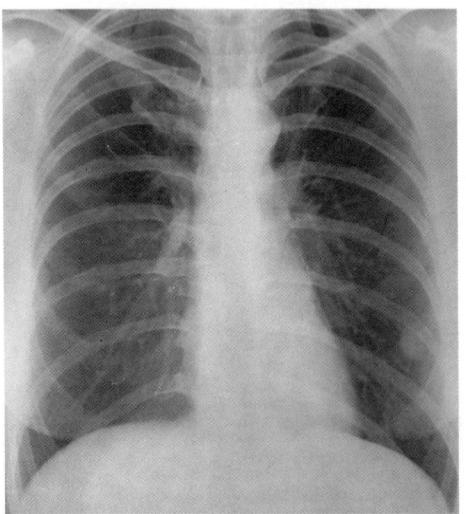
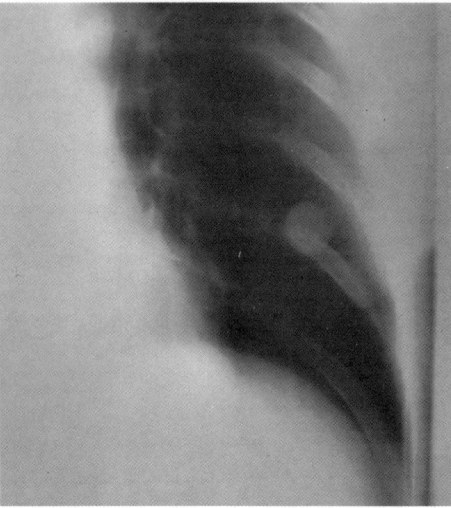

Fig. 5.15 Cryptococcoma. There is a rounded homogeneous density in the left lower lobe on this routine chest radiograph (left) in an asymptomatic 37-year-old woman. The tomogram (right) shows that the opacity lies posteriorly; it does not contain any calcification and has a smooth outline.

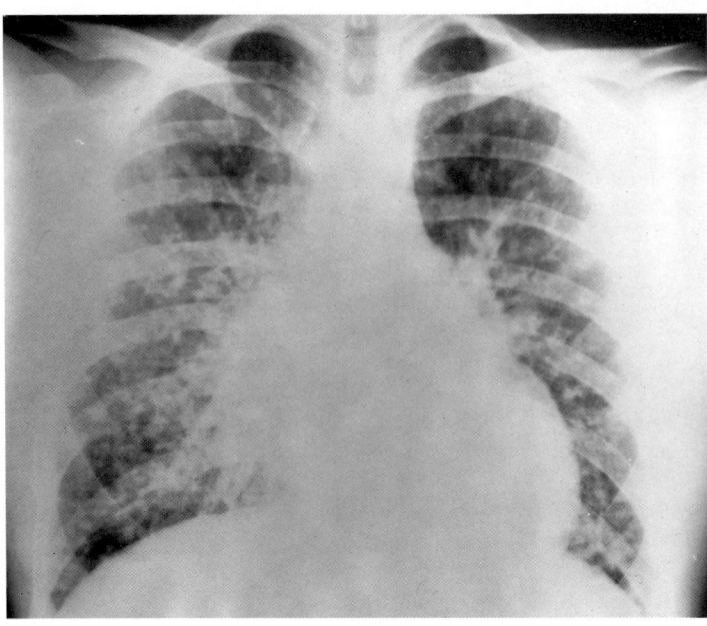

Fig. 5.16 *H. capsulatum* bronchopneumonia. The lesions are small and nodular. This is the most common appearance of acute histoplasmosis at presentation.

Protozoa

Pneumocystis carinii is a protozoon that may be found as a commensal in the upper respiratory tract. In immuno-compromised patients the organism may become invasive and cause a widespread interstitial pneumonia. In the past, this occurred most frequently in patients with acute lymphoblastic leukaemia or lymphoma who had received prolonged cytotoxic chemotherapy and corticosteroids (Fig. 5.20). The organism has assumed greater importance again with the increasing incidence of the acquired immune deficiency syndrome (AIDS).

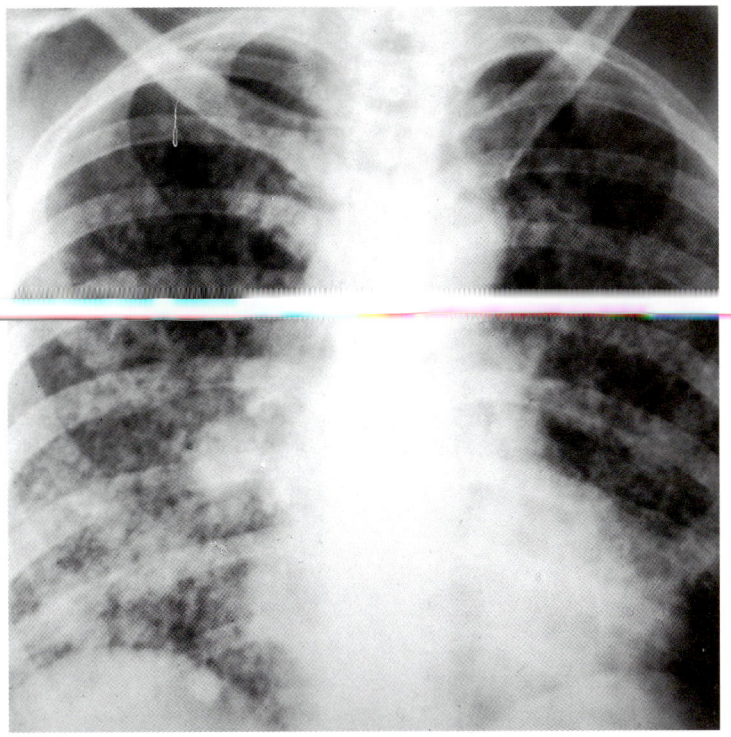

Fig. 5.17 Coccidioidomycosis. In this primary infection there are small interstitial infiltrates and prominent right hilar and paratracheal lymphadenopathy.

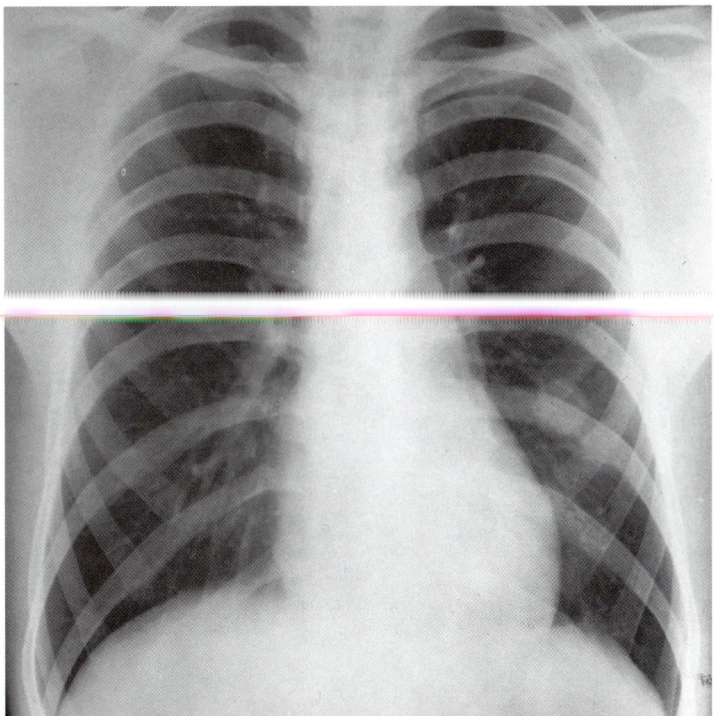

Fig. 5.18 Coccidioidoma. This routine chest radiograph shows a homogeneous round shadow in the left mid-zone. The coccidioidin skin test was strongly positive.

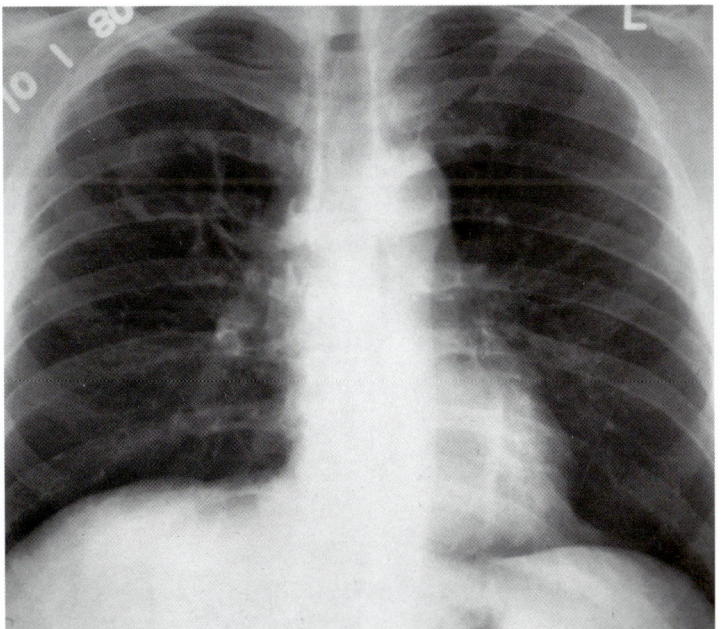

Fig. 5.19 Blastomycosis. A cavity persists in the right upper lobe after successful treatment with amphotericin B for subacute pneumonia.

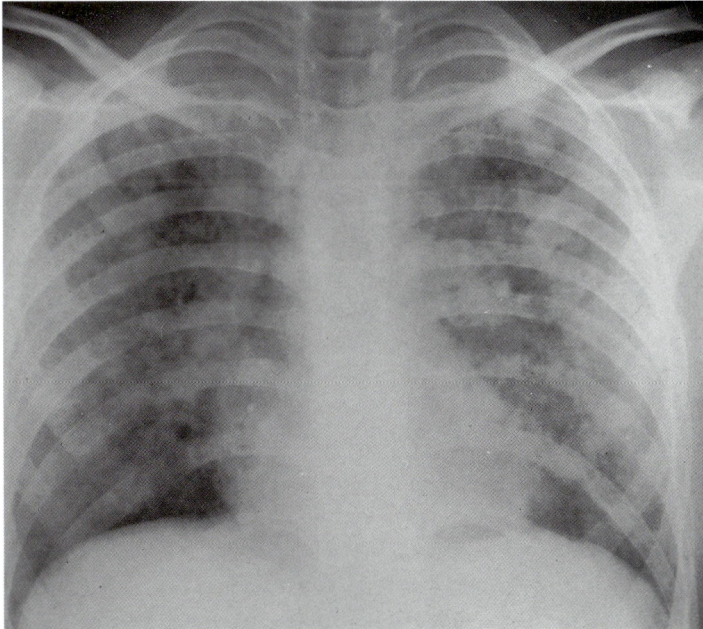

Fig. 5.20 *Pneumocystis carinii* pneumonia. There is bilateral dense interstitial shadowing. This 8-year-old boy had received two years of maintenance chemotherapy for acute lymphoblastic leukaemia.

Pneumocystis carinii gives rise to an interstitial pneumonia with a copious alveolar exudate, and the chest radiograph shows widespread interstitial shadowing, frequently with an air bronchogram. Sometimes there is sparing of one or more lobes of the lung.

Viruses

Viral pneumonia is generally of the interstitial type, with involvement of the alveolar walls and the production of an intra-alveolar exudate. On the chest radiograph there is widespread homogeneous shadowing and there may be an air bronchogram because the airways remain patent and contrast with the consolidation.

In normal individuals herpes simplex virus produces a localized lesion or 'cold sore', but in immunocompromised patients the sore may spread and a viraemia may occur, followed by the development of pneumonia. In other cases, HSV pneumonia may develop without any preceding

cutaneous manifestation (Fig. 5.21).

Varicella/zoster virus usually manifests itself first as cutaneous, vesiculating lesions which may become haemorrhagic if the patient is thrombocytopenic. This may be followed or accompanied by the development of pneumonia. Varicella pneumonia may also complicate severe chickenpox in normal individuals; this is unusual in children but quite frequent in adults, when the pneumonia may develop two to five days after the rash. The chest radiograph shows diffuse small nodular infiltrations (Fig. 5.22) which may eventually leave widespread small calcified nodules.

The radiographic appearances of cytomegalovirus are similar to those of other viral pneumonias.

The measles virus sometimes causes interstitial pneumonia (Fig. 5.23) in immunosuppressed children who have not had measles previously or who have not maintained adequate anti-measles virus antibody titres as a result of their immunosuppression.

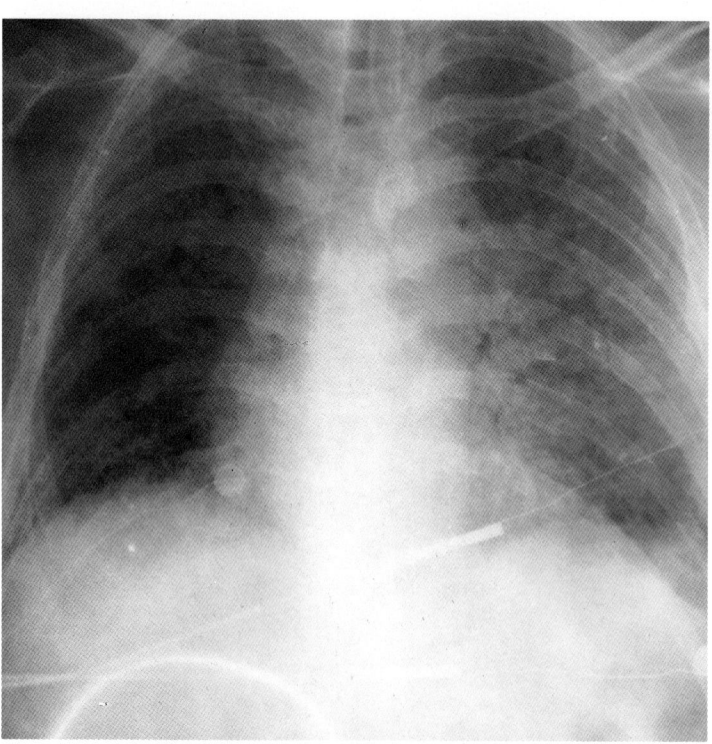

Fig. 5.21 HSV pneumonia. The chest radiograph of a man aged 55 who had received a high dosage of corticosteroids for cryptogenic fibrosing alveolitis. The bilateral interstitial pneumonia has a rather patchy appearance. HSV was isolated from his sputum.

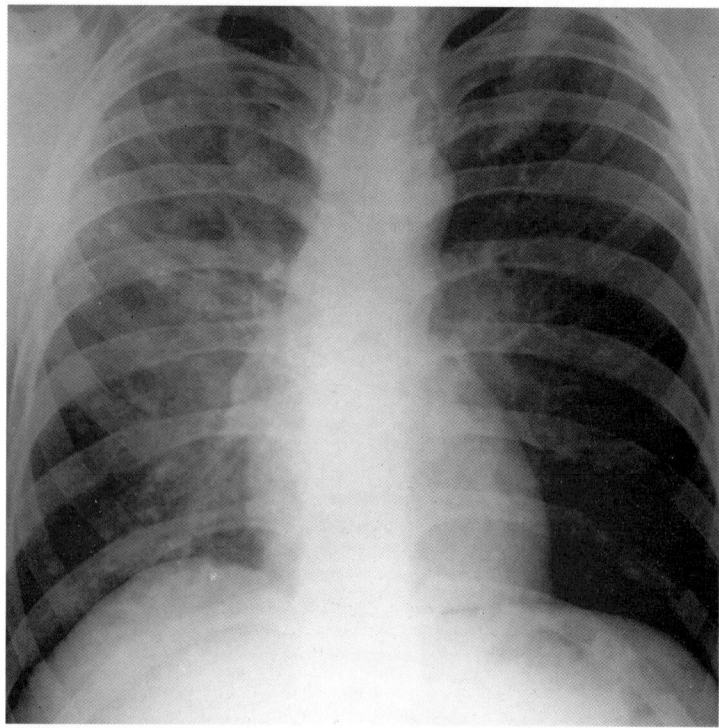

Fig. 5.22 Varicella/zoster virus pneumonia. This 30-year-old man presented with severe chickenpox. The chest radiograph shows typical confluent nodular infiltrates, mainly in the right mid-zone. After six days of treatment with acyclovir the chest radiograph showed almost complete resolution.

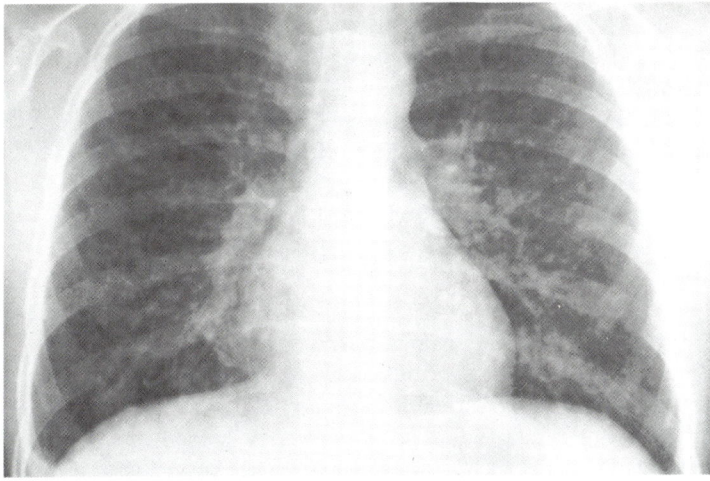

Fig. 5.23 Measles pneumonia. This radiograph of a 4-year-old boy with acute lymphoblastic leukaemia shows poorly defined patchy shadowing throughout both lungs with ~~~~~~~~~~ in the left upper zone.

Tuberculosis

Primary tuberculosis

When an individual is infected with the tubercle bacillus for the first time, the tuberculin skin test becomes positive within about three or four weeks. A minority of patients will become pyrexial or develop a hypersensitivity reaction such as erythema nodosum (Fig. 5.24), epituberculosis or phlyctenular conjunctivitis.

Only about 5–15 percent of people primarily infected with the tubercle bacillus develop overt disease. The radiological appearances of primary tuberculosis include parenchymal involvement, lymphadenopathy, pleural effusions and miliary tuberculosis. The pulmonary lesion is called a Ghon focus. In a child, the predominant lesion is an enlarged hilar lymph node (see Fig. 2.31) with a small peripheral lesion in the ~~~~~~~~~~~~~~~~~~~~

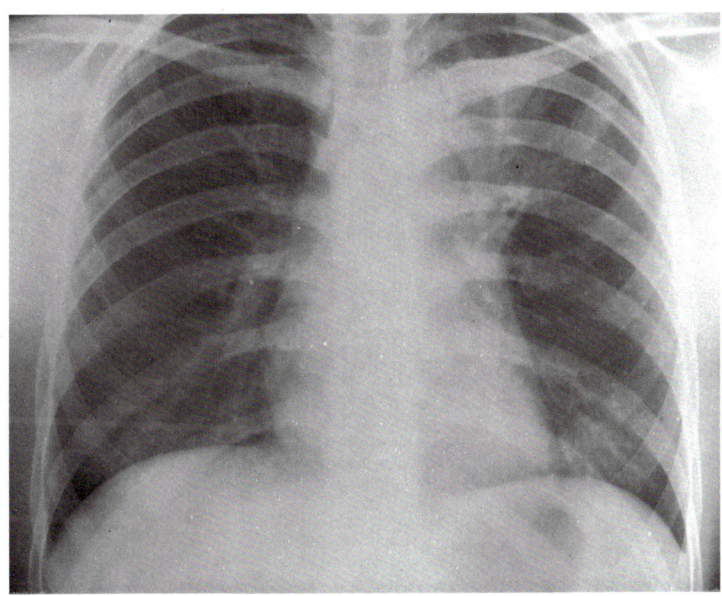

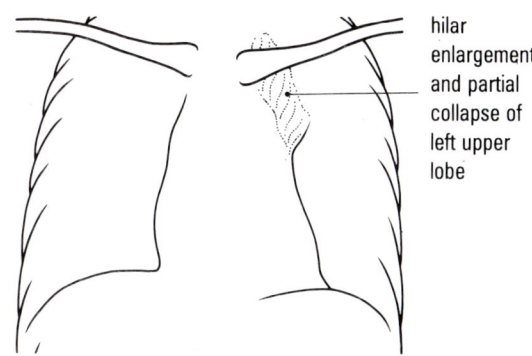

hilar enlargement and partial collapse of left upper lobe

Fig. 5.24 Chest radiograph of a 12-year-old patient, showing evidence of primary tuberculosis. There is an enlarged left hilar gland and collapse–consolidation, including part of the left upper lobe.

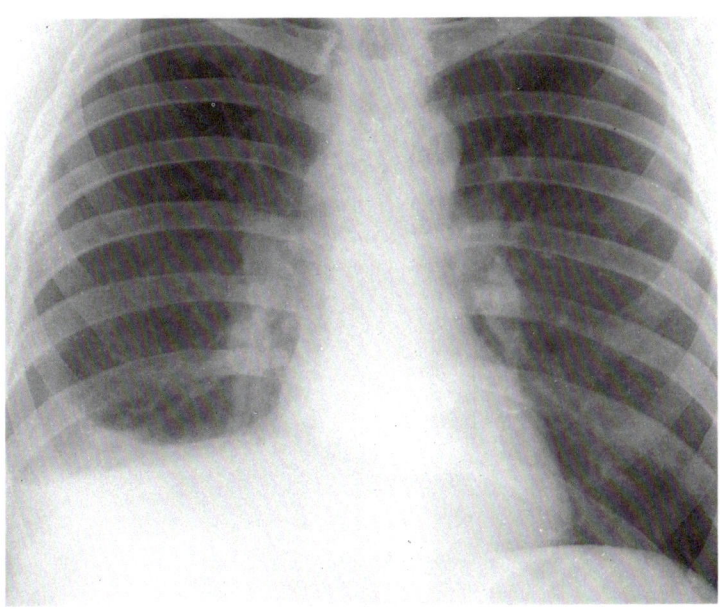

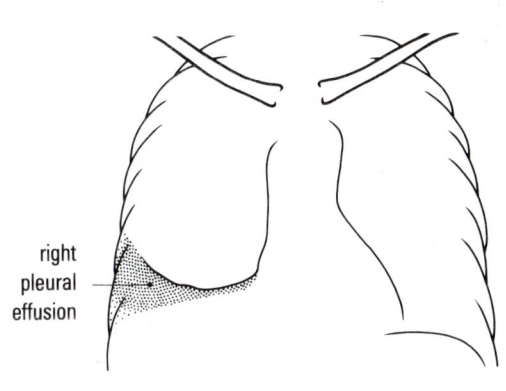

right pleural effusion

Fig. 5.25 Primary tuberculous pleural effusion.

the primary lesions heal. In the adult, the lymph nodes sometimes cause bronchiectasis or obstructive distension. Bronchial erosion, pleural effusion (Fig. 5.25) and tuberculous bronchial pneumonia may occur.

The most serious complications of primary tuberculosis are miliary tuberculosis and meningitis, which tend to occur between one and five years after primary infection.

The diagnosis of primary tuberculosis is by X-ray and positive skin hypersensitivity to tuberculin.

Miliary tuberculosis

Miliary tuberculosis is caused by acute dissemination of the tubercle bacilli via the bloodstream. It usually follows primary infection in the young. It can, however, occur in a cryptic form in the elderly or immunosuppressed patient.

In the acute form in the young person, the patient is acutely ill with a high temperature and cough, but in some cases there are no chest symptoms. The patient may have lymphadenopathy and hepatosplenomegaly. The chest X-ray is characteristic, with tubercles of 1.5–3mm evenly distributed as nodules throughout both lung fields (Fig. 5.26). The patient may have the classical choroidal tubercles. Diagnosis is by chest radiograph and a positive tuberculin test.

Postprimary tuberculosis

Postprimary tuberculosis can occur as a reactivation of a primary lesion, progression of a primary lesion or, rarely, as a case of reinfection. The patient may present with general symptoms such as weight loss, anorexia, temperature and a general feeling of ill health and/or symptoms specific to the chest such as cough, sputum, dyspnoea, haemoptysis and chest pain. A chest radiograph can reveal a number of appearances, such as pneumonia, particularly in the apical posterior segment of the upper lobe and the apical segment of the lower lobe, fibrosis, cavities, bronchogenic spread, miliary tuberculosis, tuberculomas, pleural effusions and empyema (Figs 5.27–5.30).

It should be remembered that tuberculosis can affect sites other than the lung. The most common extrapulmonary sites are the lymph nodes. When enlargement of the mediastinal lymph nodes is seen, the differential diagnoses are tuberculosis, sarcoid, lymphoma and carcinoma.

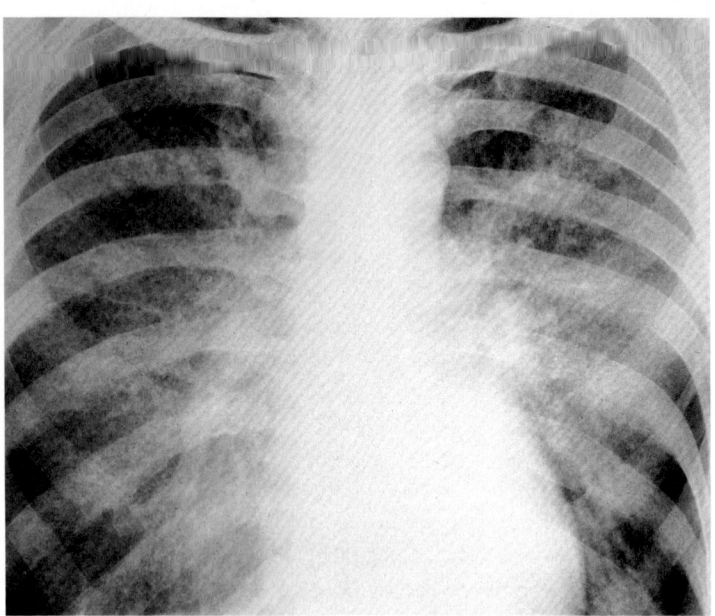

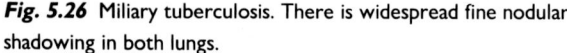

Fig. 5.26 Miliary tuberculosis. There is widespread fine nodular shadowing in both lungs.

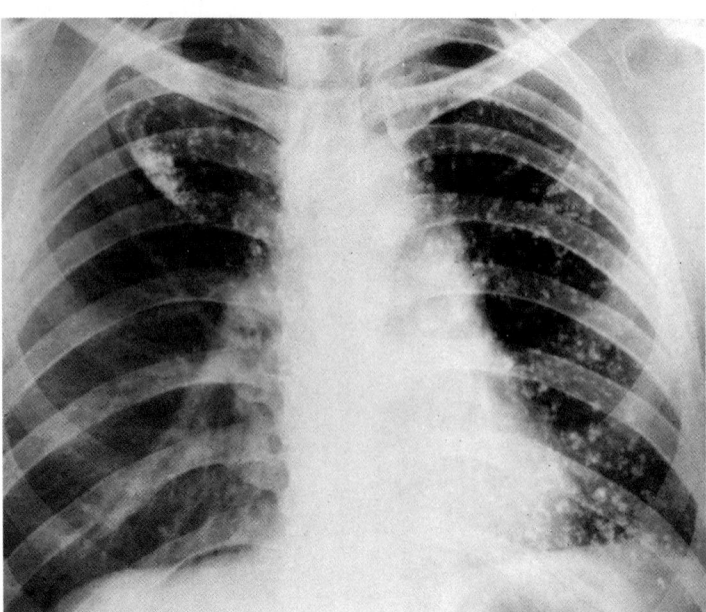

Fig. 5.27 Postprimary tuberculosis. There is widespread calcification in the left lung and right upper lobe following tuberculous infection.

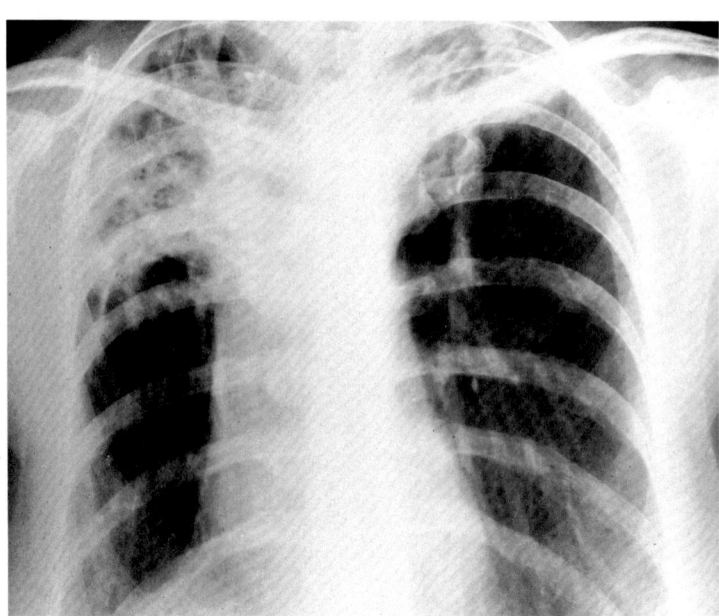

Fig. 5.28 Postprimary tuberculosis. Severe fibrosis of both upper lobes may be seen.

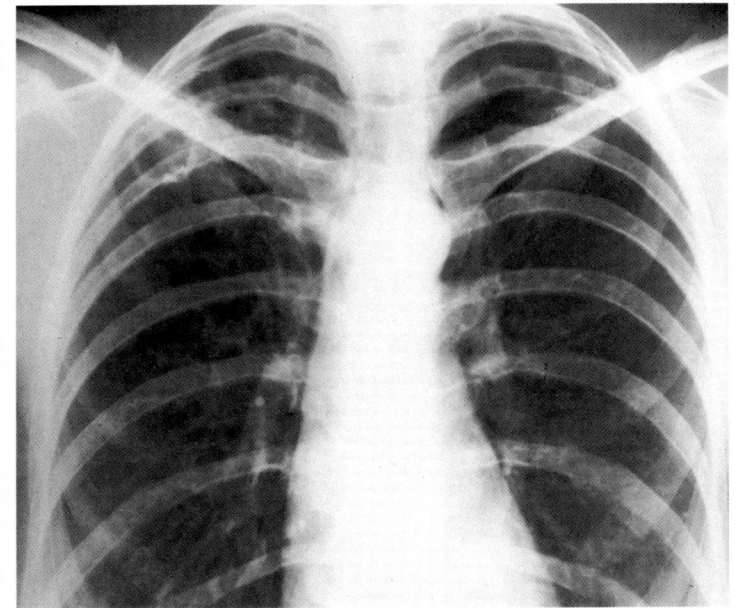

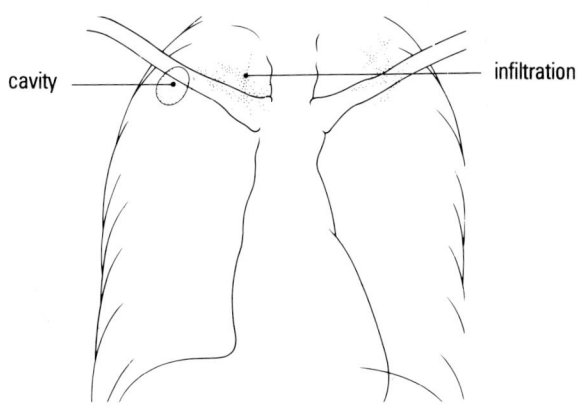

Fig. 5.29 Postprimary tuberculosis. There is infiltration at both apices and a 2cm thin-walled cavity in the right upper zone.

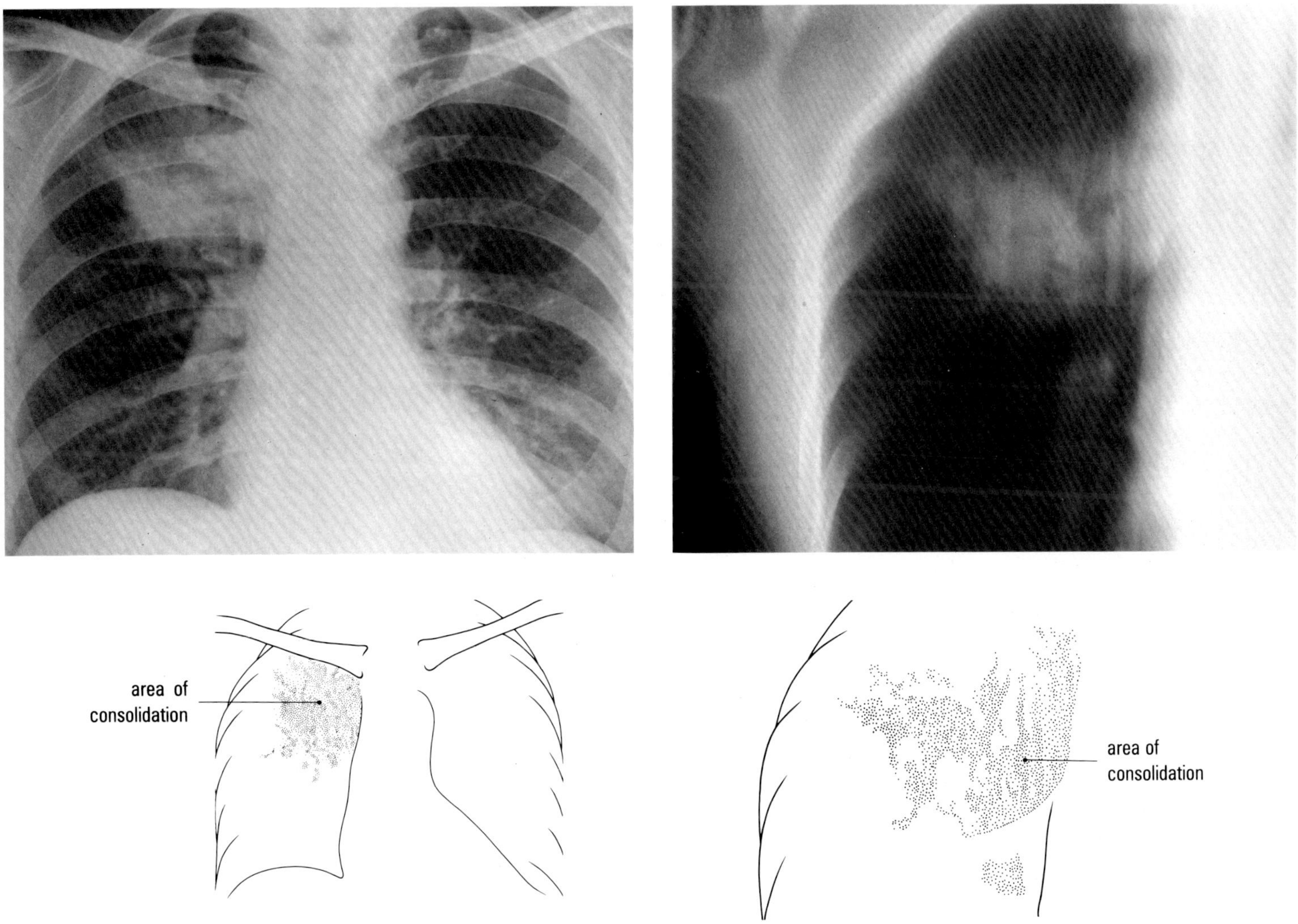

Fig. 5.30 Postprimary tuberculosis. There is an area of consolidation in the right upper lobe due to tuberculous pneumonia (left). Tomography of the same patient (right) shows an air bronchogram.

Asthma

The chest radiograph is important in asthma and often demonstrates substantial hyperinflation (Fig. 5.31). Typically this can be distinguished from destructive emphysema by a number of features. The diaphragm, although displaced downwards, often maintains its normal curvature; although there is a generalized diminution in vascular pattern towards the periphery of the lungs, there is a uniform distribution throughout both lung fields. In contrast, in emphysema some areas frequently show gross reduction of vessel calibre while others show prominent 'marker vessels' as seen in most normally perfused lungs.

The pattern of asthma reflected in ventilation–perfusion scans is important. Confusion with pulmonary emboli may arise if only perfusion scans are undertaken. In asthma the peripheral areas of poor perfusion are matched on a simultaneous ventilatory scan by similar areas of under-penetration by inhaled radiolabelled gas (Fig. 5.32). For this reason, perfusion scans by themselves are only helpful in the exclusion of pulmonary emboli when the scan is completely normal.

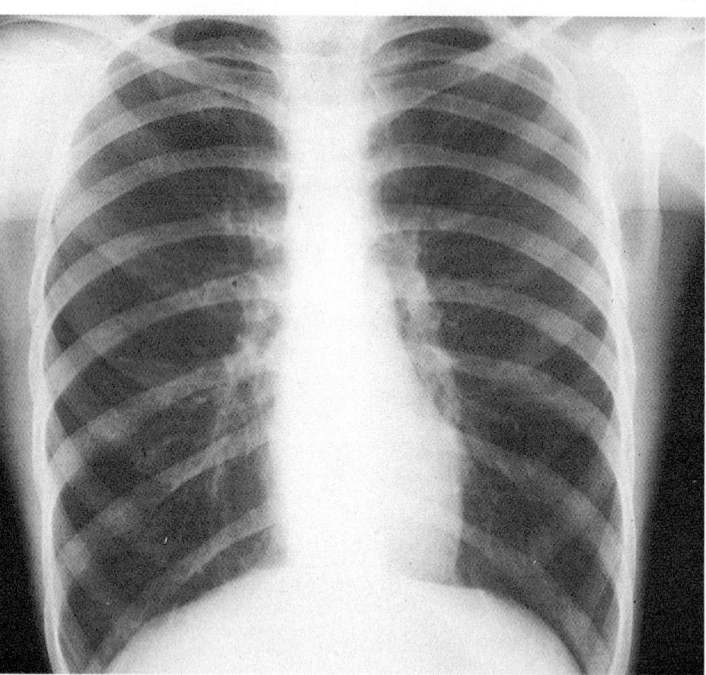

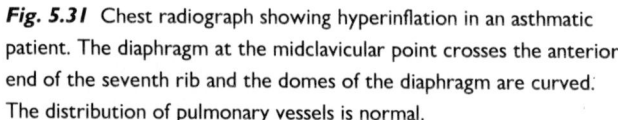

Fig. 5.31 Chest radiograph showing hyperinflation in an asthmatic patient. The diaphragm at the midclavicular point crosses the anterior end of the seventh rib and the domes of the diaphragm are curved. The distribution of pulmonary vessels is normal.

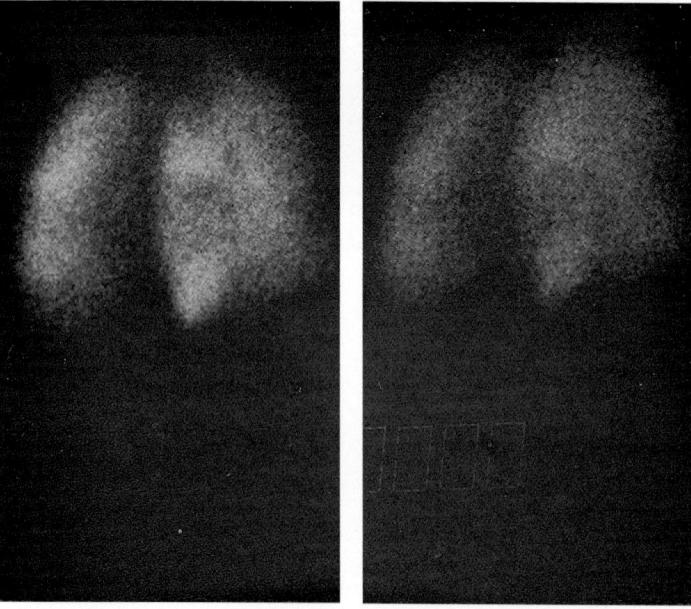

Fig. 5.32 A ventilation–perfusion scan showing matched defects where ventilatory and blood form impairment occur at the same sites.

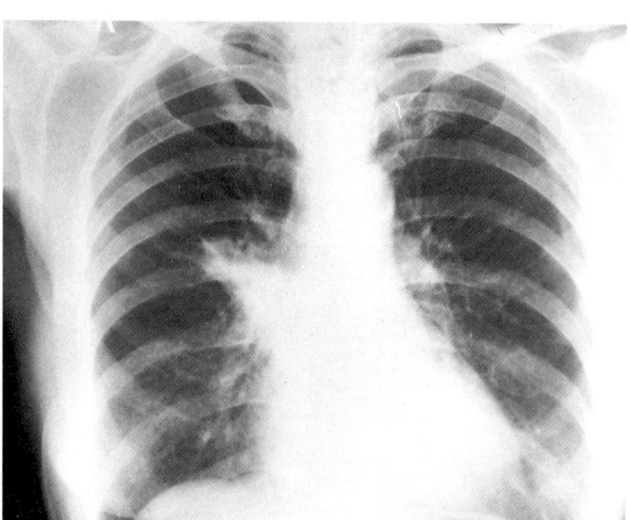

Fig. 5.33 Bronchopulmonary aspergillosis. There was a transient shadow at the right hilum in this patient with atopic asthma and a positive skin prick test to *A. fumigatus*.

Pulmonary Eosinophilia

Bronchopulmonary aspergillosis

The diagnosis of bronchopulmonary aspergillosis may be suspected in an atopic individual with a blood eosinophilia and radiographic shadows in whom the skin prick test to *A. fumigatus* is positive. Total serum IgE is usually substantially raised and the eosinophilia in the order of 1000–2000 IU/ml, although on some occasions it may be higher.

Radiographs show a variety of features and, in addition to the typical transient shadows, chronic cases can be identified. The most typical appearance is that of transient non-segmental infiltrates which appear first in one lung and then in the other, in either the upper or lower lobes (Fig. 5.33). In some instances recurrent shadows occur over very many years; in other cases one or more shadows occur in rapid succession but then do not recur. This variable history makes management of the condition difficult. As radiographic shadows recur, so proximal bronchial wall damage develops and this determines a very characteristic radiographic appearance (Fig. 5.34). In other cases the radiographic shadow presents as a more homogeneous density similar to a mucocele (Figs 5.35 and 5.36). Mucus

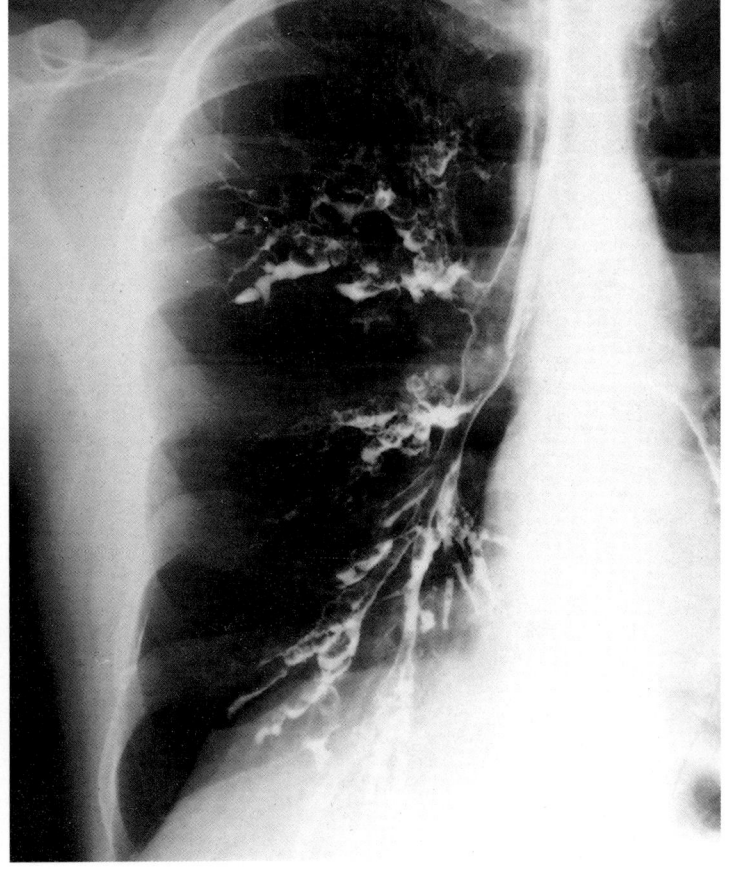

Fig. 5.34 Bronchopulmonary aspergillosis. Bronchogram showing proximal bronchiectasis with normal peripheral bronchi.

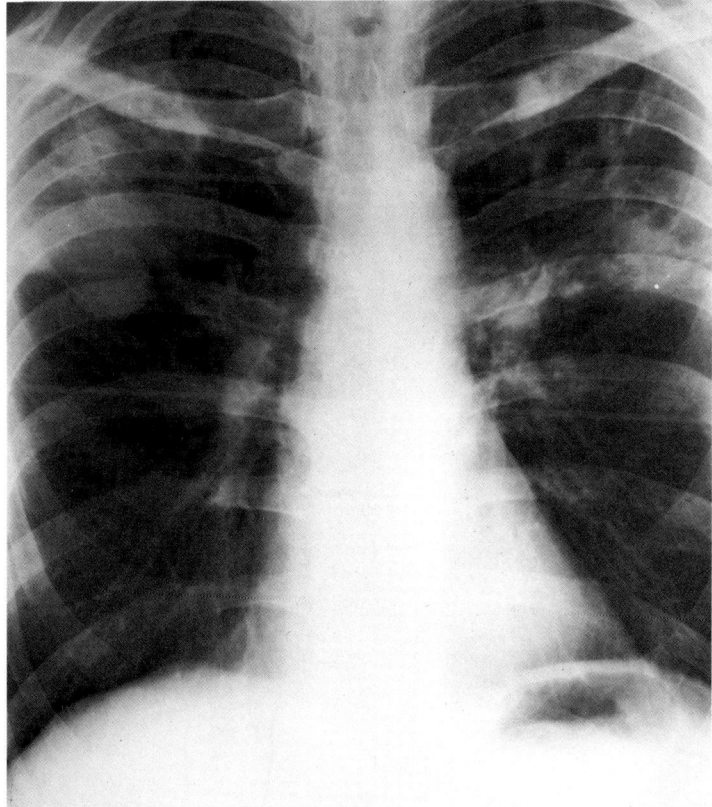

Fig. 5.35 Bronchopulmonary aspergillosis with atopic asthma. The radiograph shows bilateral upper zone infiltrates and a dense, well-defined homogeneous shadow suggestive of a mucocele in the right upper zone.

impaction of this type represents a mucus plug dilating enormously the relatively proximal bronchus. In other cases mucus impaction causes a segmental lobar or whole lung collapse. These cases clearly present a difficult diagnostic problem; the blood eosinophilia and an immediate skin prick test response to *A. fumigatus* are of diagnostic value and appreciation of their significance should avert surgical resection.

When a transient shadow together with bronchial wall damage have recurred over many years, irreversible lung changes develop. In their most typical form these are seen as contracted upper lobes and when cases are seen only at this stage they are often misdiagnosed as tuberculosis (Fig. 5.37). Less frequently recognized appearances may also be found. For example, widespread fixed nodular reticular shadows with some peribronchial thickening may be seen; a limited bronchogram may demonstrate widespread peripheral bronchiectasis. Occasionally cases present which simulate fibrosing alveolitis but haematological and bronchographic examination implicate *A. fumigatus*.

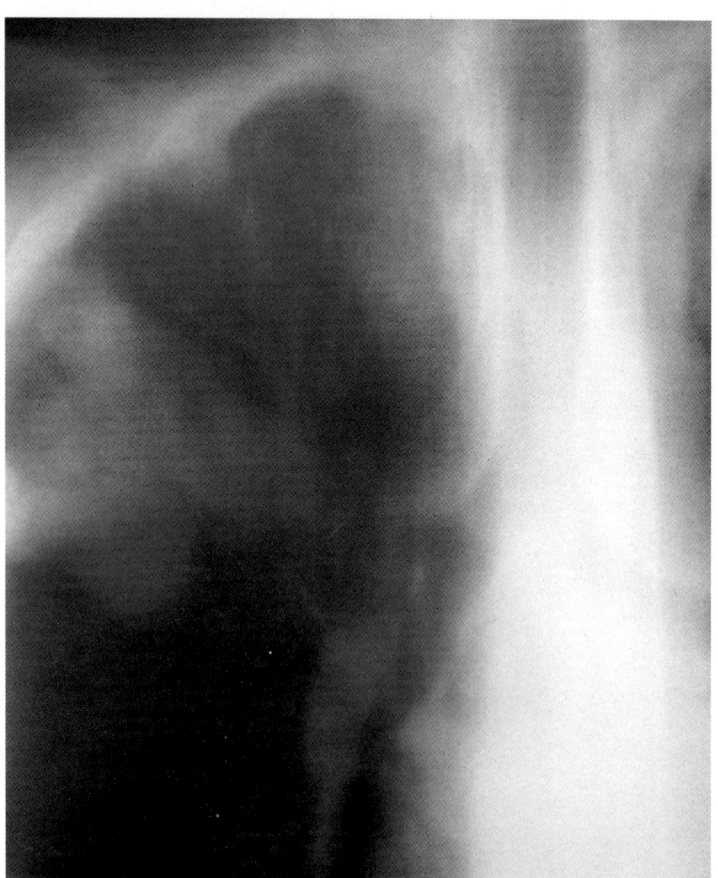

Fig. 5.36 Bronchopulmonary aspergillosis. Tomogram of the patient in Fig. 5.35 after further clearing of the infiltrates. The tomogram shows the 'gloved finger' appearance of the mucus impaction in the right upper zone.

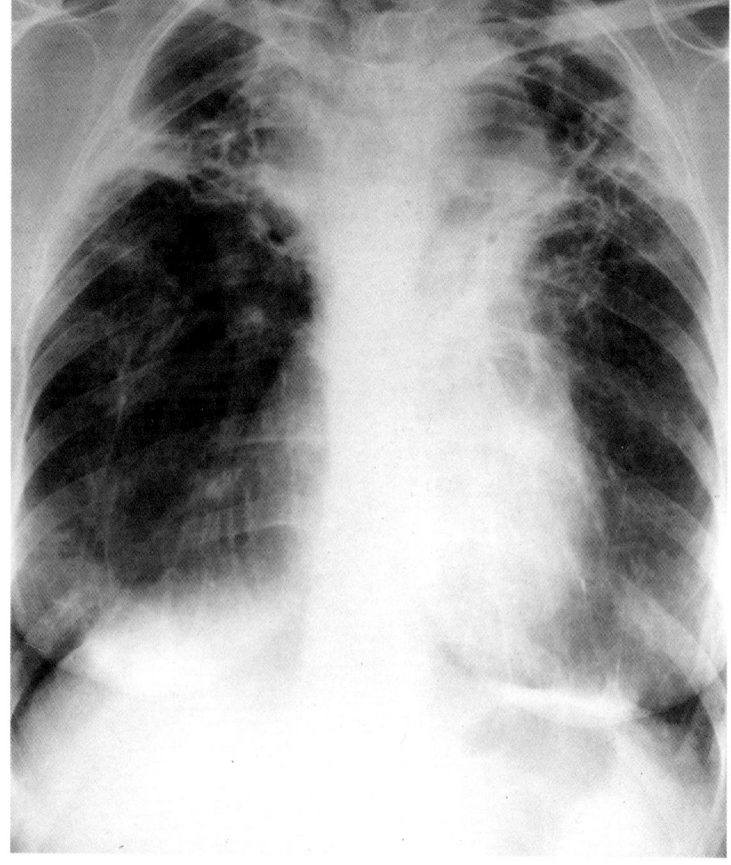

Fig. 5.37 Bilateral upper lobe contraction resulting from long-term bronchopulmonary aspergillosis with recurrent transient shadows in a lifelong asthmatic. The appearances simulate tuberculosis.

Cryptogenic pulmonary eosinophilia

The chest radiograph most typically shows peripheral bilateral shadowing, predominantly in the upper zones (Fig. 5.38). In contrast to bronchopulmonary aspergillosis, the bronchogram is normal. The extent of the shadowing varies greatly, from a localized unilateral lesion to gross and extensive bilateral shadows. The shadowing usually clears dramatically with relatively small doses of corticosteroids.

Churg–Strauss syndrome

This uncommon syndrome is characterized by asthma, a blood eosinophilia and eosinophilic infiltrates of a number of organs including the lung, pericardium, pleura and skin, giving rise to pericardial and pleural effusions (Fig. 5.39). A definite diagnosis is made on the basis of the histological appearances.

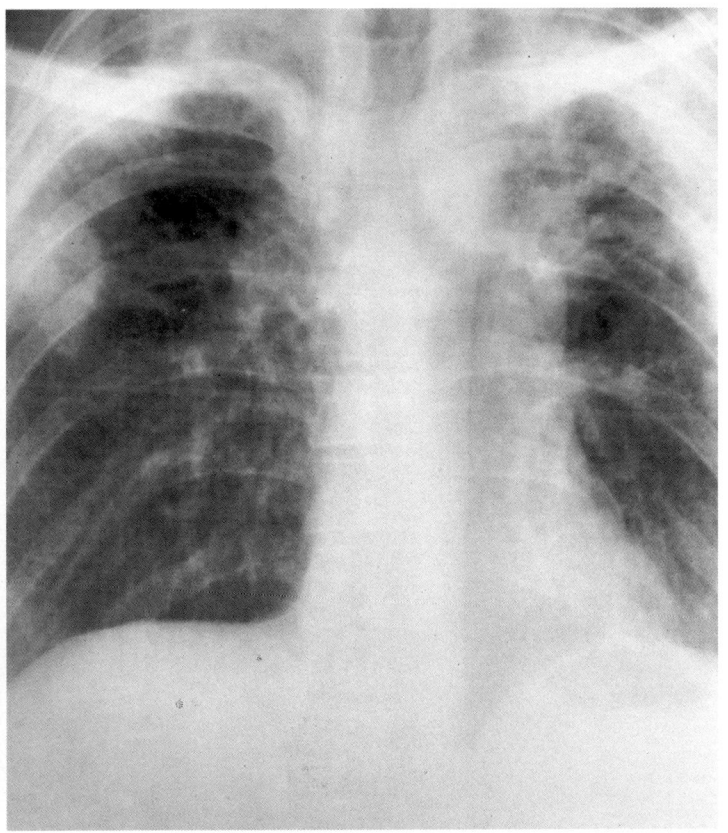

Fig. 5.38 Cryptogenic pulmonary eosinophilia. The chest radiograph shows characteristic bilateral upper zone peripheral shadows.

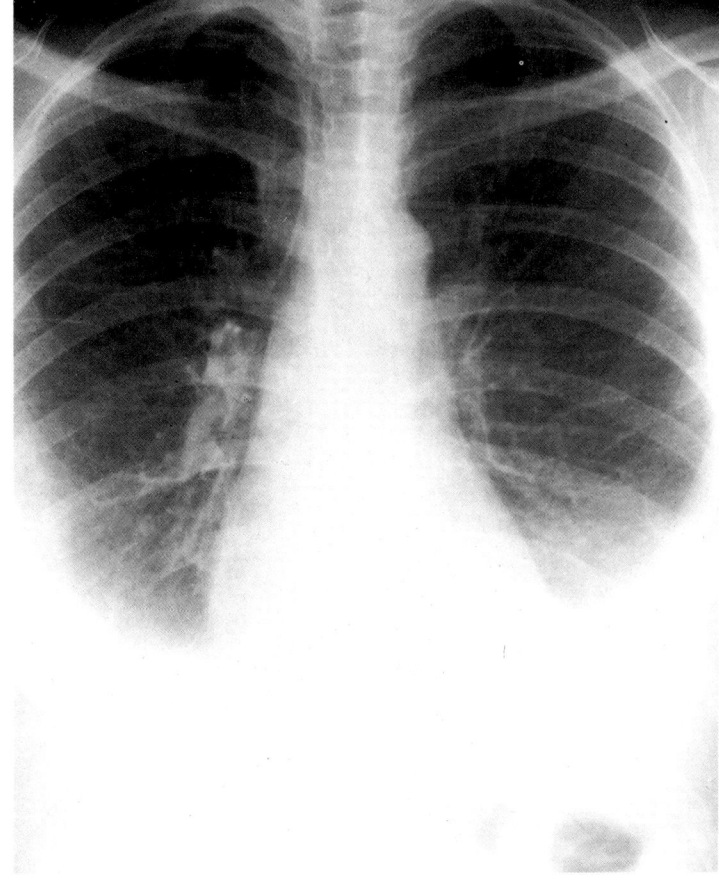

Fig. 5.39 Churg–Strauss syndrome. The chest radiograph shows pericardial and pleural effusions.

Polyarteritis nodosa

It is probable that many cases previously classified as polyarteritis nodosa fit more appropriately into the category of cryptogenic pulmonary eosinophilia or Churg–Strauss syndrome. However, occasionally blood eosinophilia and pulmonary infiltrates occur (Fig. 5.40) when there is good evidence of a necrotizing vasculitis, and the diagnosis of polyarteritis nodosa is then applicable. Most typically these patients have larger vessel involvement; the kidneys, skin and central and peripheral nervous system are commonly involved. Mesenteric artery angiograms may be of diagnostic value in demonstrating vascular aneurysms of the medium-sized vessels.

Extrinsic Allergic Alveolitis

Extrinsic allergic alveolitis (EAA) (or hypersensitivity pneumonitis) is a granulomatous inflammatory response in the peripheral gas exchanging parts of the lung which is the outcome of a specific immunological response to a variety of organic dusts.

Acute allergic alveolitis characteristically follows heavy antigen exposure. The typical abnormality on the chest radiograph is micronodular (less than 3mm) shadows which may be widespread or more prominent in the lower zones (Fig. 5.41). The nodules can merge into areas of patchy shadowing. In the absence of further exposure these radiographic abnormalities may take one or more months to resolve.

Chronic allergic alveolitis differs from acute by the development of irreversible pulmonary fibrosis. This may follow prolonged exposure to antigen in low concentration (typically the budgerigar fancier) or after several episodes of acute alveolitis (typically the pigeon fancier). Chronic irreversible changes can be seen on the chest radiograph. Linear shadows, honeycombing and lung shrinkage develop primarily in the upper lobes with compensatory dilatation of the lower lobes (Fig. 5.42). Unlike tuberculosis, calcification and cavitation do not occur.

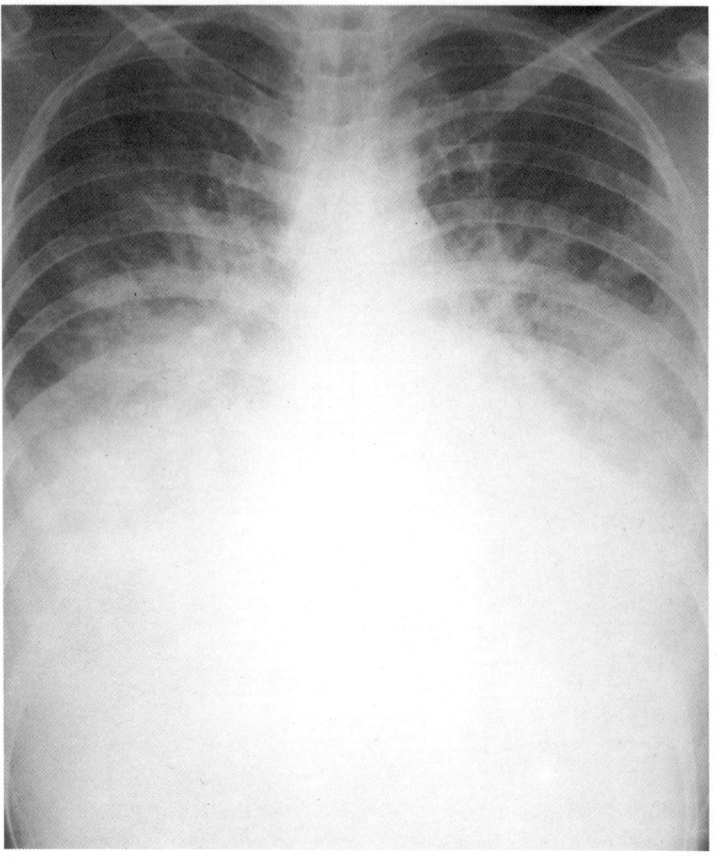

Fig. 5.40 Polyarteritis nodosa and pulmonary eosinophilic infiltrates.

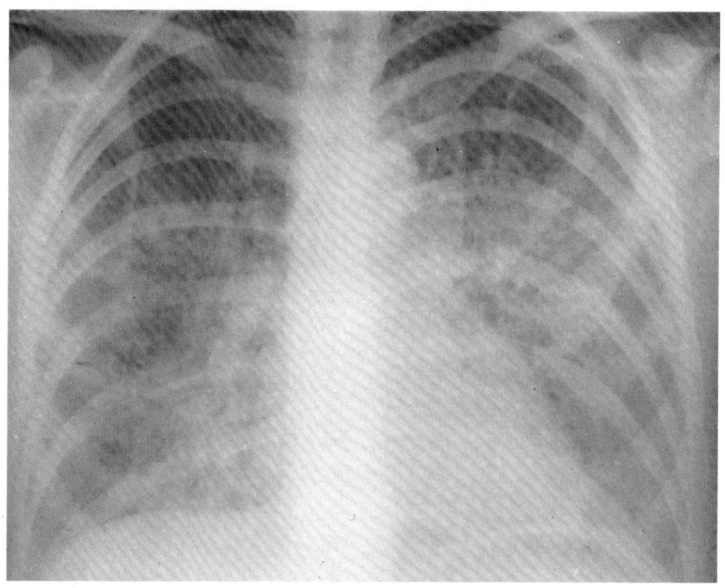

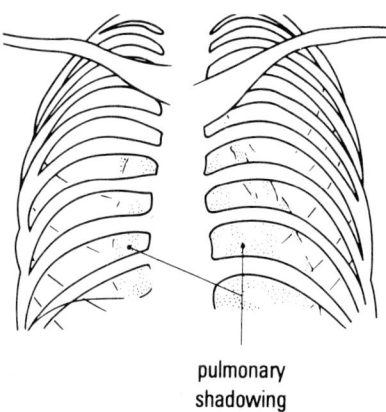

pulmonary
shadowing

Fig. 5.41 Acute extrinsic allergic alveolitis in a bird fancier: widespread pulmonary shadowing.

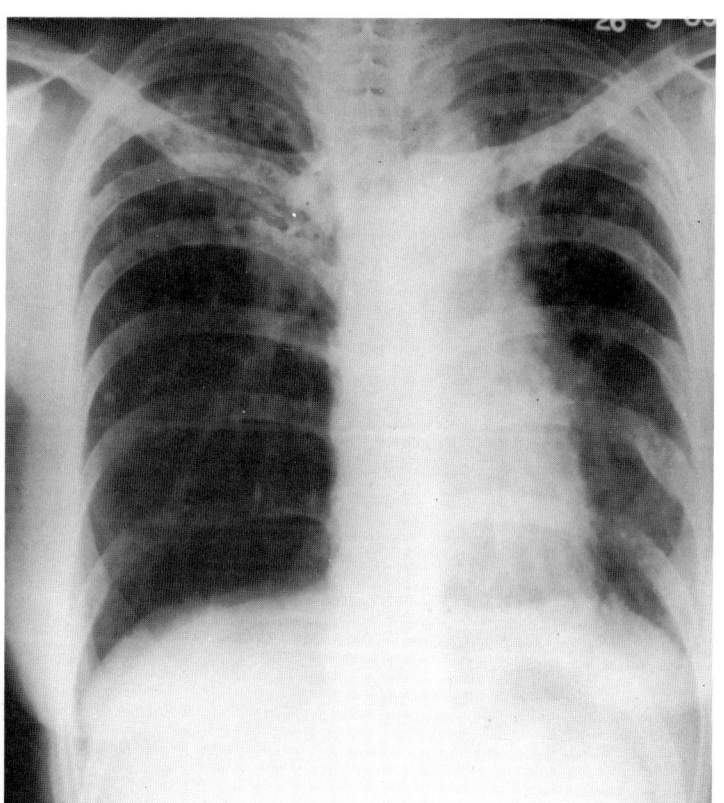

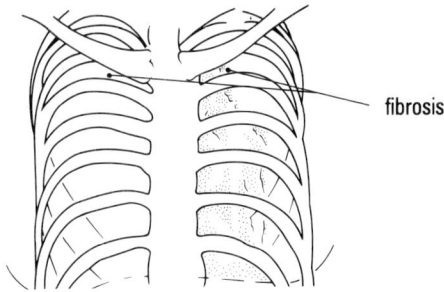

fibrosis

Fig. 5.42 Chronic extrinsic allergic alveolitis in a bird fancier. Fibrosis and contraction primarily involving the upper lobes.

6

Vascular Diseases, Diseases of Unknown Cause and Pulmonary Manifestations of Systemic Diseases

Pulmonary Vascular Disease

Pulmonary embolism

Plain chest radiography

The chest radiograph is not a reliable method of diagnosing pulmonary embolism. It may show infarcts and, if the embolism is massive, oligaemic zones (Westermark's sign) where the vessels are reduced in size and number (Fig. 6.1). Its main value is in eliminating other possible causes of this clinical picture.

Infarcts appear as ill-defined areas of consolidation more often in the lower than the upper zones and always abut a pleural surface. A common site is in the costophrenic sulcus (Fig. 6.2). The size of the area of consolidation varies from 2cm up to 10cm. An air bronchogram is rarely seen in an infarct. Cavitation is extremely rare and usually indicates septic emboli. Infarcts rarely show the classical truncated cone shape and are variable in shape. They are occasionally round in one projection. As they become organized they become better defined, and if they do not resolve rapidly they contract slowly to leave a linear scar. Plate atelectasis and areas of collapse are often associated with infarcts, as are pleural effusions.

The diaphragm is often elevated on the side of a major embolism whether there is infarction or not.

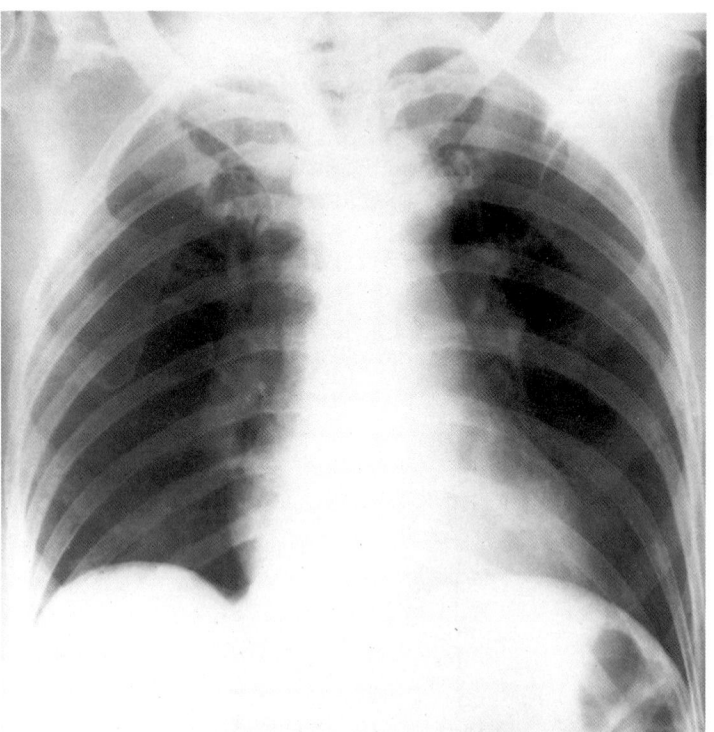

Fig. 6.1 Chest radiograph of a patient with acute massive pulmonary embolism. A paucity of normal vessel shadows is noted in the right mid and lower zones, and throughout the left lung. Angiography showed that only the right upper zone was being perfused normally, the remaining vessels being occluded or severely narrowed by emboli.

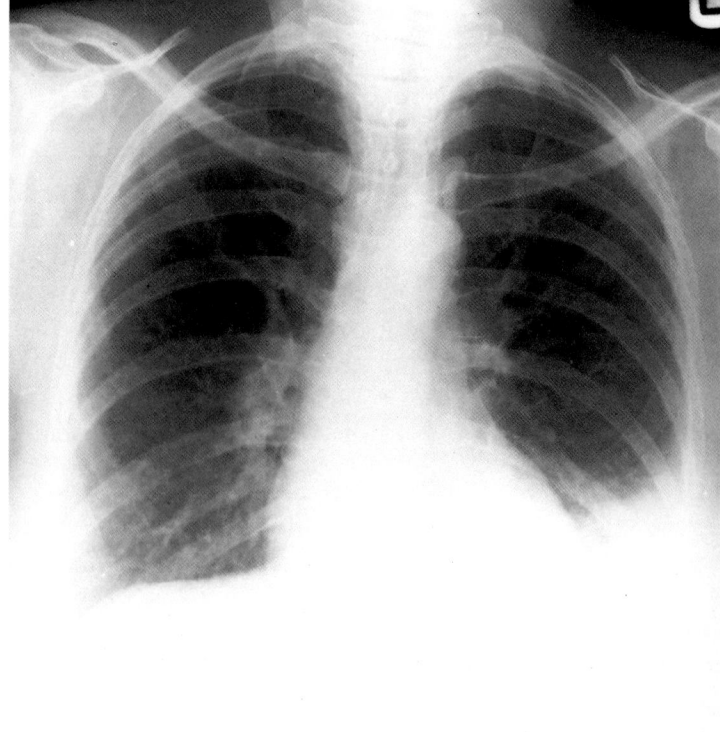

Fig. 6.2 Pulmonary infarct in the left costophrenic angle.

decreased. Alternatively, it may be classified according to the site at which the abnormality occurs: pre-capillary (including those conditions causing increased flow); capillary or post-capillary. Pulmonary hypertension is considered to be present when the pulmonary artery systolic pressure exceeds 30mmHg.

The effect of prolonged pulmonary hypertension is hypertrophy of the right ventricle leading to cardiomegaly and heart failure. In the lungs, the vascular bed is greatly distorted. Many arterioles are occluded, whilst some are dilated. The proximal pulmonary arteries and pulmonary trunk are dilated. The chest radiograph, or arteriogram, shows large hilar and proximal vessels, with reduction in vascular shadows in the mid and peripheral lung fields. Vessels which can be seen are frequently tortuous and truncated so that the periphery appears avascular.

Pulmonary hypertension — pre-capillary level

Left to right shunt. The increase in pulmonary artery pressure as a result of increased flow in congenital heart disease in which there is a left to right shunt is usually not severe. However, if normal fetal resistance does not fall, or there is progressive increase in the resistance as a result of the shunt, then pulmonary artery pressure may eventually reach systemic pressure and the shunt reverse causing the patient to become cyanotic (the Eisenmenger syndrome). The Eisenmenger syndrome includes all cases of pulmonary hypertension with reversed shunt irrespective of the site of the defect (Fig. 6.6). It occurs earlier in life in ventricular septal defect (VSD), persistent ductus arteriosus (PDA) and other aorto-pulmonary shunts, than in atrial septal defect (ASD) and partial anomalous pulmonary venous drainage. The chest radiograph shows cardiac enlargement, often gross, in cases of Eisenmenger syndrome due to ASD, but only a minor degree of enlargement in VSD, and aorto-pulmonary shunts. The pulmonary trunk is large and proximal pulmonary arteries at the hilum dilated. Mid-lung vessels are less dilated and peripherally they are considerably pruned.

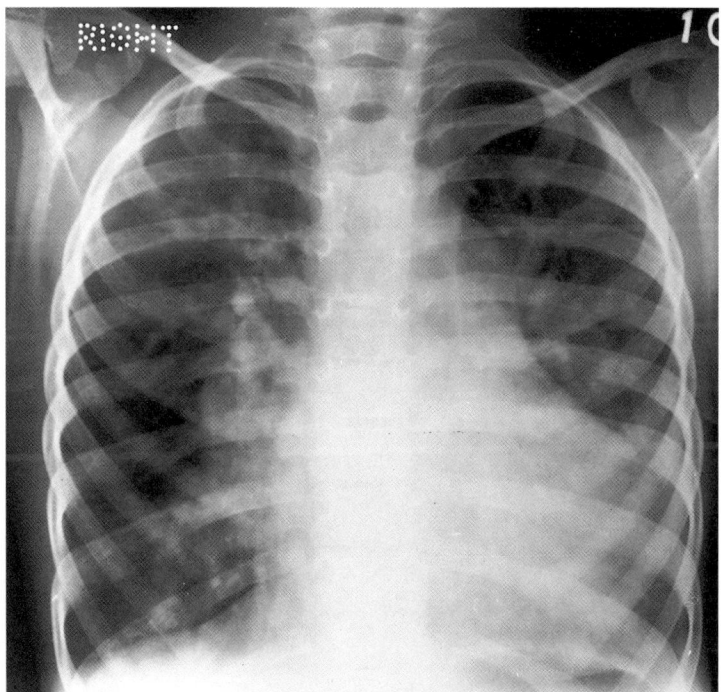 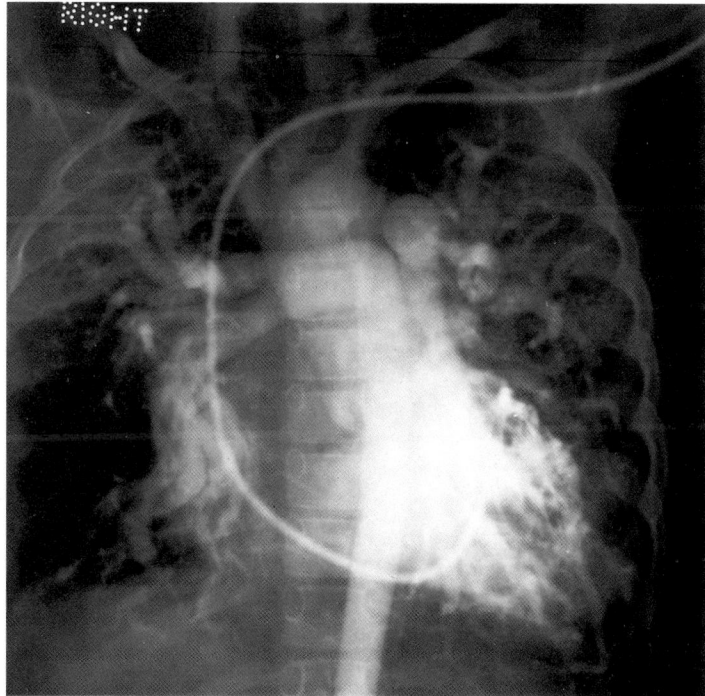

Fig. 6.6 Eisenmenger ventricular septal defect. This five year old, with a heart murmur since birth, had become intermittently cyanosed. The plain chest radiograh shows an enlarged heart, pulmonary plethora and pruning of peripheral vessels. A large pulmonary trunk and proximal pulmonary arteries are also present. The arteriogram following injection of contrast medium into the right ventricle, shows hypertrophy of the right ventricle and infundibulum, large and tortuous proximal pulmonary arteries and evidence of a right to left shunt at ventricular level as the aorta has filled early. Right ventricular pressure was 72/2mmHg and pulmonary vascular resistance, 19 units.

91

Primary pulmonary hypertension. The cause of this disease is unknown. Some regard it as a late manifestation of persistent fetal circulation and others, a result of multiple recurrent microembolism. However, it is a clearly defined clinical entity which occurs mainly in young women, sometimes with a strong family history suggesting a possible genetic transmission. The chest radiograph and arteriogram show dilatation of the proximal trunk and proximal pulmonary arteries with reduction in mid-lung and peripheral arteries, the vessels tapering in a uniform manner (Fig. 6.7). Unlike thromboembolic disease, the changes are equally in all zones and not patchy. The disease is usually progressive and the prognosis is poor, even with treatment.

Pulmonary hypertension — capillary level

Chronic anoxia of any cause may cause pulmonary hypertension. There is reflex constriction of pulmonary arteries when the lung or part of the lung, becomes anoxic.

Extrapulmonary causes include: high altitude sickness (Fig. 6.8); chronic obstruction of the upper airways; obesity; neuromuscular disease causing diaphragmatic and chest wall weakness; chest wall deformity as in kyphoscoliosis and thoracoplasty (Fig. 6.9); and extensive chronic pleural thickening.

Pulmonary causes include: chronic bronchitis and emphysema — this is the commonest cause of pulmonary hypertension and cor pulmonale; fibrosing conditions of the lungs such as cystic fibrosis, sarcoidosis, fibrosing alveolitis and pneumoconiosis; chronic infection such as pulmonary tuberculosis and bronchiectasis; and alveolar proteinosis, microlithiasis alveolaris and idiopathic haemosiderosis.

Some of these conditions cause pulmonary hypertension, not only by anoxic vasoconstriction but by destruction of the capillary bed, for example emphysema.

Pulmonary hypertension — post-capillary level

Pulmonary venous hypertension is caused by any cause of elevation of left atrial pressure such as cardiomyopathy (Fig. 6.10), coronary artery disease, aortic valve disease, systemic hypertension, mitral stenosis and regurgitation,

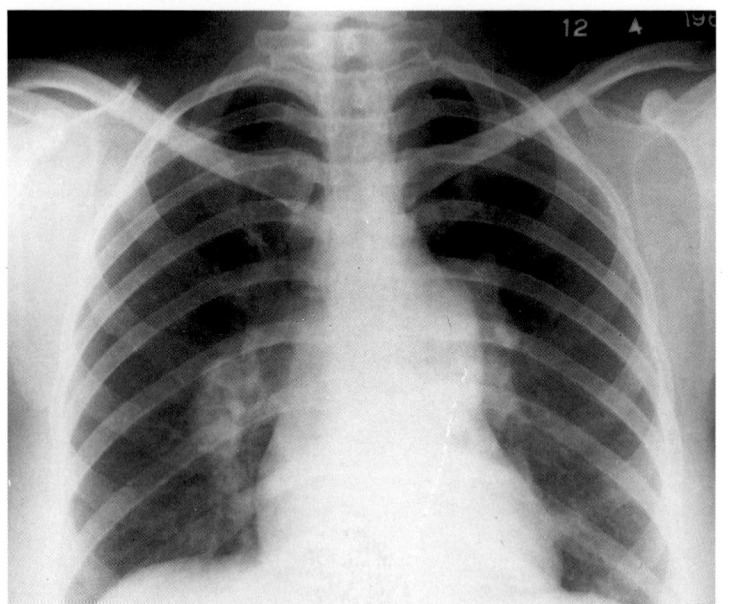 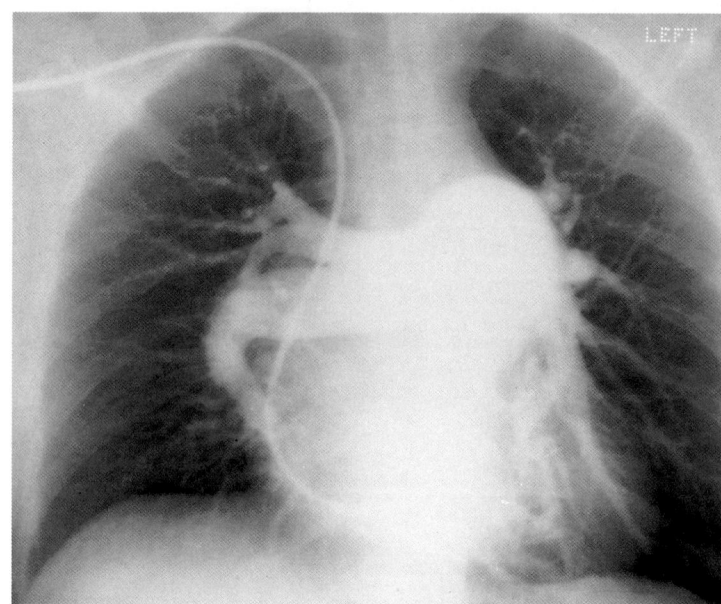

Fig. 6.7 Primary pulmonary hypertension. a) Plain radiograph. b) Pulmonary arteriogram. There is marked dilatation of the main pulmonary trunk and proximal pulmonary arteries but uniform reduction in mid-lung and peripheral vessels.

cardiac tumours and dysrhythmias. It is also caused by obstruction of the pulmonary veins as in some cases of total anomalous pulmonary venous drainage, constrictive pericarditis, and in veno-occlusive disease. Veno-occlusive disease is a rare condition of unknown cause, in which the walls of the intrapulmonary veins are thickened and the veins thrombose.

When pulmonary venous pressure reaches 25mmHg the balance of fluid in the extravascular tissue is so upset that it begins to accumulate and interstitial oedema develops. Interlobular septae become thickened to such an extent that they become visible on a radiograph. They are seen as 1–2cm horizontal lines up to 4mm in thickness, extending inwards from the pleural surface best seen in the costo-phrenic sulci or in the lateral view behind the anterior chest wall. Interstitial oedema also causes the vessel shadows to become less distinct due to perivascular fluid. Acute elevation of pulmonary venous pressure above 30mmHg, in addition to interstitial oedema, causes intra-alveolar oedema, in which there is opacification of the lungs, often with a strikingly perihilar distribution causing a 'bats wing' opacification of both lungs. Chronic pulmonary venous hypertension, in addition to signs of interstitial oedema, may cause deposition of haemosiderin in the lungs, which results in nodules which may calcify or even ossify.

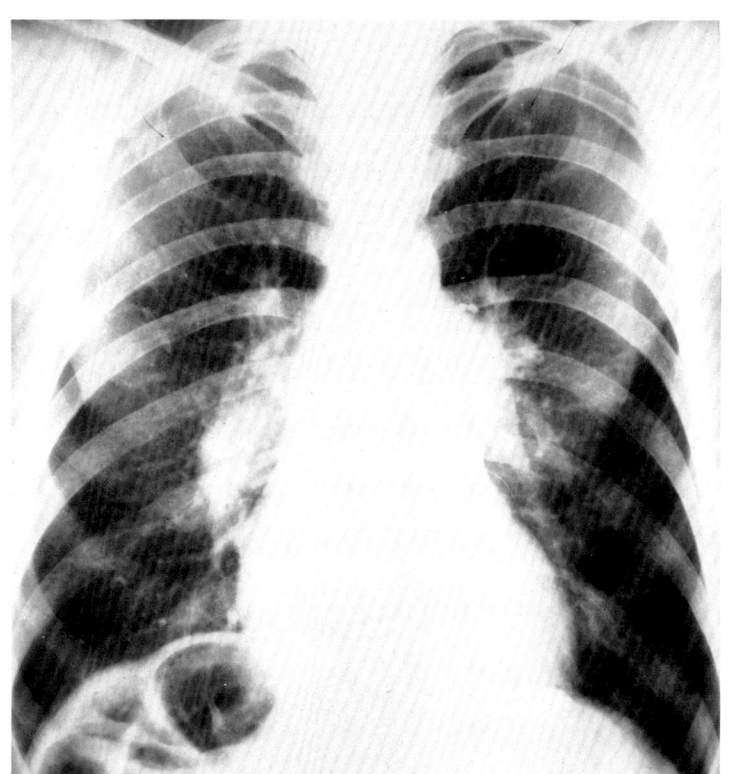

Fig. 6.8 High altitude pulmonary hypertension in a patient who dwells high in the Himalayas.

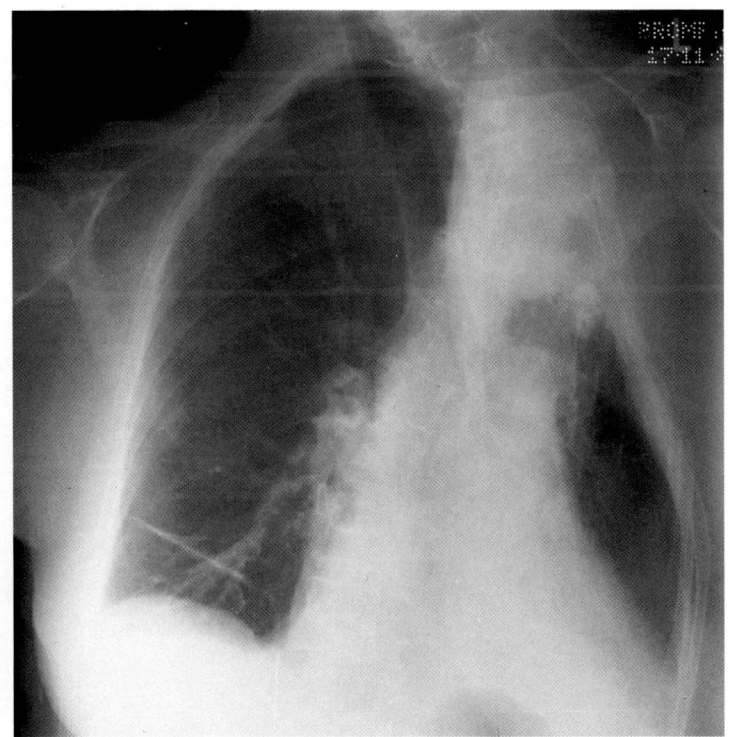

Fig. 6.9 Extensive left thoracoplasty for pulmonary tuberculosis. The heart has increased in size over the past few years indicating cor pulmonale.

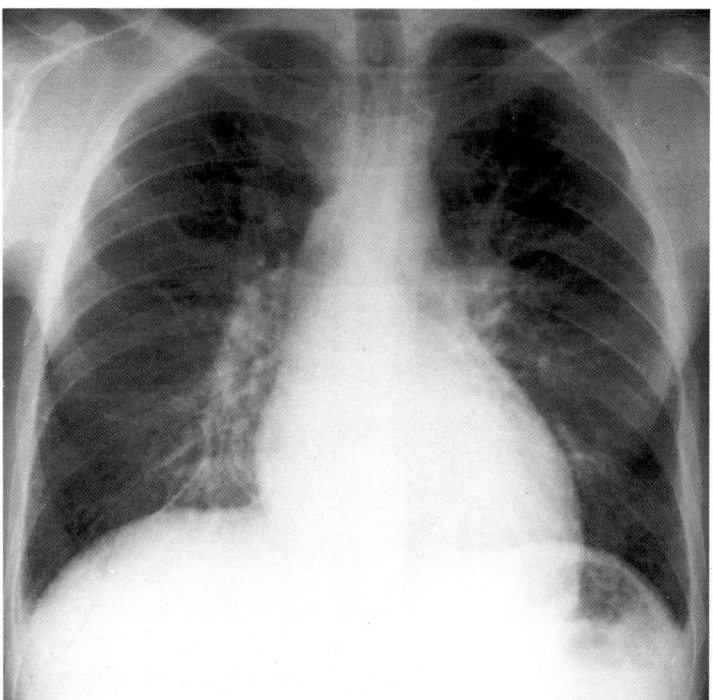

Fig. 6.10 Raised pulmonary venous pressure due to a cardiomyopathy. Upper lobe vessels are dilated as are the proximal pulmonary arteries. Septal lines indicating interstitial oedema are present at both bases. Pulmonary artery pressure was 50/30mmHg and the mean pulmonary wedge pressure 33mmHg.

Arteriovenous fistula

The commonest vascular fistula in the lung is between a pulmonary artery and pulmonary vein (Fig. 6.11). Less common is a fistula between a systemic artery and a pulmonary vein though systemic to pulmonary connections are usually present in cyanotic congenital heart disease.

In pulmonary to pulmonary fistula there is usually a round or oval mass within the lung visible on a chest radiograph. At least one large feeding artery, and one large draining vein are present.

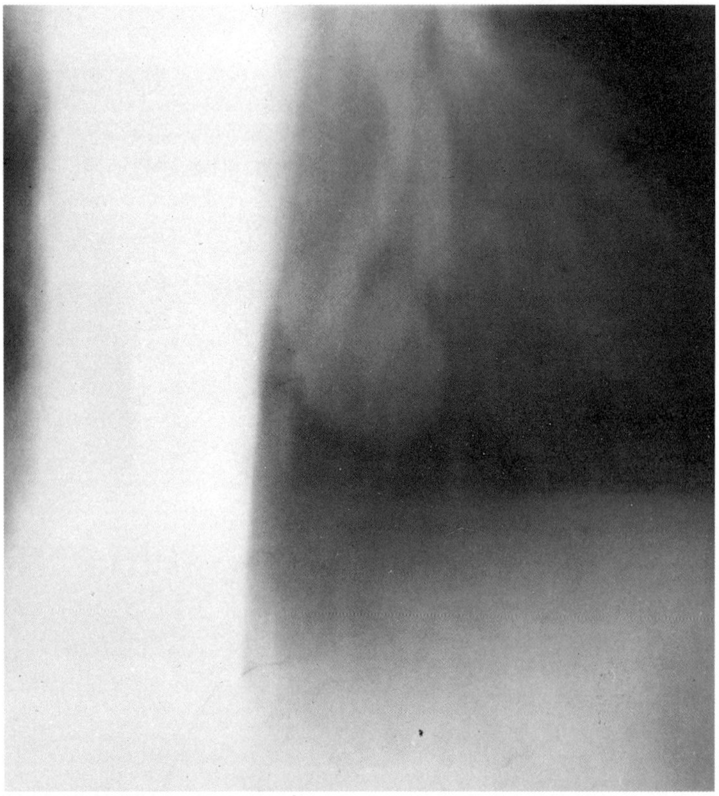

Pulmonary Exudates

Exudation of intravascular fluids and cells from pulmonary capillaries into the alveolar walls and spaces is perhaps the most important acute event compromising gas exchange in the lung.

Acute pulmonary oedema of hydrostatic origin

The chest radiograph shows widespread bilateral shadows (Fig. 6.12) which often predominate in the mid-zones, with relative sparing of the apices and bases; this is the classical 'batwing' distribution but the appearances are very variable and may change rapidly with posture. The presence of Kerley B lines, reflecting fluid accumulation in septa and lymphatics (Fig. 6.13 and see Fig. 6.10), supports the diagnosis, and blood diversion to the upper lobes may also be seen.

It is important to recognize the chronic consequences of pulmonary oedema, because they are often mistaken for separate, coexisting fibrosing pulmonary disease.

Idiopathic pulmonary haemosiderosis

This unusual condition is characterized by episodic or recurrent haemorrhage into the lung. These episodes range from life-threatening massive haemorrhages, especially common in, but not exclusive to, children, to small recurrent 'fleck' haemoptysis associated more commonly with adult idiopathic haemosiderosis. The chest radiograph

Fig. 6.11 Arteriovenous fistula in the left lower lobe (tomogram).

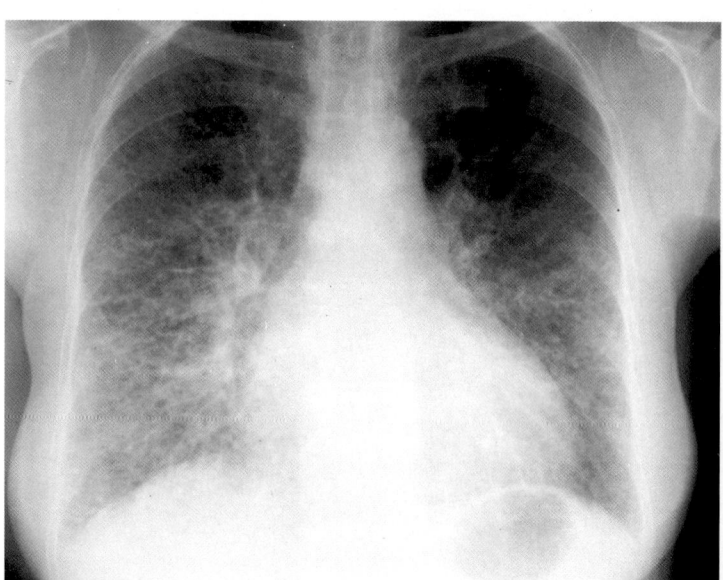

Fig. 6.12 Acute pulmonary oedema. Chest radiograph showing the typical 'batwing' distribution of prominent mid-zone shadowing spreading from the hilar regions, with relative sparing of the apices and bases.

the parenchymal shadows are often predominant in the upper zones, showing elevation of the hilar shadows and horizontal fissures (Fig. 6.19).

A number of less typical radiographic appearances may be seen and must be recognized. For example, a radiograph may show more confluent lesions (Fig. 6.20) without hilar node enlargement. Parenchymal shadows may be more localized and nodular, and are particularly difficult to diagnose if they occur in the absence of hilar node enlargement (Fig. 6.21) or if they show cavitation (Fig. 6.22).

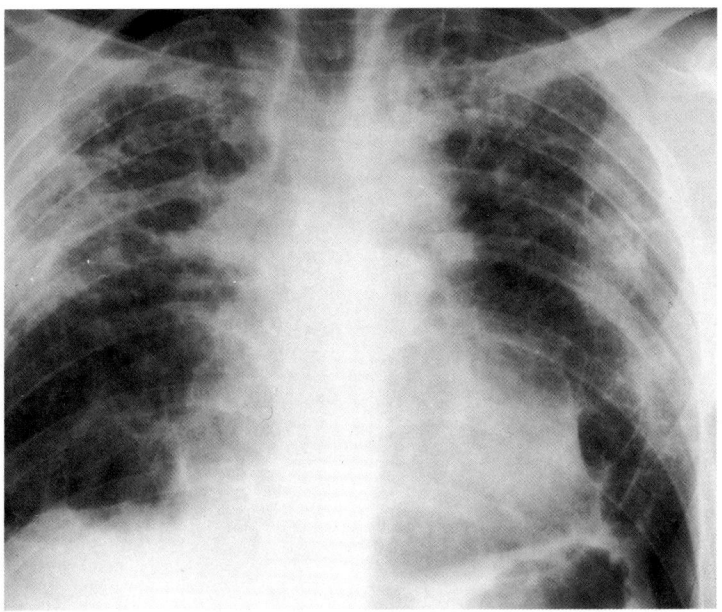

Fig. 6.19 Massive shadowing can be seen in both lungs, with a tendency to predominate in the upper zones. There is elevation of both hilar shadows and evidence of linear shadowing reflecting parenchymal distortion.

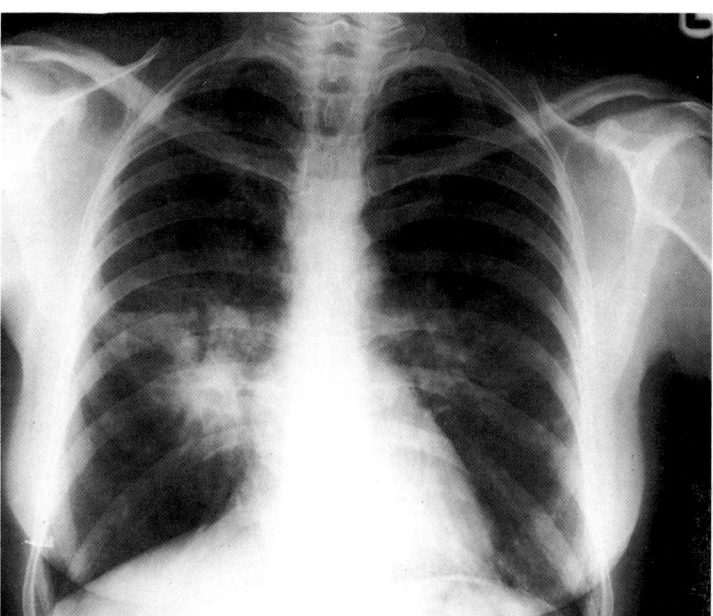

Fig. 6.20 The chest radiograph shows coarse confluent lesions. In such cases the assessment of hilar node enlargement is difficult.

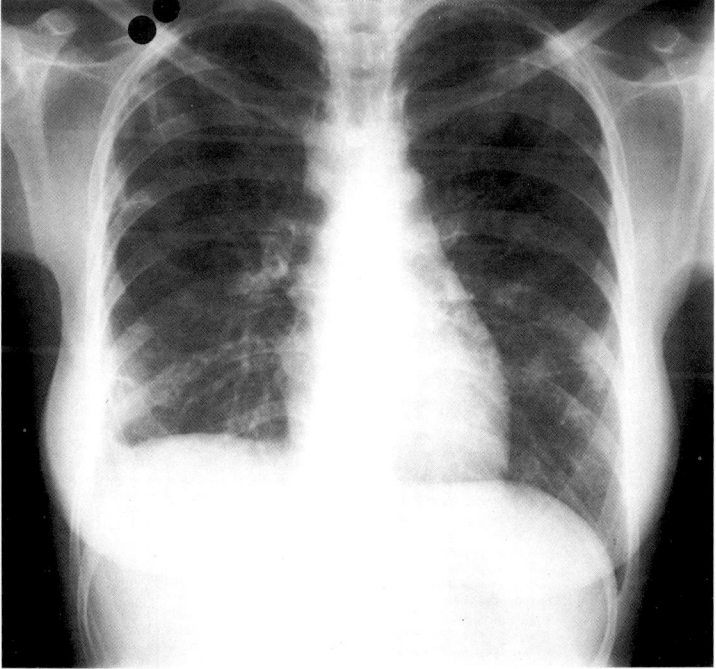

Fig. 6.21 The chest radiograph shows peripheral lesions with evidence of pleural involvement. Some lesions are cavitated. Open lung biopsy showed sarcoid granulomas and central necrosis but no caseation. The Kveim–Silzbach test was strongly positive, as was the gallium-67 scan.

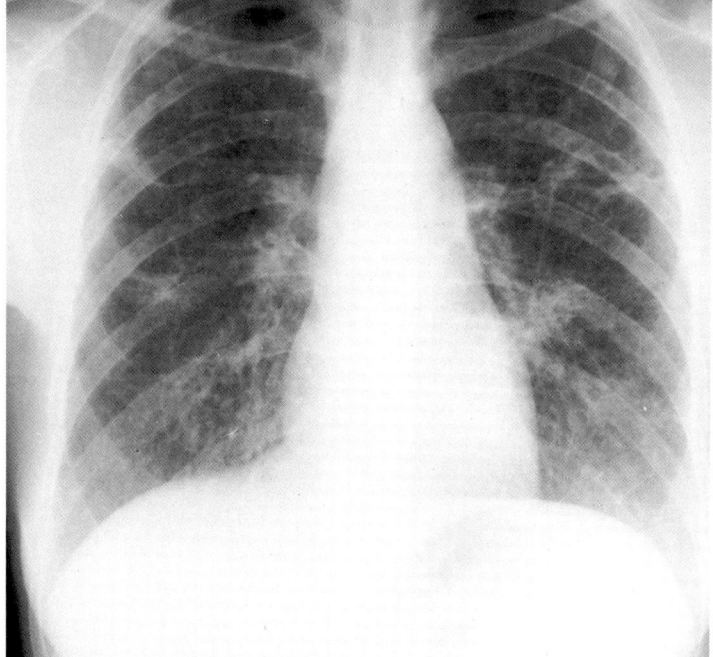

Fig. 6.22 Chest radiograph of proven sarcoidosis with linear shadows in both mid-zones and some evidence of cavitation, seen most easily in the third left interspace. The presence of cavities was confirmed by tomography.

Even more uncommon are pleural effusions and very occasionally pleural biopsy will demonstrate the presence of sarcoid granulomas. Occasionally diagnosis is difficult because lung function tests show an irreversible obstructive defect which may be caused by bronchial stenoses.

Rarely, lesions characteristic of sarcoidosis are seen on radiographs of the hands (Fig. 6.23); such lesions may occur with or without pulmonary involvement.

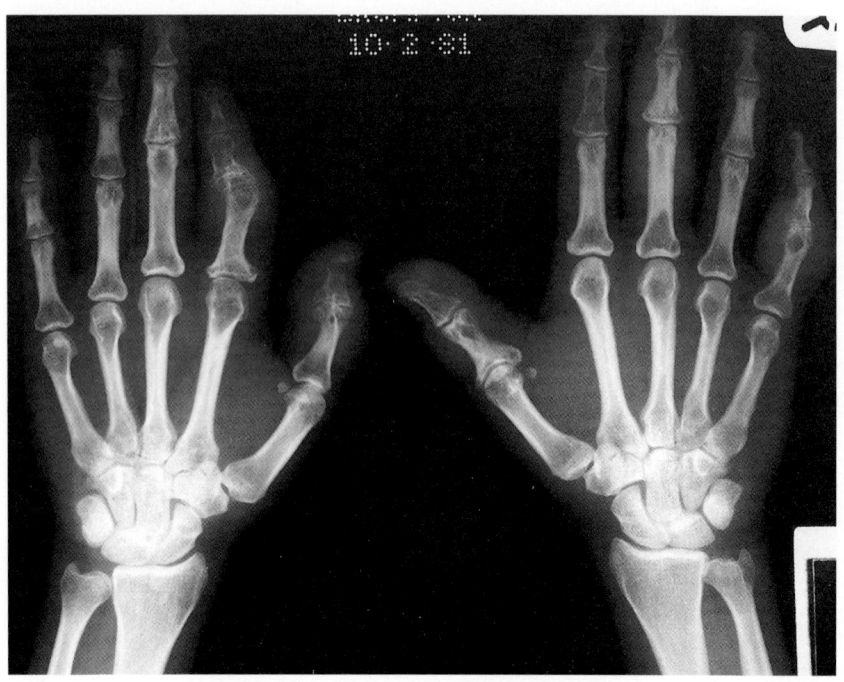

Fig. 6.23 Hand lesions in sarcoidosis. The radiograph shows multiple cystic appearances with bony distortion in the metacarpals and phalanges. The extent of soft tissue involvement can also be seen.

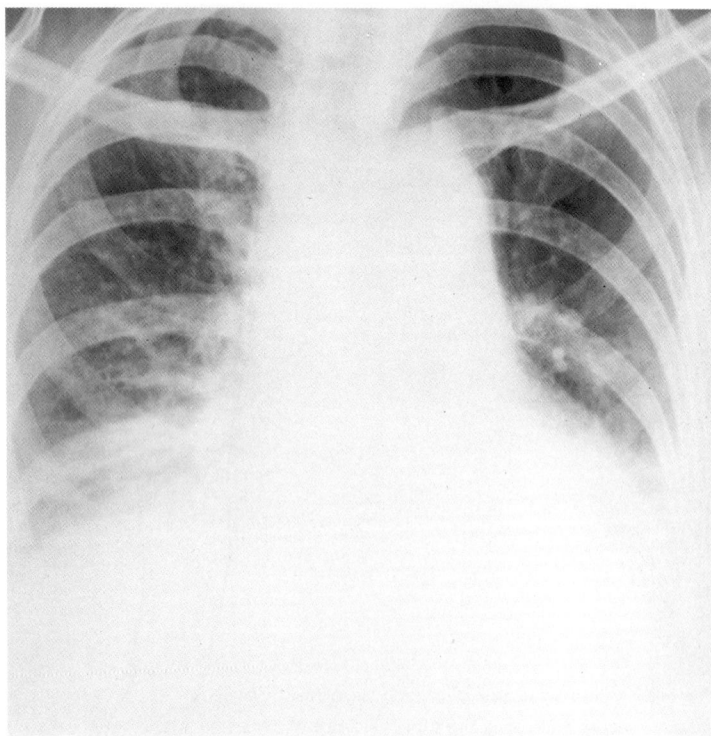

Fig. 6.24 Cryptogenic fibrosing alveolitis. This chest radiograph shows bilateral and predominantly basal irregular shadows.

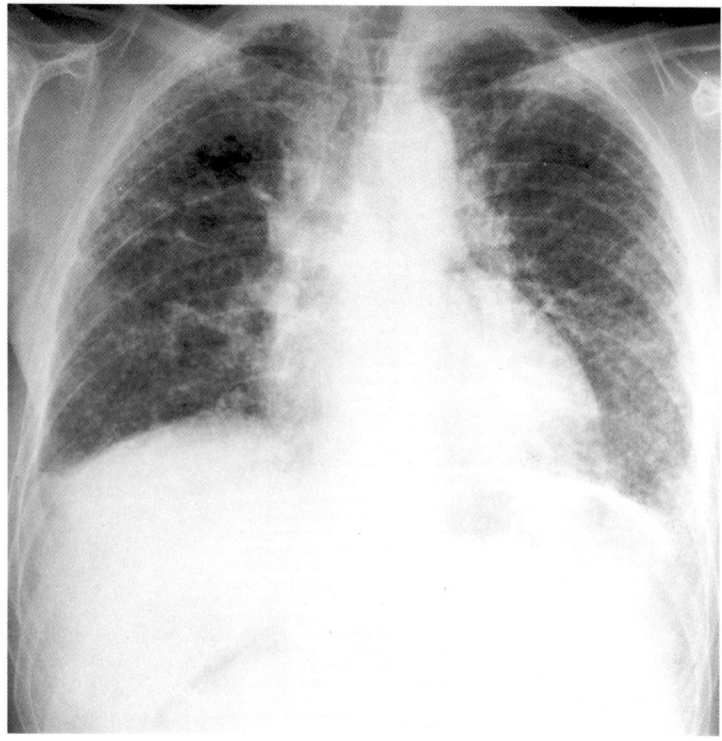

Fig. 6.25 Cryptogenic fibrosing alveolitis. There are widespread irregular shadows throughout all zones of both lungs.

Cryptogenic Fibrosing Alveolitis

Cryptogenic fibrosing alveolitis (CFA) may be defined in descriptive terms as a condition of unknown cause, characterized by an inflammatory exudate of the alveolar wall with a tendency to fibrosis.

The chest radiograph shows bilateral shadows, predominantly basal in distribution (Fig. 6.24), but occasionally affecting all zones (Fig. 6.25). The radiographic appearance is variable: sometimes the shadows are small and irregular, sometimes more confluent (Fig. 6.26). One lung may be more extensively involved than the other (Fig. 6.27). In advanced cases small ring shadows (honeycombing) are visible, usually in the area of greatest radiographic abnormality (Fig. 6.28). The radiographic lung volumes are typically diminished unless there is associated emphysema.

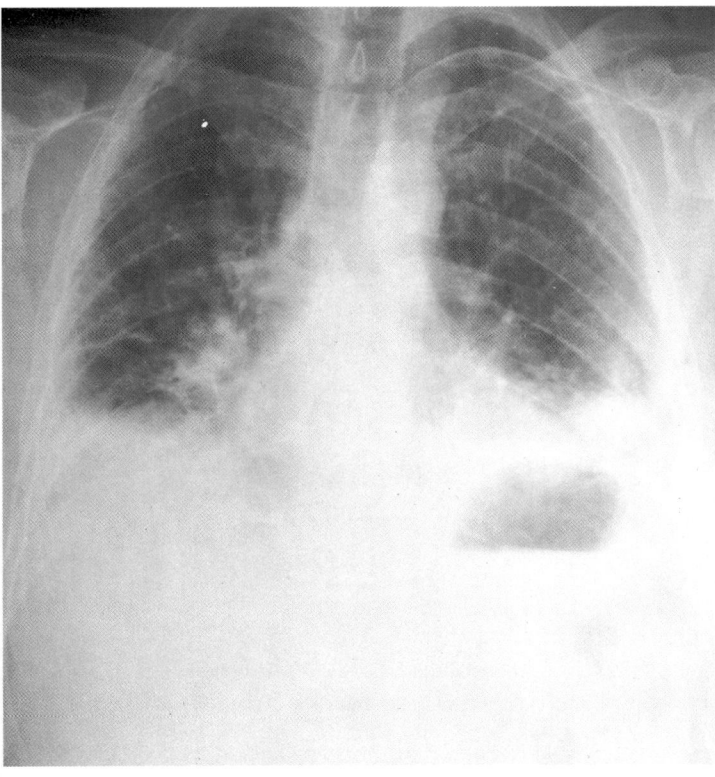

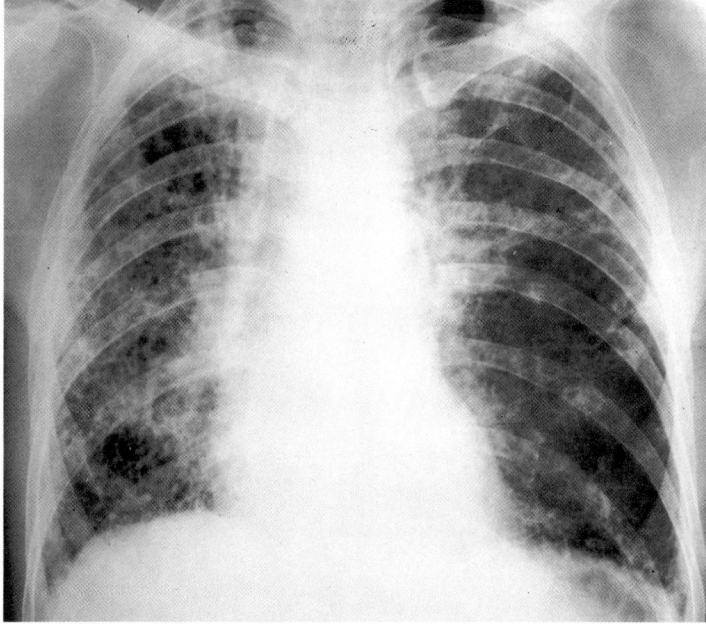

Fig. 6.26 Cryptogenic fibrosing alveolitis. There are basal confluent shadows; the pleural reaction in the right lung resulted from lung biopsy. Pleural involvement is unusual in fibrosing alveolitis.

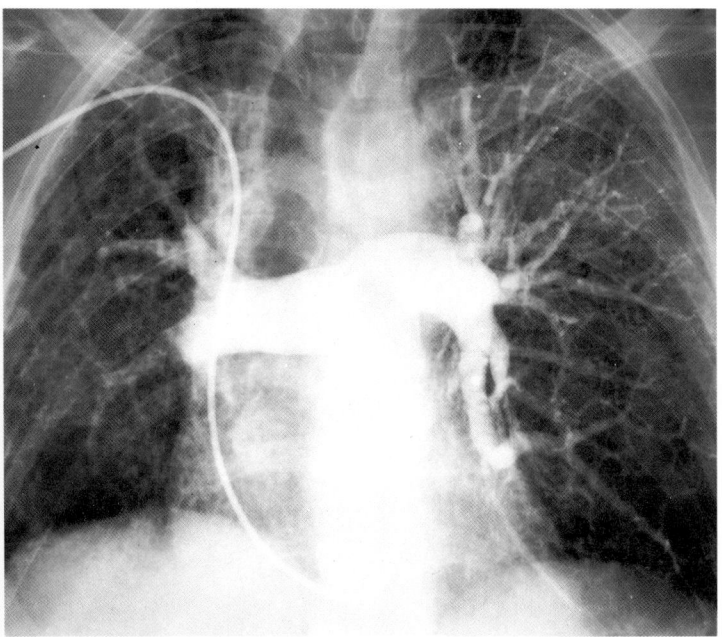

Fig. 6.27 Cryptogenic fibrosing alveolitis. The radiograph showed unequal involvement of the right and left lungs. The pulmonary angiogram shows upper lobe diversion and attenuation of the pulmonary vessels in the lower lobe.

Fig. 6.28 Cryptogenic fibrosing alveolitis. This radiograph shows widespread shadowing and clearly visible honeycombing.

Fibrosing alveolitis, whether cryptogenic or associated with rheumatoid arthritis (see Fig. 6.41) or systemic sclerosis, has been shown to have a characteristic CT appearance. There is a crescentic subpleural distribution in the lower lobes (Fig. 6.29) and changes may be demons-trable by CT when the plain radiograph is normal (Fig. 6.30). As the fibrosis progresses a widespread coarse reticular pattern supervenes resulting in a non-specific appearance of end-stage pulmonary fibrosis (Fig. 6.31).

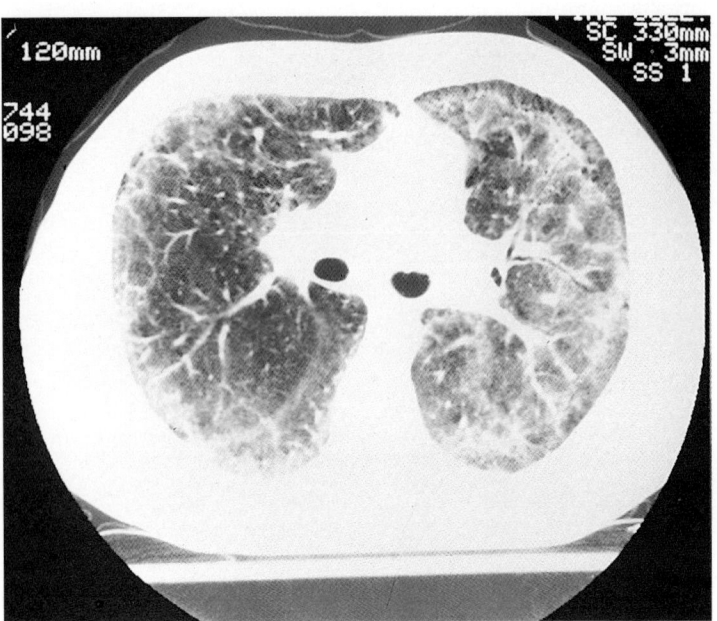

Fig. 6.29 High resolution CT (3mm slice) in cryptogenic fibrosing alveolitis showing predominant subpleural disease, though most of the lung is affected by fibrosis.

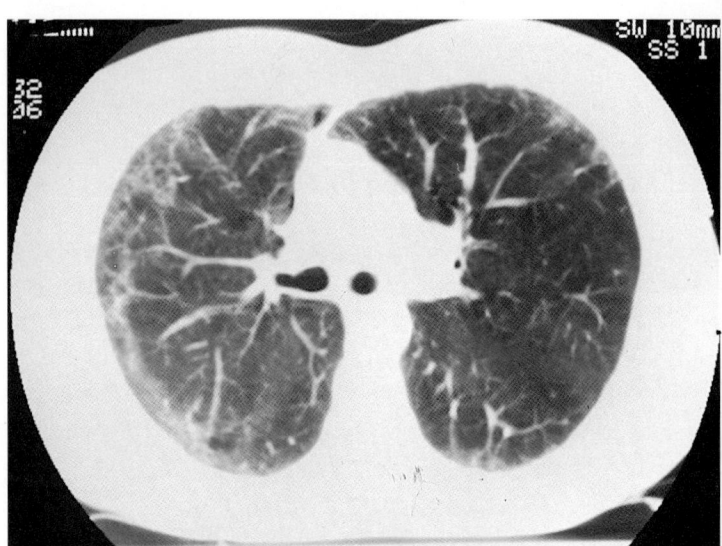

Fig. 6.30 CT in cryptogenic fibrosing alveolitis showing the characteristic subpleural area of the disease. The plain chest radiograph in this patient was normal.

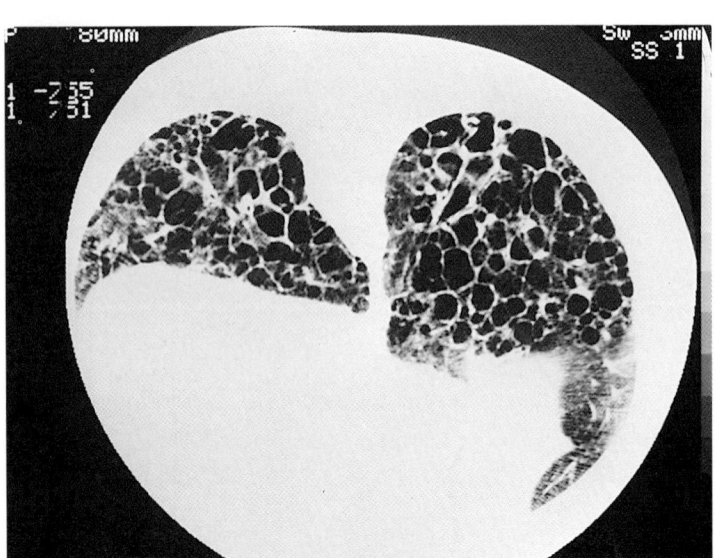

Fig. 6.31 High resolution CT (3mm slice) of late stage pulmonary fibrosis with an extensive honeycomb pattern.

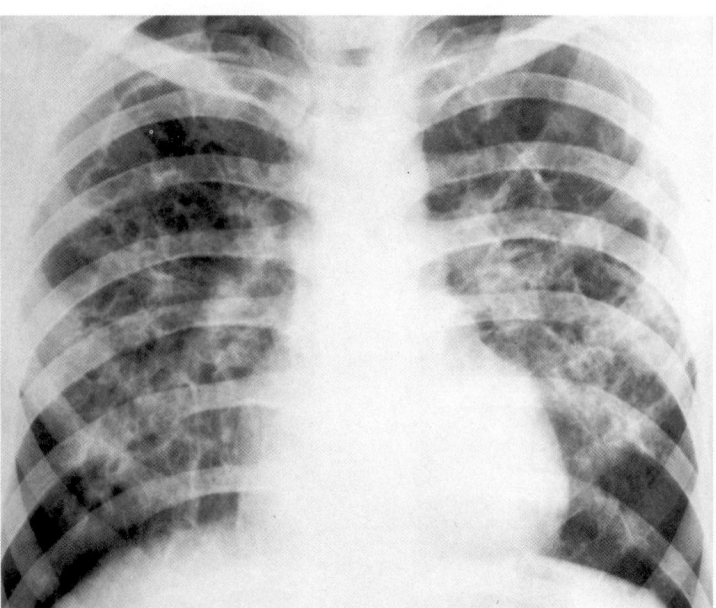

Fig. 6.32 Eosinophilic granuloma. Chest radiograph showing extensive cystic changes in the upper zones. The lung bases are often, though not invariably, spared.

Eosinophilic Granuloma

Eosinophilic granuloma affects particularly the lungs and bones, the patient presenting with dyspnoea and widespread shadows on the chest radiograph (Figs 6.32 and 6.33). The lesions often affect the upper and middle zones, with relative sparing of the costophrenic angles. In their acute stages the lesions may be confluent or irregular in shape, but in the later stages they form cystic spaces (honeycomb lung) and on occasion much larger cysts may form, particularly in the upper zones. A characteristic feature of eosinophilic granuloma is the development of pneumothoraces which may cause life-threatening breathlessness and which may be particularly difficult to treat.

Lymphangioleiomyomatosis

In this very rare disorder there is an overgrowth of smooth muscle affecting lymphatic channels, small vessels, pulmonary veins and small airways. The patients, usually premenopausal women, present with breathlessness and very widespread radiographic shadows (Fig. 6.34). Radiographs may show cystic areas, perhaps due to obstruction of airways. The macroscopic appearance of the lung is that of honeycombing. Chylous pleural effusions may develop due to obstruction of the lymphatic channels.

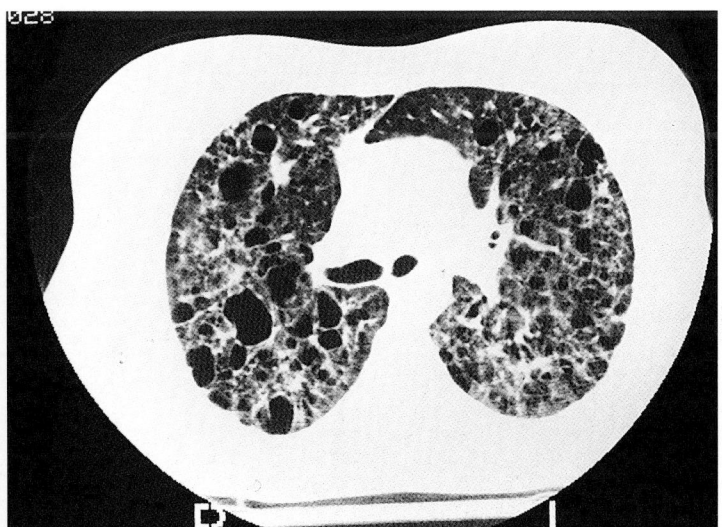

Fig. 6.33 High resolution CT (3mm slice) in eosinophilic granuloma. Note the large cystic spaces with thickening of their walls and associated pulmonary fibrosis. In contrast emphysematous bullae have very thin walls.

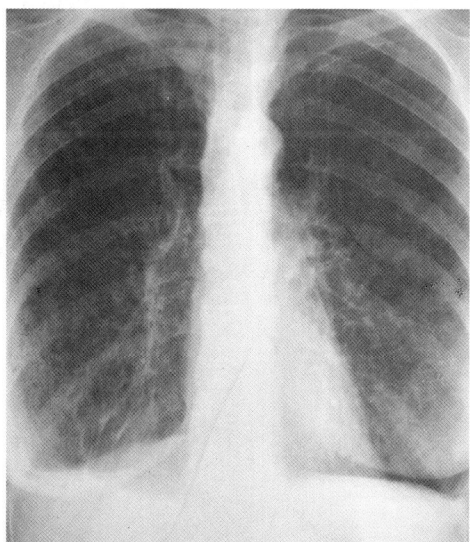

Fig. 6.34 Lymphangioleiomyomatosis. Chest radiographs showing 'honeycomb' lung with large cysts at the apices. There is hyperinflation reflecting the often severe airflow limitation.

Microlithiasis

Alveolar microlithiasis is a very rare condition that usually presents as an incidental radiographic finding in an asymptomatic individual (Fig. 6.35). The histological appearance shows whorls of amorphous calcification filling the airspaces, with remarkably little effect on the lung architecture which remains largely normal. For this reason symptoms are often slight compared to the radiographic abnormality.

Pulmonary Manifestations of Systemic Disorders

Systemic lupus erythematosus

Intrathoracic organs may be affected in a number of ways. Pleurisy is common, with or without effusion on one or both sides. Dyspnoea is the commonest symptom: it may be due to pleural involvement, diaphragmatic weakness (often suggested by elevation of the diaphragm), and various

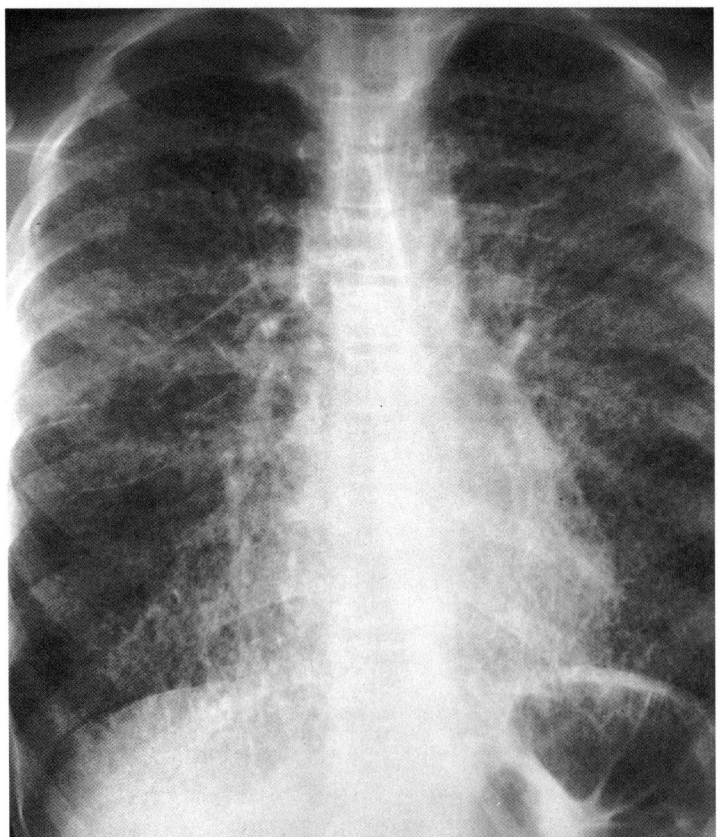

Fig. 6.35 Microlithiasis. Chest radiograph showing dense pinhead lesions widely distributed throughout the lungs.

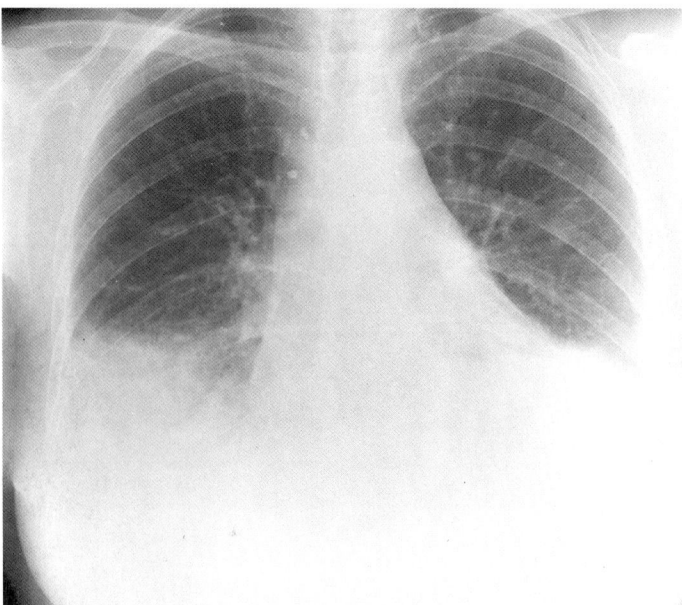

Fig. 6.36 Systemic lupus erythematosus. Chest radiograph showing bilateral pleural effusion.

intrapulmonary lesions. Bilateral pleural effusion (Fig. 6.36) not only causes dyspnoea, but can obscure the lung bases so that it is not possible to identify or exclude intrapulmonary involvement from the chest radiograph alone.

Bilateral lower-zone linear shadows, often associated with elevation of the diaphragm, are common. The linear shadows sometimes represent earlier infarction, associated perhaps with pulmonary vasculitis, but they much more often reflect atelectasis.

Elevation of the diaphragm alone can be a rather characteristic abnormality (Fig. 6.37) and computerized tomography can be used to confirm the absence of intrapulmonary disease (Fig. 6.38). Pulmonary infiltrates which may proceed to fibrosing alveolitis are well described, and in these cases the chest radiograph is indistinguishable from 'lone' cryptogenic fibrosing alveolitis. Rarely, intrapulmonary haemorrhage is a presenting feature, the chest radiograph showing confluent lesions so massive that they simulate pulmonary oedema. Haemoptysis of variable size may give a clinical clue to the true nature of the pathology (Fig. 6.39).

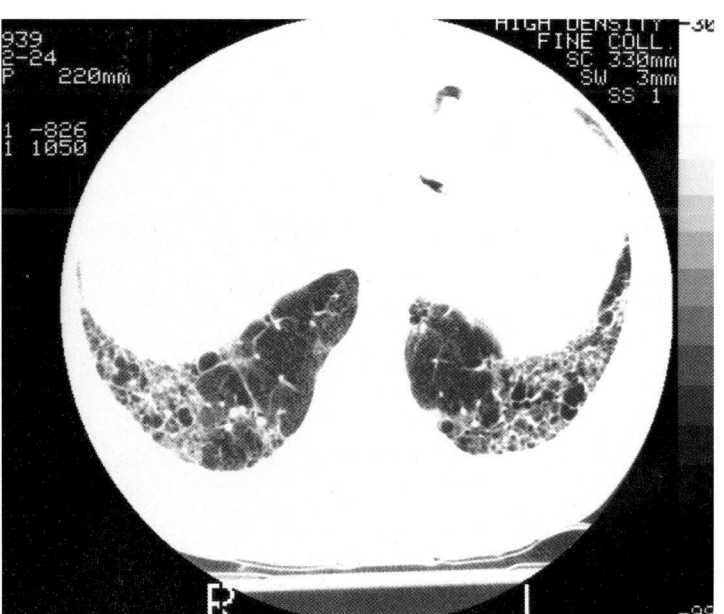

Fig. 6.37 Systemic lupus erythematosus. Chest radiograph of a patient who presented with dyspnoea, showing the characteristic feature of elevation of the diaphragm but no intrapulmonary lesion. A diaphragmatic muscle study illustrated bilateral impaired function.

Fig. 6.38 Systemic lupus erythematosus. The chest radiograph showed bilateral but scanty widespread small irregular shadows, predominantly in the middle and lower zones. Histology verified the presence of fibrosing alveolitis. The CT scan shows the true extent of the disease.

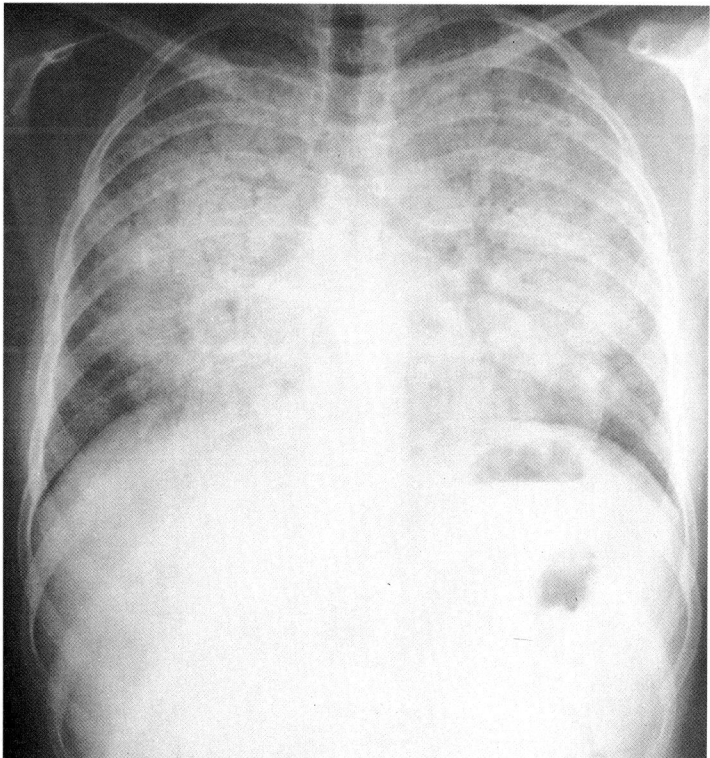

Fig. 6.39 Systemic lupus erythematosus. Chest radiograph of a patient who presented with life-threatening dyspnoea, respiratory failure and haemoptysis. The shadows represent the haemorrhage.

Rheumatoid arthritis

Intrathoracic involvement in rheumatoid arthritis (RA) is variable in type and can include, in order of frequency, fibrosing alveolitis, pleural effusion, necrobiotic nodules and obliterative bronchiolitis.

Where fibrosing alveolitis complicates rheumatoid arthritis (Figs 6.40 and 6.41), it tends to develop within a few years of onset of the disease, and only rarely involves patients with very longstanding RA. The clinical, radiographic and histological features of fibrosing alveolitis associated with RA are usually indistinguishable from 'lone' cryptogenic fibrosing alveolitis (CFA).

Pleural effusion may be small and transient or large and recurrent, and may be unilateral or bilateral (Fig. 6.42).

Necrobiotic nodules are a rare manifestation of RA. They may occur as solitary nodules (see Fig. 2.11) and are difficult to distinguish from bronchial carcinoma, hence they are often resected; however, with the more frequent use of percutaneous biopsies for solitary lesions, their true nature may be identified. They may be multiple (Fig. 6.43)

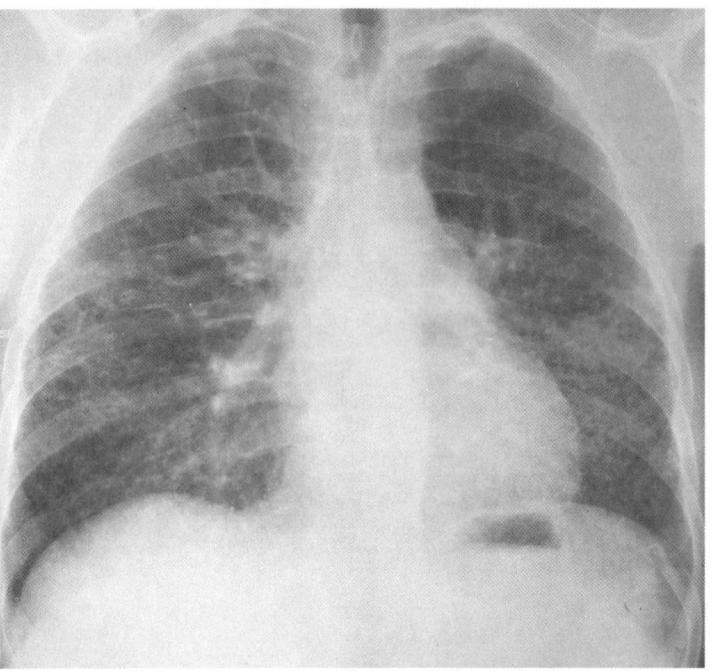

Fig. 6.40 Rheumatoid arthritis. Chest radiograph of a 33-year-old man with RA of three years' duration, showing widespread shadowing, the histology of which confirmed typical fibrosing alveolitis.

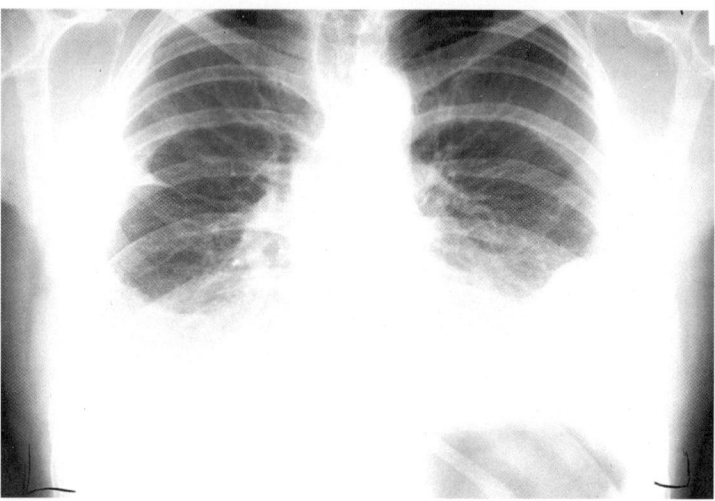

Fig. 6.42 Rheumatoid arthritis. Chest radiograph showing extensive bilateral pleural effusions. These persisted in spite of treatment with corticosteroids.

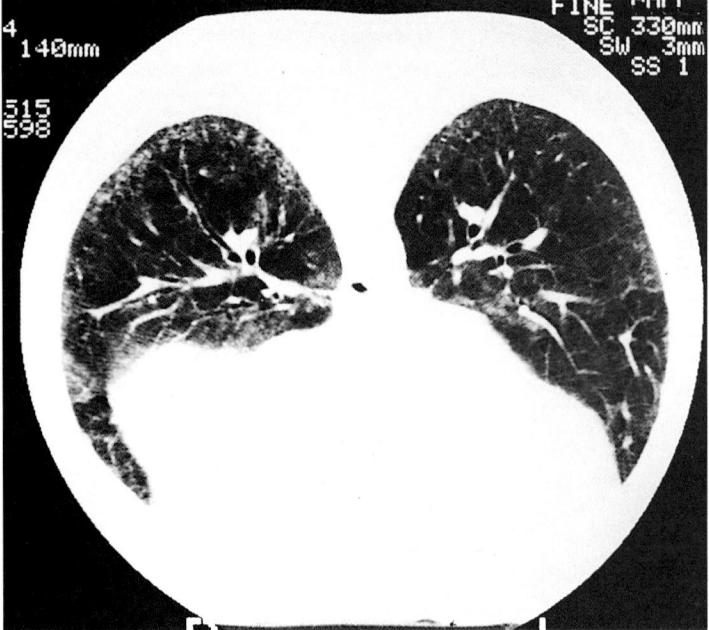

Fig. 6.41 High resolution CT (3mm slice) in rheumatoid disease. The appearance of the subpleural opacification is identical with that seen in other conditions in which there is a fibrosing alveolitis, such as cryptogenic fibrosing alveolitis and systemic sclerosis.

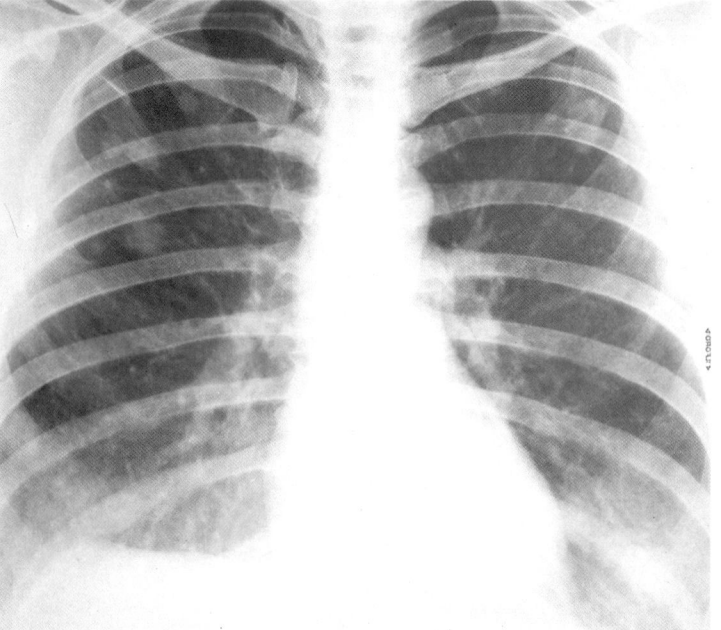

Fig. 6.43 Rheumatoid arthritis. Chest radiograph showing multiple bilateral upper zone nodules.

and may thus be mistaken for metastases. The nodules may recur, first in one lung and then in the other, and may cavitate. The histological structure is similar to that of a rheumatoid nodule occurring at any other site. The main significance of an intrapulmonary nodule is in the differ-ential diagnosis, and this is especially difficult in those very rare cases where a rheumatoid nodule precedes the development of RA.

Systemic sclerosis

When the lungs are affected this usually represents a fibrosing alveolitis. While it has often been said that this condition is particularly fibrotic in type, with little inflam-matory cell infiltrate, it has to be recognized that cases are seen covering the whole spectrum from more cellular to more fibrotic histology. The chest radiograph may show very scanty basal lesions that remain stable for long periods (Fig. 6.44), or a rather aggressive pattern of fibrosis. More confluent shadows on the chest radiograph may be caused by spillover of the oesophageal contents as a consequence of dyskinetic changes in the oesophagus.

Wegener's granulomatosis

This multisystem disorder is characterized by necrotizing granulomas, particularly affecting the cartilage and soft tissues of the nose, lungs, skin, kidneys and other organs.

The lungs are often involved, with massive confluent shadows (see Fig. 2.12) which may excavate giving rise to ragged-wall cavitatory lesions (Fig. 6.45). The macroscopic appearance of the lungs shows large areas of haemorrhagic necrotic tissue and histology reveals extensive areas of necrosis.

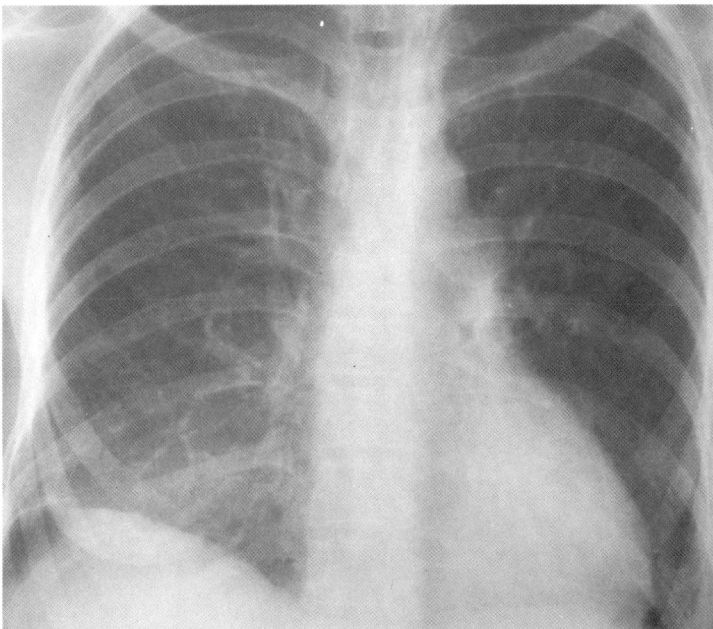

Fig. 6.44 Systemic sclerosis. Chest radiograph showing minimal shadowing in the lower lobe.

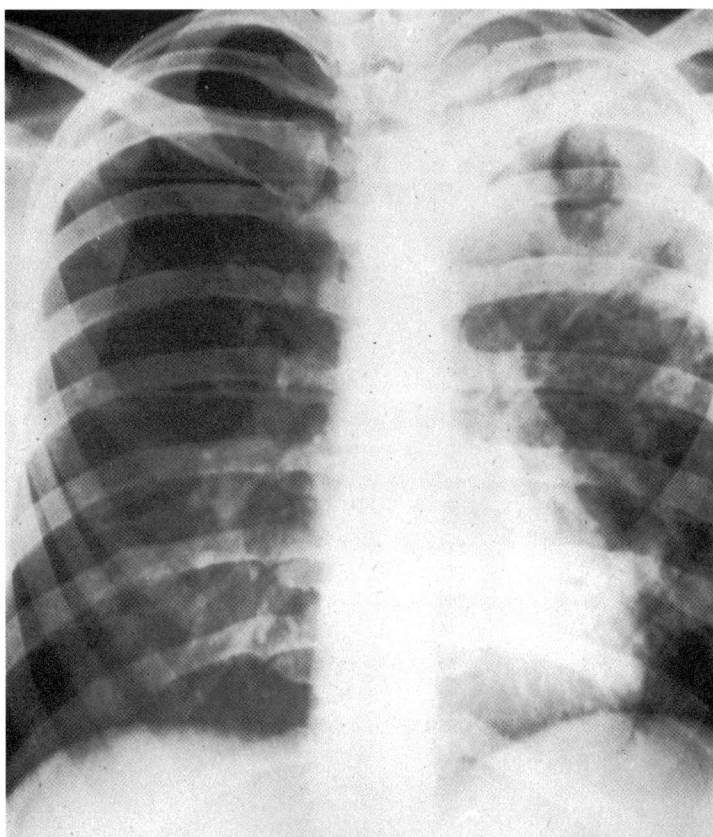

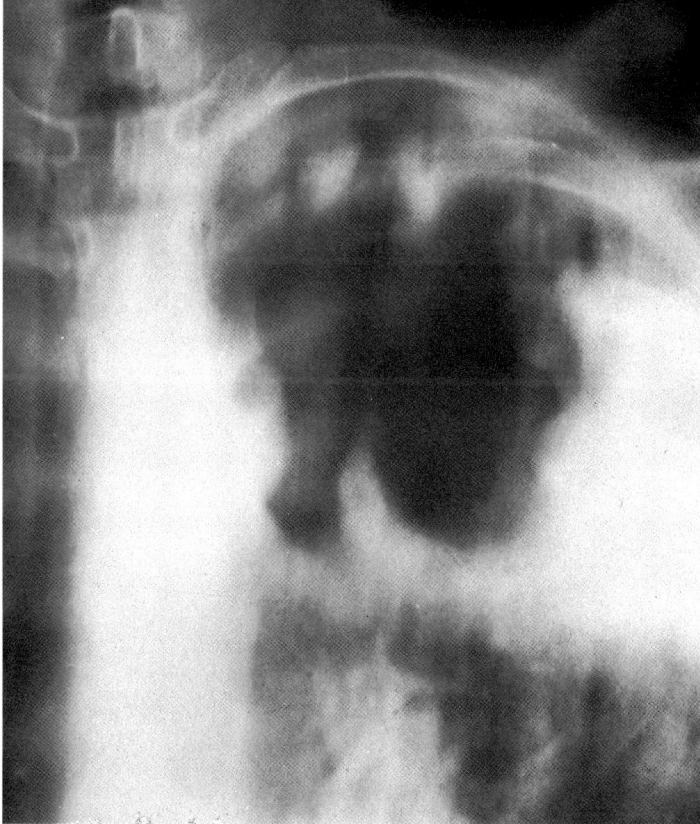

Fig. 6.45 Wegener's granulomatosis. The chest radiograph shows a large lesion in the left apex, with extensive necrotic cavitation. The tomogram demonstrates the extent of the ragged left upper zone cavity.

Limited Wegener's granulomatosis is a condition presenting with pulmonary lesions only. These may occur as confluent shadows but are frequently multiple, and often massive, cavities (Fig. 6.46).

Lymphomatoid granulomatosis

This is a very rare condition, the chest radiograph often showing extensive confluent shadows similar to Wegener's granulomatosis.

Behçet's syndrome

When the lungs are affected this is mainly due to the presence of pulmonary infarcts (Fig. 6.47); these may be recurrent and, indeed, fatal. The symptoms are those of pulmonary infarction and patients commonly present with pleuritic pain and haemoptysis.

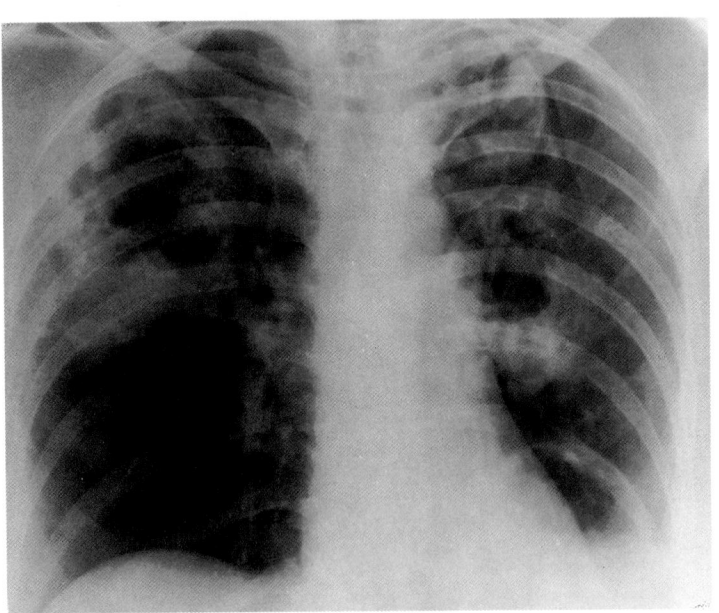

Fig. 6.46 Wegener's granulomatosis. Chest radiograph of a patient presenting with bilateral multiple cavities and no evidence of systemic disease. The lesions cleared fairly quickly over one month on treatment with prednisolone and cyclophosphamide. Further clearing occurred slowly over the next two years.

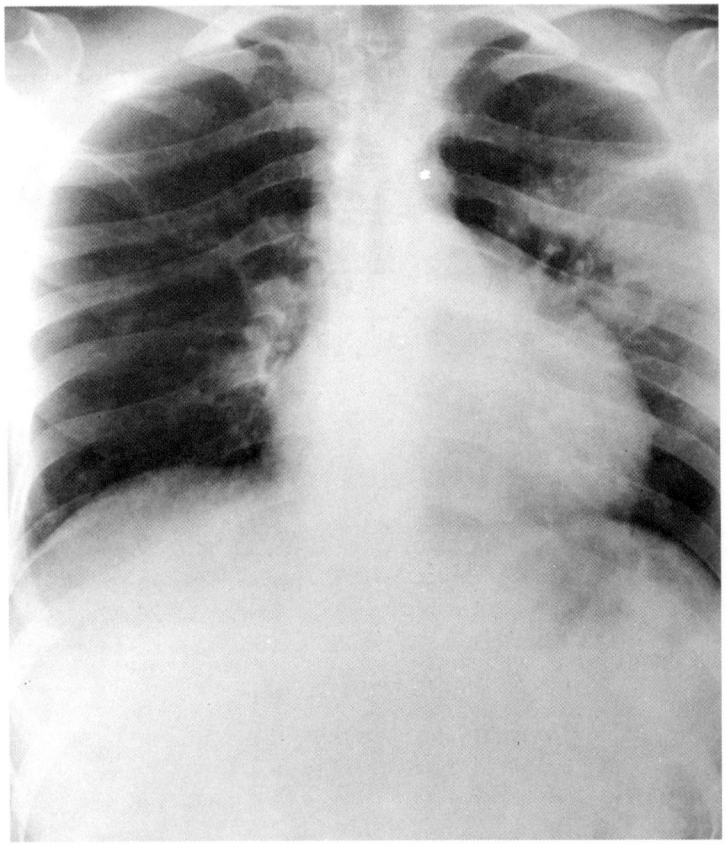

Fig. 6.47 Behçet's syndrome. The confluent shadow in the left lung represents an extensive infarct; these are often due to vasculitic lesions in the pulmonary vessels.

7

Occupational Lung Disease, and Diseases of the Pleura, Diaphragm and Chest Wall

Occupational Lung Disease

Respiratory irritants

A wide variety of materials which an individual may have contact with at work are toxic to respiratory epithelial cells. The site of damage is primarily dependent upon the solubility of the agent in the predominantly water-based lining of the respiratory tract. Water-soluble gases such as sulphur dioxide and ammonia are dissolved in the moist mucosal surfaces of the eyes, upper respiratory tract and proximal bronchi where they cause immediate toxic damage. Gases which are insoluble in water such as phosgene and fumes such as cadmium oxide are not dissolved in the upper respiratory tract and can therefore penetrate into the alveoli where they cause pulmonary oedema (Fig. 7.1).

Fibrogenic dusts

Dusts whose aerodynamic diameter is sufficiently small (roughly less than 5μm diameter for a spherical particle and 3μm for a fibre) can penetrate into the alveoli, where they are taken up into alveolar macrophages. Inhaled in small amounts the macrophage can clear them from the alveoli, but if the clearance capacity is overcome, macrophages with their retained particles accumulate in alveoli in the respiratory bronchioles. If the dust is not fibrogenic this accumulation will not impair lung function or shorten life, but may, for dusts such as tin oxide and iron oxide which absorb X-rays, cause nodules on the chest radiograph (Fig. 7.2).

Fibrogenic dusts such as coal, silica and asbestos when retained in sufficient amounts cause pulmonary fibrosis, impair lung function and shorten life. Silica causes nodular fibrosis in the lungs (silicosis) (Fig. 7.3), whereas asbestos

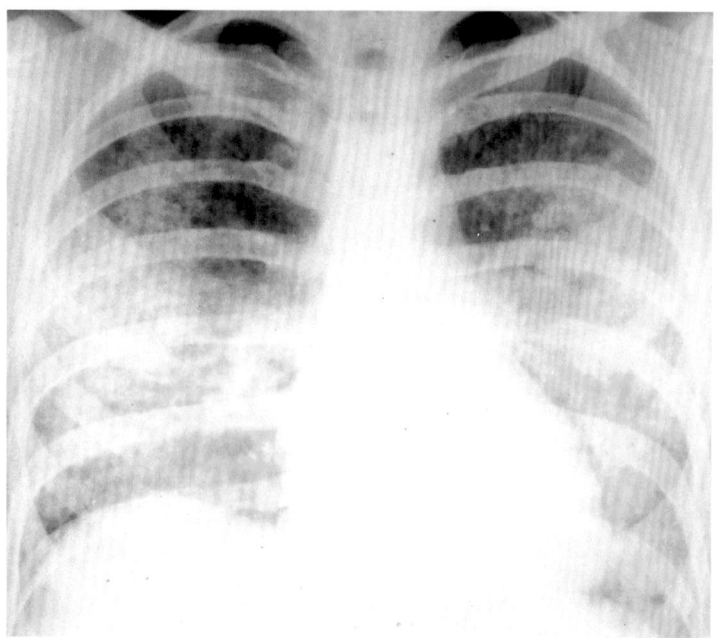

Fig. 7.1 Pulmonary oedema caused by inhaled chlorine.

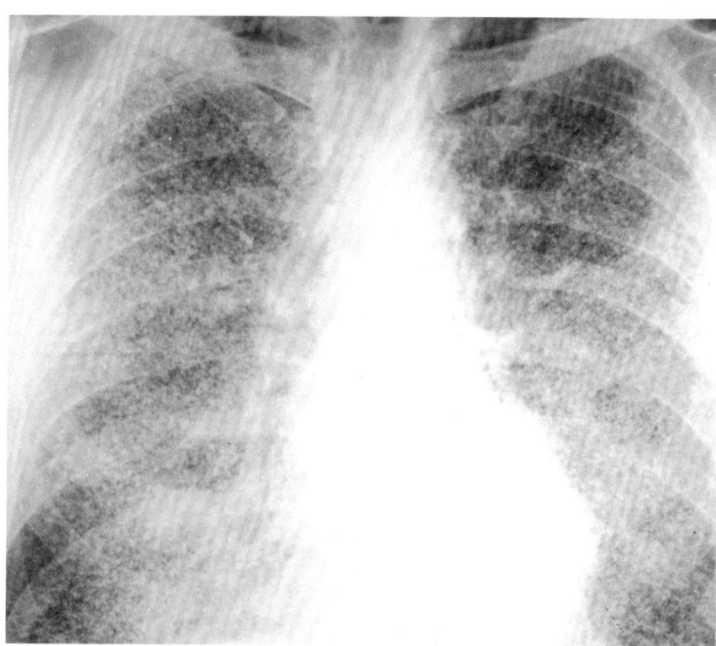

Fig. 7.2 Stannosis in a tin smelter. Widespread nodules due to retained tin oxide are present.

causes diffuse interstitial fibrosis of the lungs (asbestosis) (Figs 7.4 and 7.5). Retained coal dust causes little adverse effect on the lungs unless it provokes progressive massive fibrosis (see Fig. 2.7) in which large masses of scar tissue form in the lungs. These can progress in the absence of any further exposure to coal dust. Silicotic nodules may also coalesce to form areas of progressive massive fibrosis.

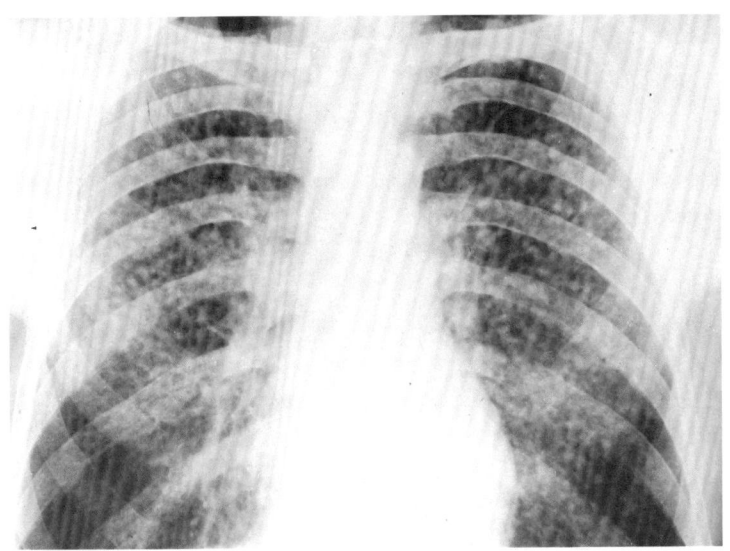

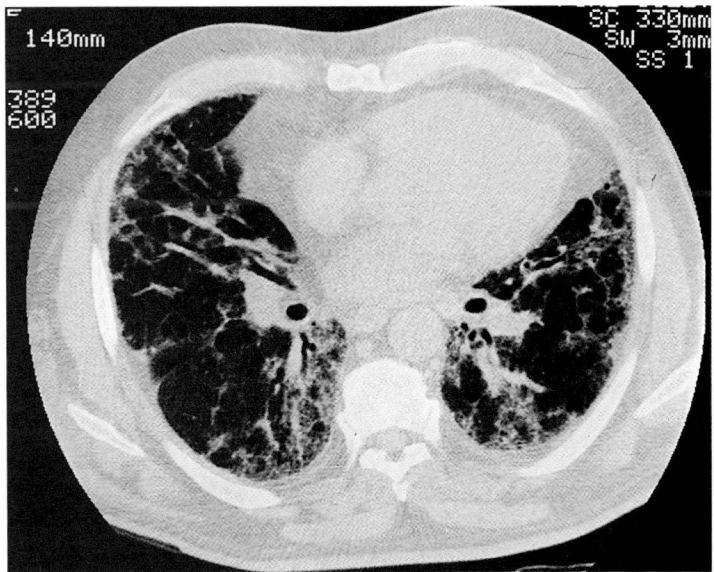

Fig. 7.3 Silicosis. Widespread nodules caused by nodular fibrosis in the lungs.

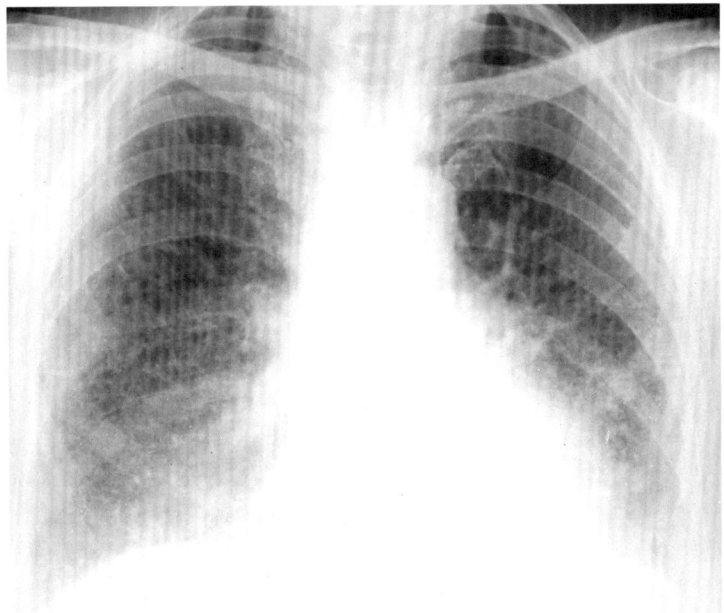

Fig. 7.4 Asbestosis. Predominantly basal irregular shadows with associated calcification of diaphragms caused by inhaled asbestos.

Fig. 7.5 High resolution CT (3mm sections) in asbestosis. There is subpleural predominance as in cryptogenic fibrosing alveolitis, but there is pleural involvement causing triangular opacities peripherally with attachment to the pleura. The pleura is thickened, particularly posterolaterally.

Progressive massive fibrosis caused by coal dust and silica can cause considerable impairment of lung function and respiratory disablement and shortens life. In addition patients with silicosis have an increased risk of developing pulmonary tuberculosis. Patients with asbestosis have a greatly increased risk of developing lung cancer.

Carcinogens: lung cancer and mesothelioma

Numerically the most important occupational cause of lung cancer is asbestos. All the major types of asbestos used commercially — chrysotile (white), crocidolite (blue) and amosite (brown) — seem able to cause lung cancer.

Mesothelioma of the pleura (see Figs 2.4 and 7.17) and

peritoneum, however, seem particularly associated with the long straight fibres (amphiboles) — crocidolite, amosite and tremolite — and less, if at all, with the airway serpentine chrysotile.

Allergens and haptens

Inhalation of protein laden dusts or aerosols or dusts or fumes containing complex biological materials or synthetic chemicals which can bind to body proteins to act as haptens, can cause an allergic response in the airways — asthma, or alveoli — extrinsic allergic alveolitis (extrinsic allergic alveolitis is discussed in more detail in Chapter 5).

The major concern with both occupational asthma and

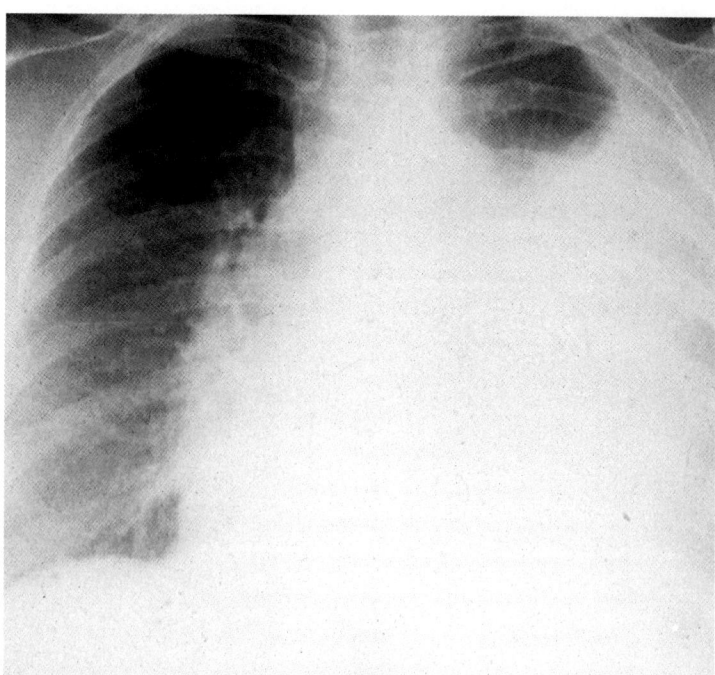

Fig. 7.7 A very large left sided pleural effusion.

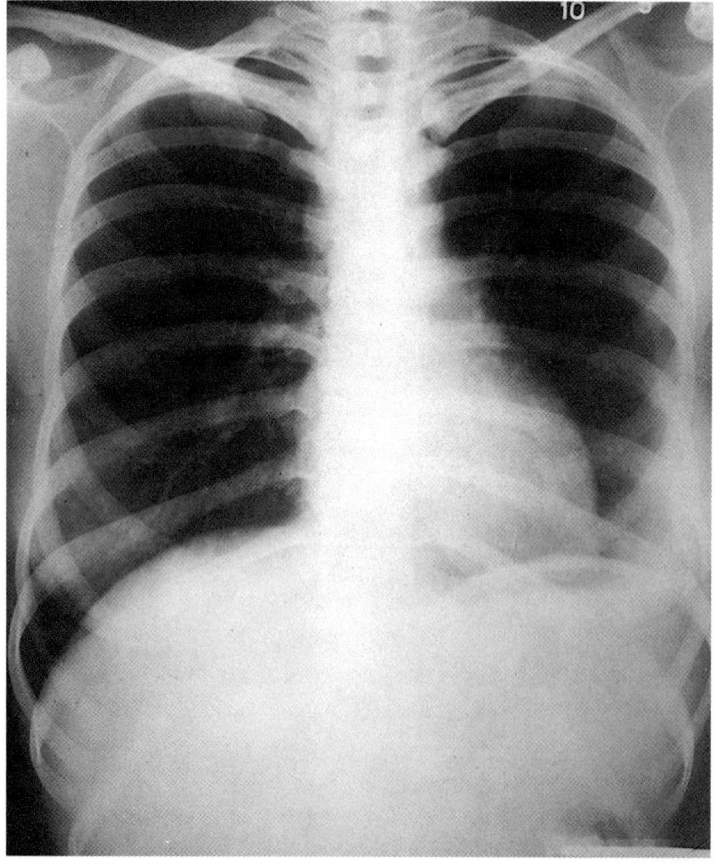

Fig. 7.6 Pleural effusion. There is a left side pleural effusion following the contour of the greater fissure and filling in the left costophrenic angle.

allergic alveolitis is the development of chronic damage to the lungs. Many cases of asthma induced by an occupational cause become chronic persisting after avoidance of exposure to their initiating cause. Similarly patients with allergic alveolitis may develop pulmonary fibrosis.

Abnormalities of the Pleura

Pleural effusions

Radiological appearances vary with the size of the effusion. A small effusion may only obliterate the costophrenic angle (Fig. 7.6) but effusions of any size will produce a homogeneous density in the lower hemithorax, with a concave upper margin. A large effusion may fill the whole hemithorax (Fig. 7.7) and cause the mediastinum to shift towards the opposite side. Effusions may be bilateral and the radiograph may reveal underlying disease. In circumstances where it is difficult to be certain if a pleural effusion is present, a lateral decubitus film may be helpful (Fig. 7.8). This is also helpful when the effusion is subpulmonary, that is between the lower surface of the lung and the diaphragm. Ultrasound and CT demonstrate effusions well.

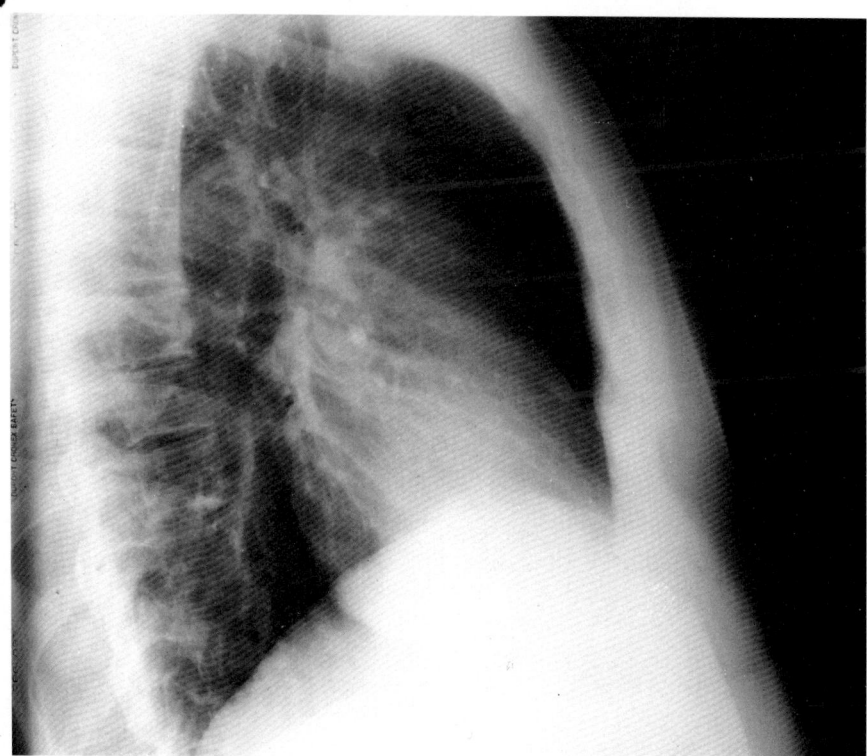

Fig. 7.8 Pleural effusion. PA, minimal pleural shadowing at the right costophrenic angles. (Top), pleural fluid along the right lateral chest wall (bottom).

Empyema

Empyema may be acute or chronic and is a purulent pleural effusion. Infection has reached the pleural space through the blood stream, the chest wall or the bronchial tree and the cause may be pneumonia, lung abscess, bronchiectasis, tuberculosis (Fig. 7.9) or a penetrating chest wall wound. If the empyema is untreated it may rupture through into a bronchus causing a bronchopleural fistula and a pyopneumothorax. Oesophageal pleural fistulae may also occur.

The radiological appearances are those of a pleural effusion, and diagnosis depends on the aspiration of purulent fluid.

Haemothorax

Haemothorax is usually the result of severe chest wall trauma, a complicated pneumothorax or the rupture of an aortic aneurysm, but may occur spontaneously (Fig. 7.10). The signs are those of a pleural effusion and may be accompanied by those of shock due to blood loss. Diagnosis is confirmed by aspiration. It is often necessary to perform a thoracotomy to stop the bleeding.

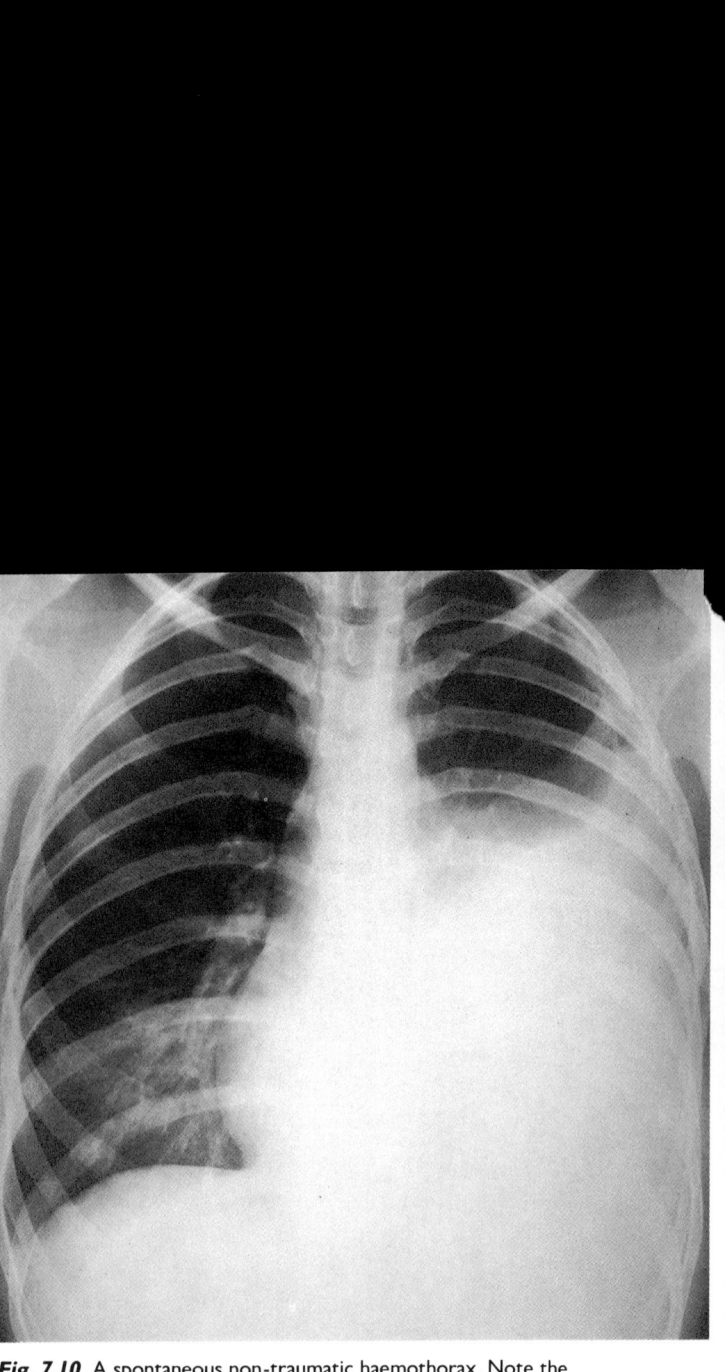

Fig. 7.9 Empyema. There was an air fluid level to the left of the heart, pleural thickening with calcification at the left apex, calcified old tuberculous infiltration of both lungs particularly in the upper lobes, and some pleural calcification overlying the left lung in the region of the air fluid levels. Contrast injection into the pleural cavity shows the lower part of the cavity and some contrast in the bronchial tree outlining the left main bronchus.

Fig. 7.10 A spontaneous non-traumatic haemothorax. Note the small amount of air following diagnostic aspiration.

Pneumothorax

Pneumothorax (see Figs 9.3 and 9.4) is present when there is separation of the visceral and parietal layers of the pleura by air. When a pneumothorax occurs the lung recoils downwards forming a space, unless it is held up by adhesions. If a large pneumothorax is present the mediastinum may be displaced. Air may enter the pleural space through a hole in the parietal pleura which has extended through the layers of the chest wall, or, more commonly, through the visceral pleura, air being drawn from the lung by the subatmospheric pressure in the pleural space. Closed pneumothorax is present when the hole in the pleura has closed. Open pneumothorax is present when the breach in the pleura is still present and air moves in and out during respiration; the lung will not then re-expand. If the communication is between the bronchus and the pleural space it is called a bronchopleural fistula. Tension pneumothorax occurs when the hole in the pleura acts as a valve so that air can enter the pleural space but not leave it; pressure therefore rises causing mediastinal displacement. This is an emergency situation and if not treated the patient will die from circulatory collapse and hypoxia.

The radiograph will show a zone without lung markings between the chest wall and the lung edge. A small pneumothorax is not easy to see (Fig. 7.12) but it is helpful to take a radiograph in expiration. In the case of a tension pneumothorax, mediastinal shift will be obvious on the radiograph (Fig. 7.13). If the patient has a significant pneumothorax, blood gases should be checked and any sputum should be sent for culture. The clinical picture of a large pneumothorax can be very similar to that of a pulmonary embolus or myocardial infarction. Large bullae may mimic a pneumothorax.

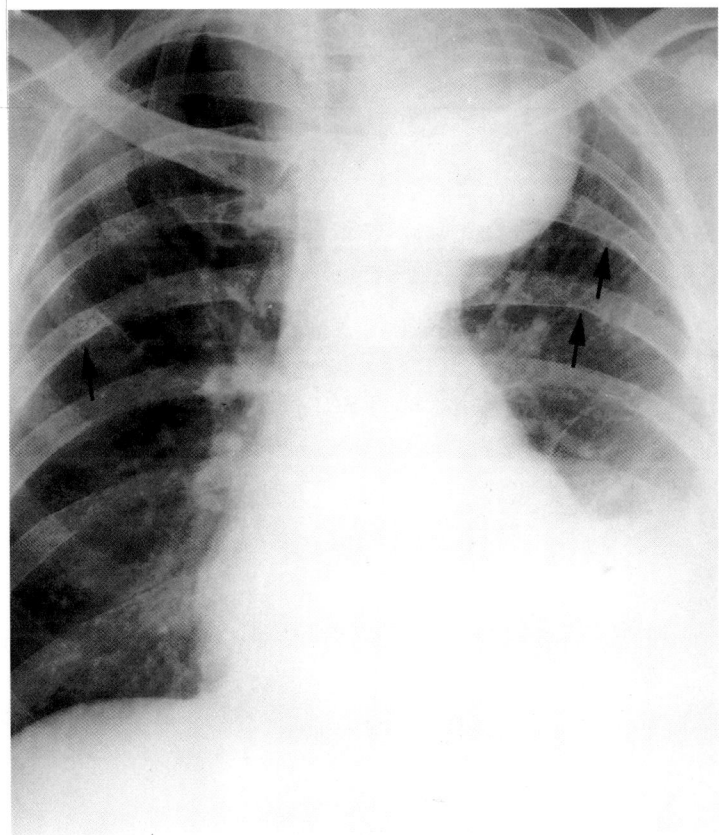

Fig. 7.11 Chylothorax. Following surgery for coarctation of aorta, note rib notching (arrowed). A mediastinal collection of fluid and a left pleural effusion are seen. On aspiration the effusion was discovered to be chyle.

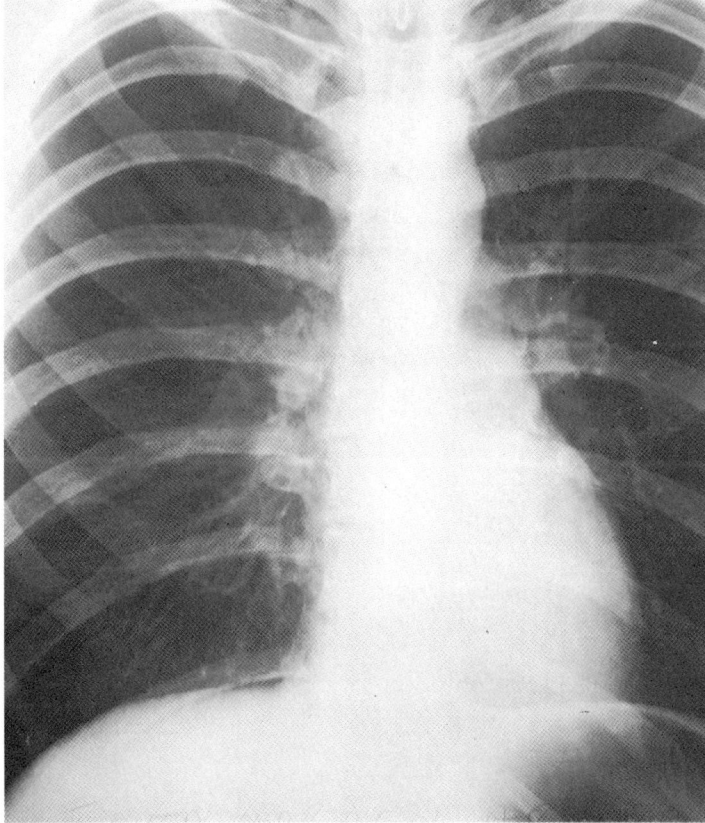

Fig. 7.12 Small right-sided pneumothorax. Note the lung edge in the right upper chest. There are no lung markings peripheral to this.

Pleural calcification

Pleural calcification (Fig. 7.14) is rarely extensive. It can be found following empyema or haemothorax, or in association with tuberculous infection, or in individuals who have worked with asbestos (Fig. 7.15).

Pleural tumours

Benign cysts of the pleura and pleural tumours are rare and often asymptomatic. Finger clubbing, hypertrophic pulmonary osteoarthropathy and some chest pain are all possible presentations in pleural fibroma (Fig. 7.16).

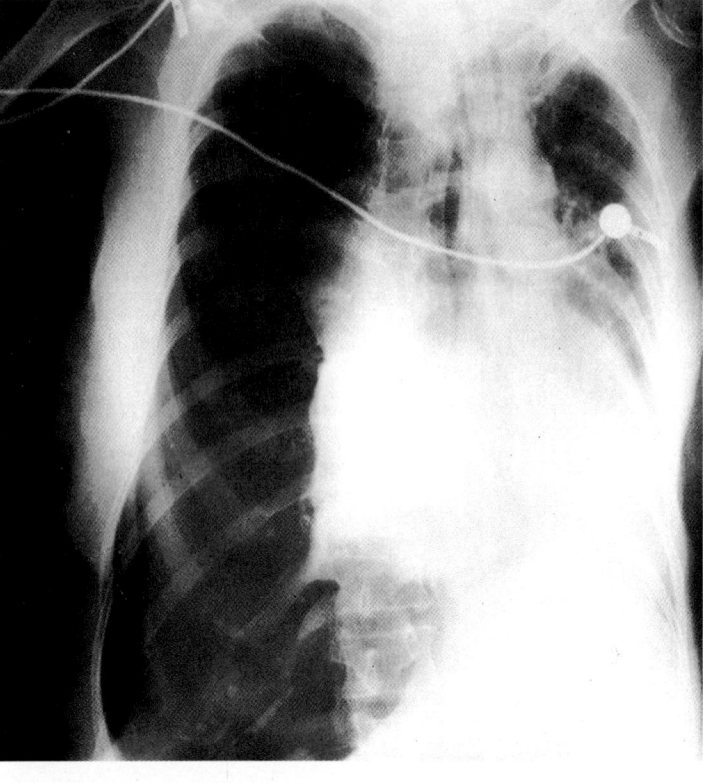

Fig. 7.13 Tension pneumothorax in a patient being artificially ventilated. Total collapse of the right lung with gross displacement of the right dome of the diaphragm and mediastinal shift to the opposite side causing collapse of the left lung.

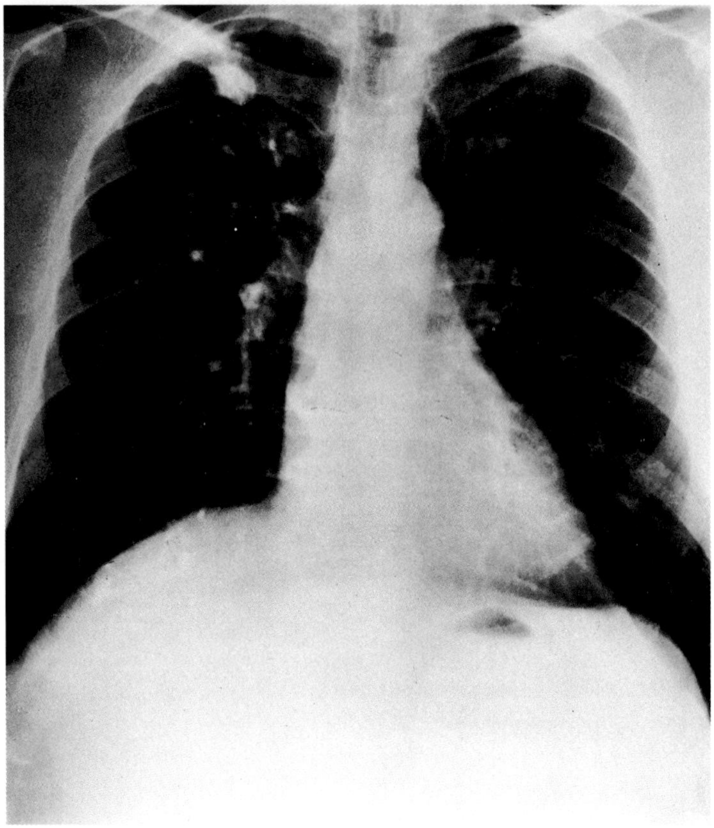

Fig. 7.14 Pleural calcification. Calcification due to tuberculosis.

Malignant mesothelioma is in most patients associated generally with a history of asbestos inhalation many years previously. Histologically the tumours may be of sarcomatous, epithelial or mixed type. The patient may present with chest pain, pleurisy or dyspnoea due to a large pleural effusion (Fig. 7.17). The diagnosis is usually made following a pleural biopsy or thoracotomy. Pleural effusions should be controlled if necessary by pleurectomy and adequate analgesia given. Treatment is very unsatisfactory; most patients die within two years.

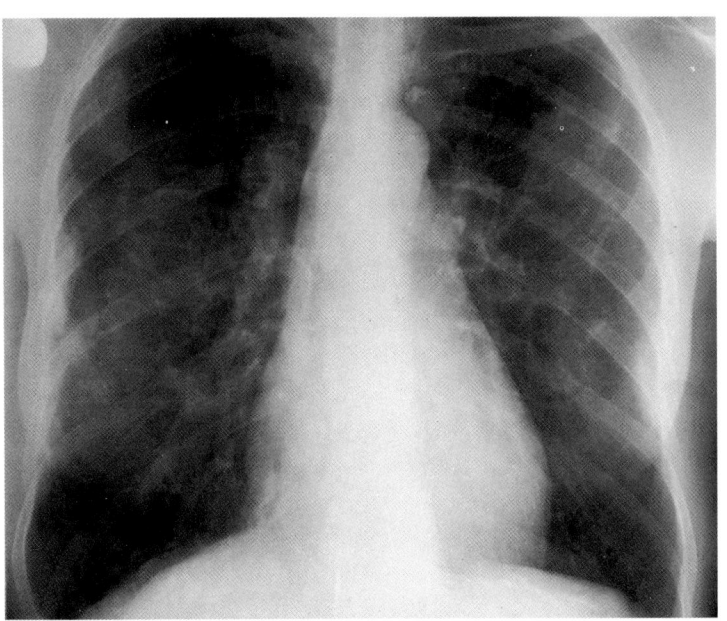

Fig. 7.15 Pleural calcification. Asbestos exposure. Pleural shadowings on the lateral chest wall and diaphragm with partial calcification typical of asbestos pleural plaques.

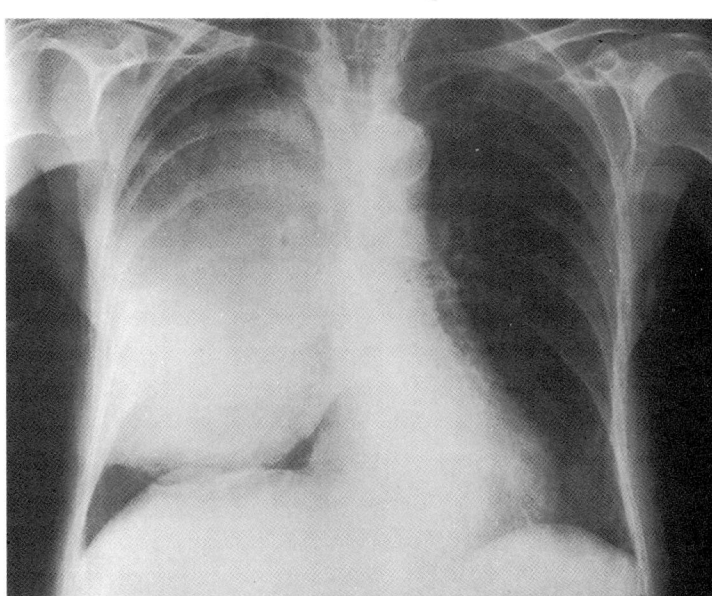

Fig. 7.16 A pleural fibroma.

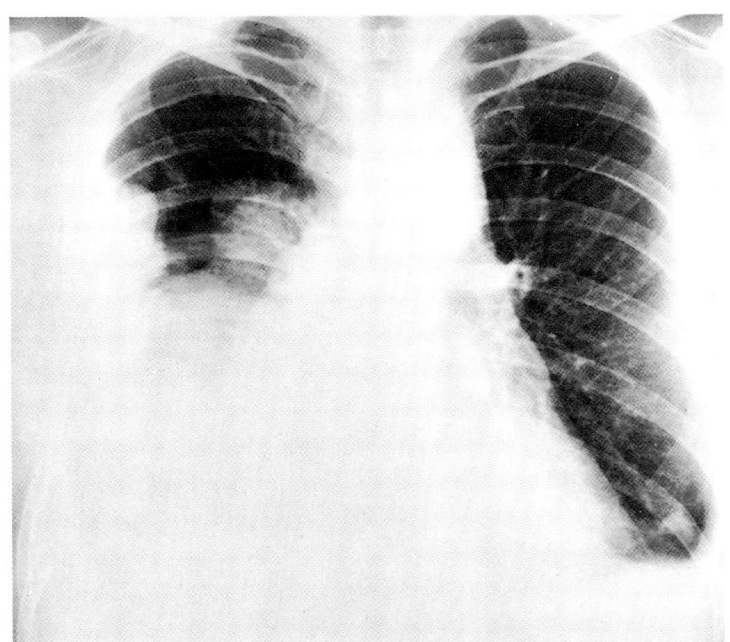

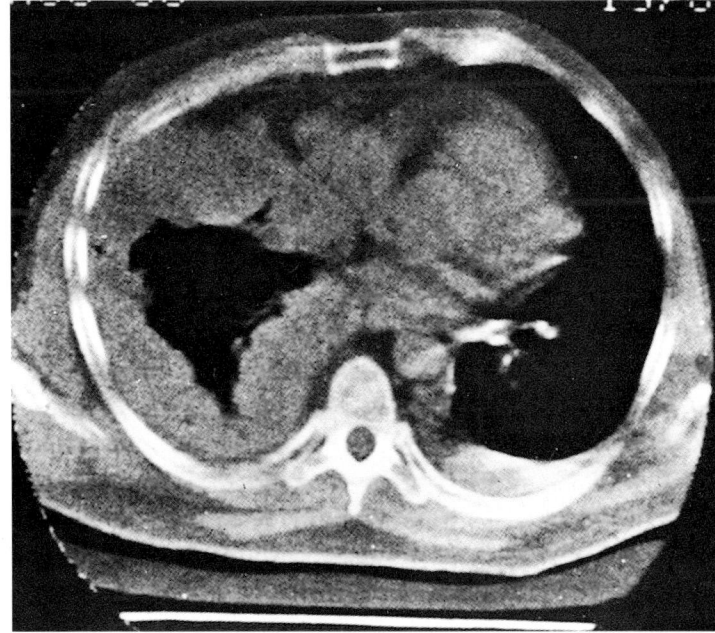

Fig. 7.17 Pleural tumour. Left, nodulated mass along the lateral chest wall and mediastinum and the right base. Appearances are of a pleural tumour. A small left pleural effusion is also present — malignant mesothelioma. Right, CT scan confirms that there is extensive pleural involvement on the right extending through medially behind the heart to the left side where there is a pleural effusion.

Diaphragm Paralysis

Unilateral paralysis of one hemidiaphragm may occur when the phrenic nerve is involved by malignancy, following surgery, and medical causes of neuropathy including neuralgic amyotrophy (Fig. 7.18). Congenital absence of the muscular part of the diaphragm (sometimes called eventration) causes a similar picture but complete absence of the hemidiaphragm is more dramatic (Fig. 7.19).

Chest X-ray (see Fig. 7.18) can show elevation of one hemidiaphragm, and unilateral paralysis can be confirmed easily at fluoroscopy. However, diffuse respiratory muscle weakness or bilateral diaphragm paralysis is much harder to identify radiologically. If weakness is severe both diaphragms are elevated with small but otherwise normal lung fields (Fig. 7.20). These appearances can be similar to those of obesity as well as failure to take a deep inspiration. Fluoroscopy can be technically difficult and the diaphragm may move apparently normally, even during sniffing, particularly in the upright posture.

If the paralysis is complete such patients may be able to

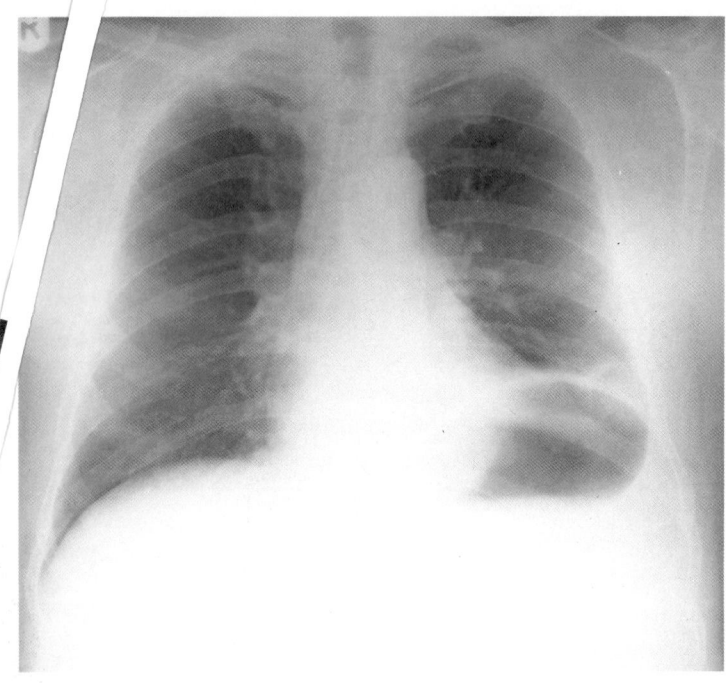

Fig. 7.18 Chest radiograph of a patient after left sided hemidiaphragm paralysis. The patient noticed sudden onset of breathlessness with epigastric discomfort. These symptoms improved spontaneously although the hemidiaphragm paralysis persisted, seen as a raised hemidiaphragm on the left above a conspicuous gastric air bubble.

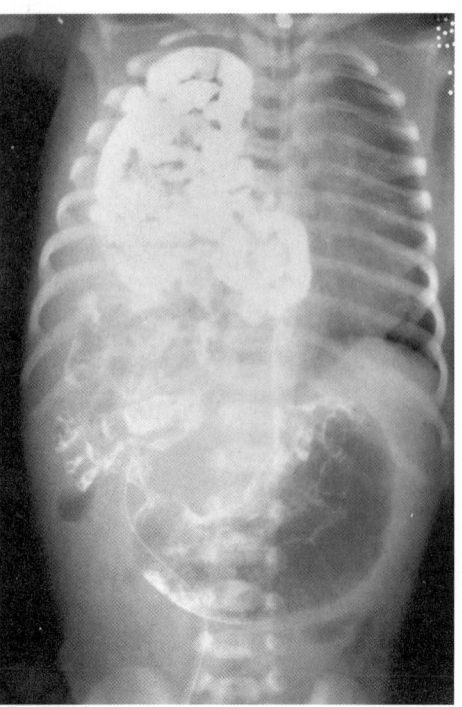

Fig. 7.19 Radiograph of chest and abdomen of a two-day-old infant with congenital absence of the right hemidiaphragm. The child swallowed barium, which outlines the small intestine occupying the right hemithorax. The heart is shifted to the left. The baby was centrally cyanosed with severe hypoxia and acidosis.

tolerate the supine position for only a brief period, but in partial weakness it may be possible to perform fluoroscopy supine, when paradoxical motion of the diaphragm may be seen — particularly during sniffing.

Chest Wall

The familiar shape of the rib cage must be distorted very substantially to cause respiratory difficulties. Thus depression of the sternum (pectus excavatum) or anterior displacement of the sternum (pigeon chest) are usually of no physiological importance. Other minor abnormalities such as cervical or bifid ribs (see Chapter 2) are usually only chance findings on chest X-ray. Fibrous dysplasia can cause abnormalities of one or more ribs but is only rarely generalized. Rarely the rib cage may be diffusely malformed, as in Jeune's syndrome (Fig. 7.21). The ribs can be involved in many pathological processes such as malignancies, infections and trauma — these are usually more important for their local or systemic effects rather than for

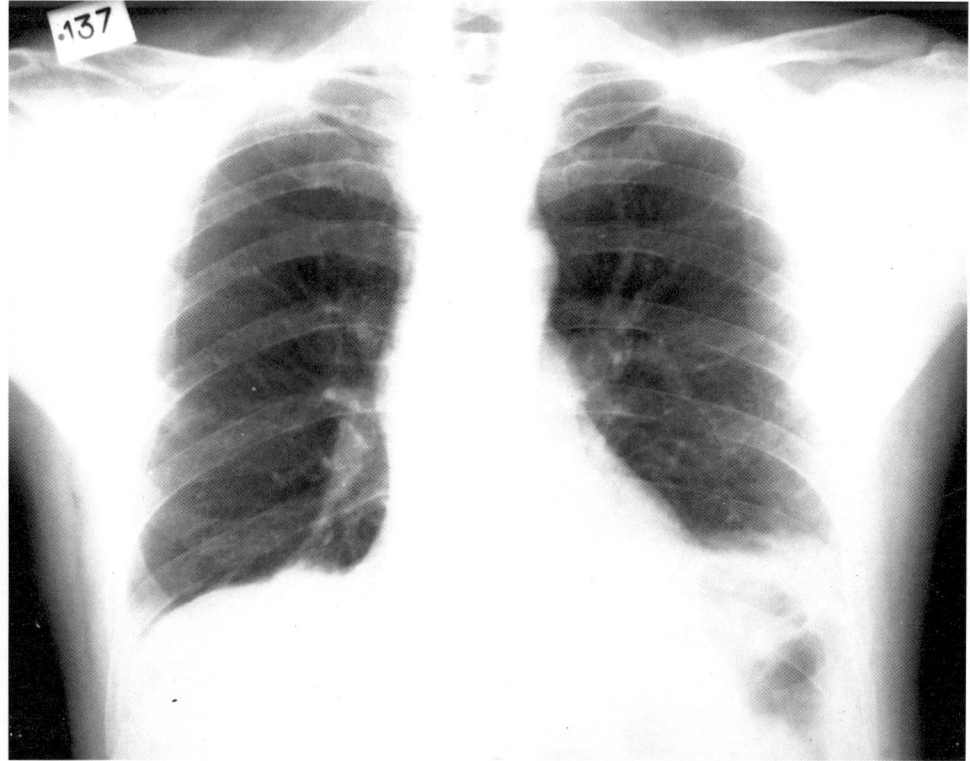

Fig. 7.20 Chest radiograph of a 42-year-old man after idiopathic bilateral paralysis of the diaphragms. The patient had a mild viral illness and developed breathlessness on exertion and severe orthopnoea. These persisted and investigations showed a vital capacity of 2.1 litres, with a 55% fall when supine. He could generate less than 10cmH$_2$O pressure across his diaphragms compared with a normal lower limit of 100cmH$_2$O. A diagnosis of neuralgic amyotrophy was made. Following paralysis the chest radiograph shows that both diaphragms are high with a little patchy collapse at both bases but otherwise the lungs are clear.

their effects on respiration. However, conditions which cause substantial destruction or distortion of the rib cage can cause hypoventilation due to restriction. These include widespread fractures (see Chapter 8), and other conditions such as osteogenesis imperfecta, ankylosing spondylitis and severe congenital or acquired kyphoscoliosis (Fig. 7.22).

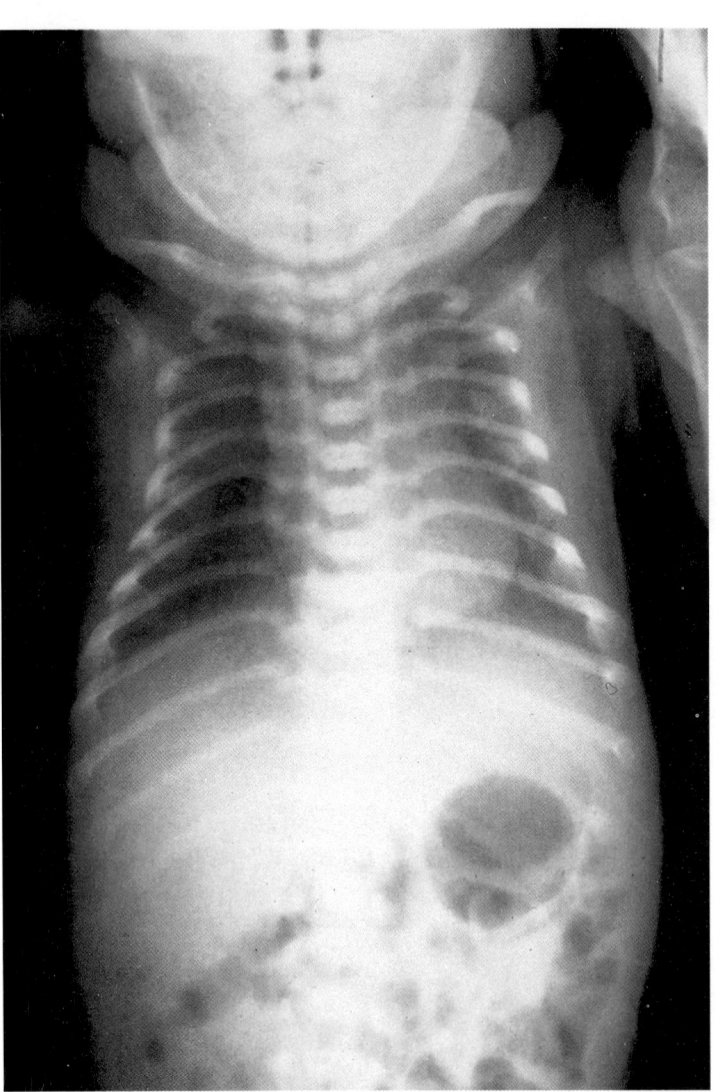

Fig. 7.21 Chest radiograph of an infant with asphyxiating thoracic dystrophy (Jeune's syndrome). There is characteristic deformity of the ribs, which are short and the ends are broadened. The rib cage is distorted and small, and may lead to respiratory failure.

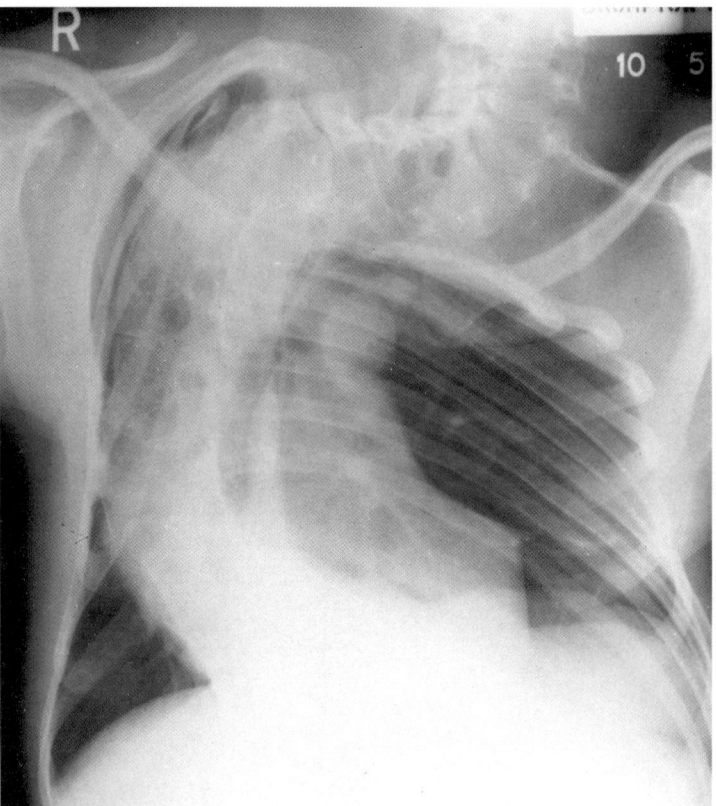

Fig. 7.22 Chest radiograph (normal PA view) of a young man with severe kyphoscoliosis. Surprisingly, severe kyphoscoliosis can be compatible with normal blood gas exchange but with age and increasing disability such patients may develop nocturnal hypoventilation and chronic respiratory failure.

8

Diseases of the Mediastinum

The mediastinum consists of those structures and organs which lie between the two lungs and extends from the diaphragm below to the thoracic inlet above and from the sternum in front to the spine posteriorly. The extrapleural paravertebral gutter on each side is usually included for convenience though it is not strictly part of the mediastinum.

For descriptive purposes the mediastinum has been divided by anatomists over the years in different ways; the usual division is into superior, anterior, middle and posterior mediastinum but different boundaries are given by different authors. The anterior mediastinum is best regarded as that region extending from the thoracic inlet to the diaphragm in front of the ascending aorta and superior vena cava. The superior region is that part of the mediastinum behind the anterior mediastinum above the aortic and azygos arches. The middle and posterior regions lie below the superior mediastinum behind the anterior mediastinum and do not have a distinct boundary separa-

ting them; the posterior mediastinum includes the paravertebral areas. The value to the clinician or radiologist in anatomical division of the mediastinum lies in the help it provides in the diagnosis of masses in the mediastinum, for example, thymic tumours are anterior and neurogenic tumours almost entirely posterior or superior (Fig. 8.1). Masses developing in the middle mediastinum are nearly always (ninety percent) malignant and masses in the anterior mediastinum at the cardiophrenic angle are nearly always benign.

The main structures lying within the mediastinum are the heart and pericardium, the aorta and venae cava, the azygos and hemiazygos venous system, the head and neck vessels, the oesophagus, the trachea, the thymus, thoracic duct and lymphatics, the vagus and sympathetic nerves, the phrenic nerves, fat, connective tissue and lymph-nodes. Diseases of the heart and pericardium, most diseases of the great vessels and diseases of the oesophagus are not within the province of this book and diseases of the airway are covered in other chapters.

In the diagnosis of mediastinal lesions fluoroscopy, oblique radiography, conventional tomography, barium swallow and angiography have almost entirely been replaced by computed tomography (CT). Not only does CT show the anatomical position and boundaries of a lesion, but it also provides information on the character of the tissue within it, i.e. whether it is fatty, cystic, solid or vascular.

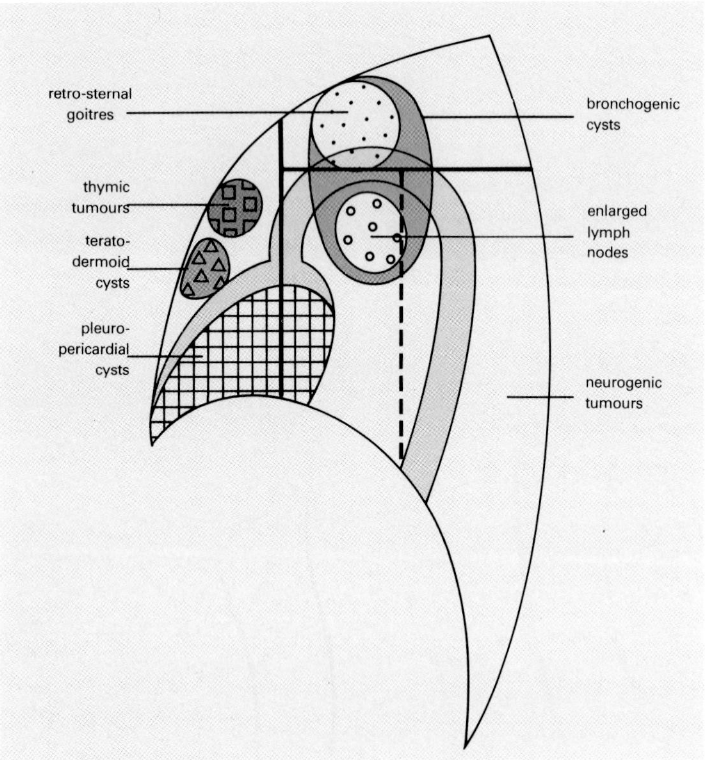

retro-sternal
goitres

thymic
tumours

terato-
dermoid
cysts

pleuro-
pericardial
cysts

bronchogenic
cysts

enlarged
lymph
nodes

neurogenic
tumours

Fig. 8.1 Typical sites of tumours in the mediastinum.

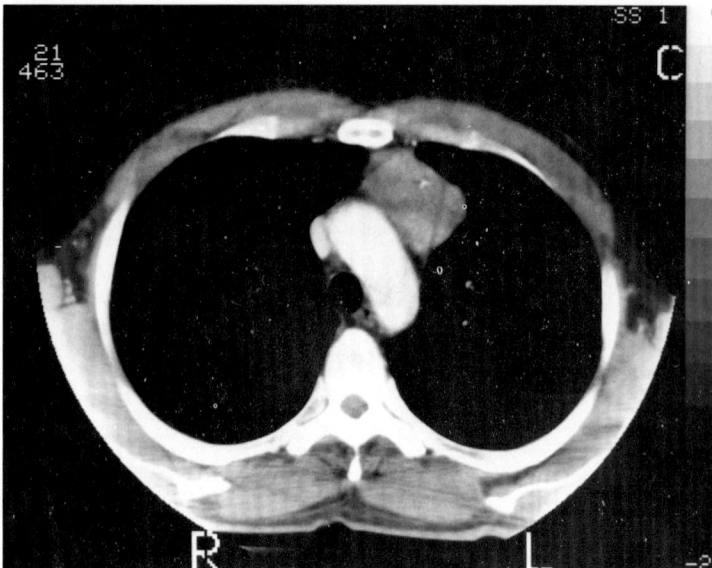

Fig. 8.2 Thymoma in a patient with myasthenia gravis. A lobulated mass is seen in the anterior mediastinum in front of the aortic arch and left hilum. CT scan.

Tumours and Cysts of the Mediastinum

It is convenient and of help in diagnosis to group these according to the site where they most commonly occur.

Anterior mediastinum
Thymic tumours

Thymoma is the commonest tumour in the anterior mediastinum (see chapter 2); nearly all occur just in front of the base of the heart. The majority are solid but about five to ten percent are cystic. Areas of necrosis and calcification are often present, the calcification frequently being sufficiently extensive to be visible on a plain chest radiograph.

Approximately half of patients with a thymic tumour have myasthenia gravis and one-fifth of patients with myasthenia have a thymic tumour. As the thymus lies in the midline, thymic tumours may be difficult to identify on frontal chest radiographs where they are hidden by the shadows cast by the spine and other mediastinal structures.

When sufficiently large they usually bulge on both sides of the mediastinal shadow. Computed tomography is of particular value in the demonstration of these tumours, especially in patients with myasthenia in whom only small tumours may be present (Fig. 8.2).

A rare (six percent) association with thymoma is hypo-gammaglobulinaemia. Even more rare is anaemia due to erythroid hypoplasia. Occasionally a fatty element of the thymus forms a large thymolipoma in which there is a capsule of thymic tissue surrounding a central tumour of fat; such tumours may become very large. Carcinoid tumours also arise in the thymus, usually in men. They tend to be more aggressive than those that arise in the lungs. Thymic carcinoids may cause Cushing's syndrome or be one component of Werner's multiple endocrine adenoma syndrome.

Malignant tumours of the thymus spread locally and into the pleura, where they may seed causing widespread pleural deposits, though most thymomas are benign.

Germ cell tumours

These tumours are derived from germ cells in the anterior mediastinum and may become very large. If benign, the lesion is usually cystic (see Fig. 2.34) with teeth (Fig. 8.3), bone and calcification within the wall, and often containing cholesterol and sebaceous debris. About thirty percent of mediastinal germ cell tumours are malignant and may become very large (Fig. 8.4; see Fig. 2.35). Some have a cell structure identical to seminoma of the testis or dysgerminoma of the ovary. Other malignant varieties consist of extra-embryonic tissue such as yolk sac or chorion. They occur mainly in young men.

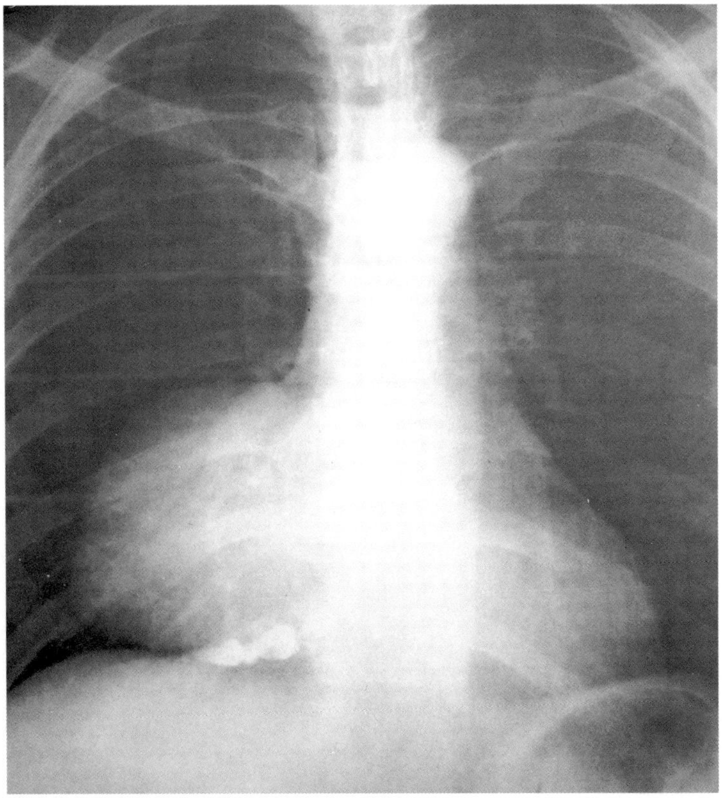

Fig. 8.3 Dermoid cyst. A frontal radiograph showing a cyst with teeth in its lower part.

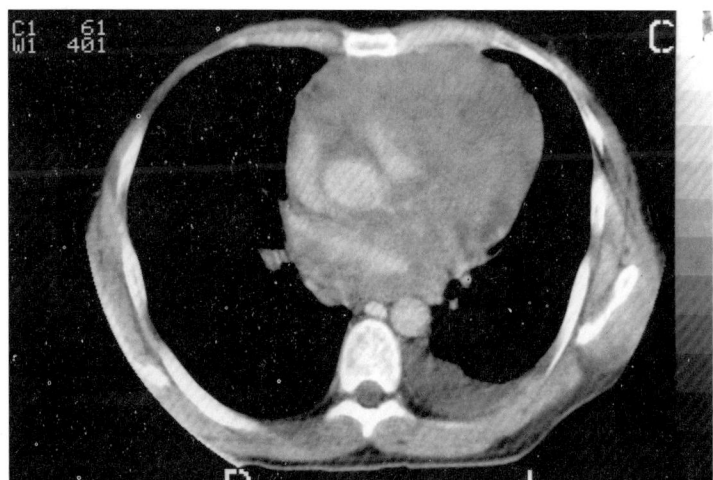

Fig. 8.4 Germ cell tumour of the mediastinum. Radiographs showed a large irregular mediastinal mass and a left pleural effusion. The CT scan at the level of the right pulmonary artery confirms the large mediastinal mass due to an infiltratory tumour surrounding the ascending aorta, pulmonary trunk and the right pulmonary artery. These last two are severely compressed and distorted. The left pleural effusion is evident.

Retrosternal goitre

In a great majority of patients with a mediastinal thyroid (see Fig. 2.32) there is a direct connection with a palpable thyroid swelling in the neck. The majority extend from the lower pole of the thyroid into the anterior mediastinum in front of the trachea, but the remainder extend from the posterior aspect of the thyroid behind the trachea and the head and neck vessels. Rarely they extend into the posterior part of the mediastinum below the level of the aortic arch and occasionally they are found as low as the pericardium in the anterior mediastinum. Histologically, mediastinal goitre is usually of the nodular colloid variety.

Radiologically, the mass is clearly defined, smooth or slightly lobulated and of uniform density, though calcification may be identified, particularly on CT (Fig. 8.5). The mass frequently displaces and compresses the trachea either from in front or from one side (see chapter 2). When posterior to the trachea, the goitre displaces the trachea forwards and the oesophagus to one side and posteriorly. Radioactive isotope studies may show the lesion and confirm the diagnosis but frequently retrosternal goitres are non-functioning and do not take up the isotope. Patients with retrosternal goitre are usually asymptomatic but may have cough, respiratory embarrassment, stridor and

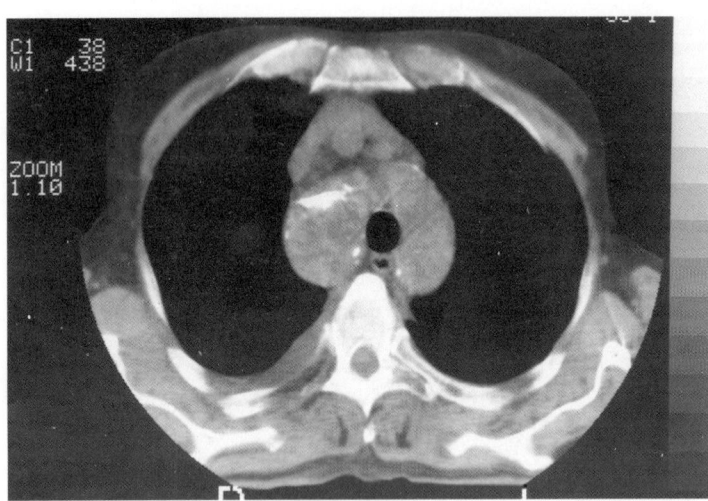

Fig. 8.5 Intrathoracic goitre. CT scan of a patient with a partially calcified intrathoracic goitre on the right of the trachea opposite the top of the aortic arch.

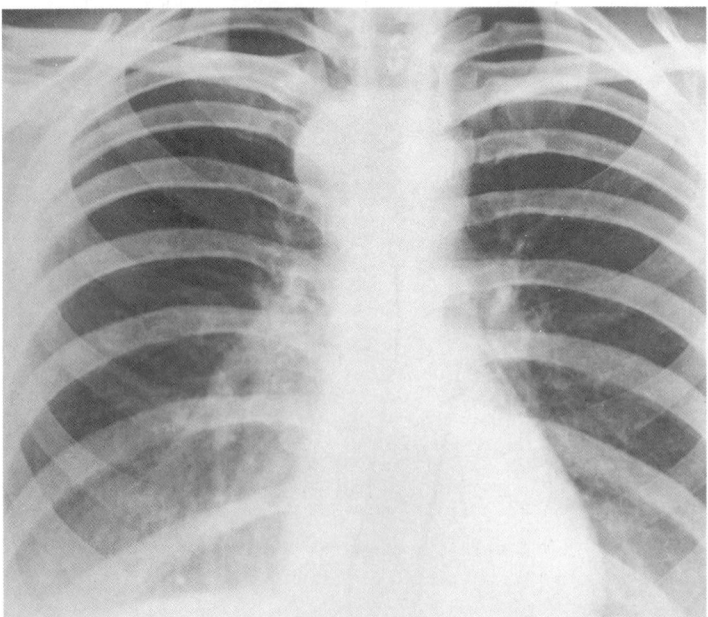

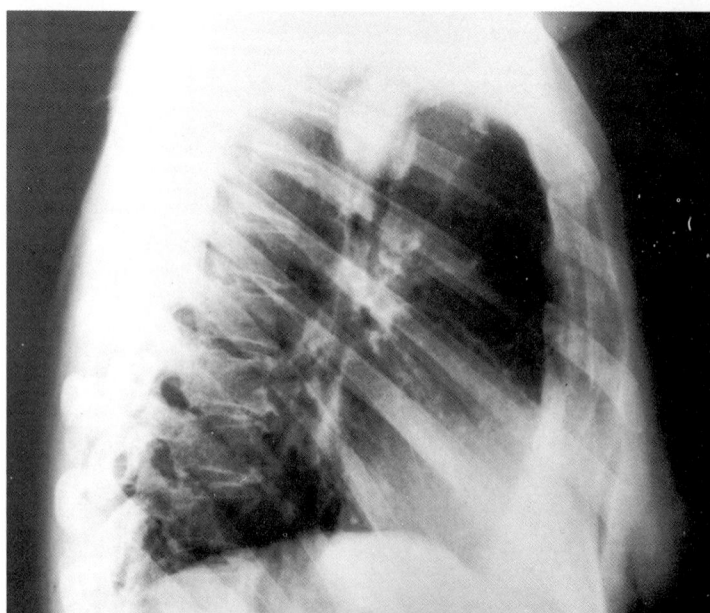

Fig. 8.6 Tuberculous lymphadenopathy. A smooth swelling is seen on the right side of the superior mediastinum due to enlarged paratracheal lymph nodes.

hoarseness due to recurrent laryngeal paralysis. The onset of symptoms may be acute due to a sudden haemorrhage into the goitre causing acute compression of the trachea.

Middle and posterior mediastinum
Lymphadenopathy

The mediastinum contains an abundance of lymph-nodes in all divisions but mainly concentrated around the major bronchi and the trachea. Evaluation of enlarged lymph-nodes is mainly radiological. At the hilum, lymphadenopathy is probably just as well detected by conventional tomography as by CT but there is no doubt that in the mediastinum CT is the examination of choice. Normal lymph-nodes are usually less than 1cm in diameter. In the staging of carcinoma of the bronchus, mediastinal lymph-nodes less than 1cm in diameter on computed tomography show histological evidence of involvement in five to six percent, but if over 1.5cm in diameter invasion by tumour is found in ninety-four to ninety-seven percent. A node over 1cm in diameter should therefore be regarded with a high degree of suspicion.

The causes of lymphadenopathy in the mediastinum are the same as elsewhere in the body.

Infection

Enlargement of nodes in the hilum and mediastinum may occur in any acute lung infection such as pneumonia, but is seldom detected except in children. Some chronic infections such as those in cystic fibrosis cause slight enlargement of hilar and mediastinal lymph-nodes. As part of the generalized infection, enlarged mediastinal nodes are rarely seen on the chest radiograph in infectious mono-nucleosis (glandular fever) but are often very large in the much rarer infection, bubonic plague (*Yersinia (Pasteurella) pestis* infection) (see Fig. 5.3). The commonest infection in which enlarged hilar and mediastinal nodes are found is tuberculosis (Fig. 8.6), often part of a primary complex (see chapter 5). Histoplasmosis and coccidioidomycosis, prevalent in the United States of America, are other infections which are associated with mediastinal lymphadenopathy. Central irregular calcification of nodes occurs in tuberculosis, histoplasmosis and coccidioidomycosis when healing occurs.

Lymphoma and leukaemia

Hodgkin's disease is the most frequent lymphoma to affect the mediastinal lymph-nodes and is one of the commonest causes of mediastinal lymph-node involvement. About seventy percent of patients with Hodgkin's disease have mediastinal lymphadenopathy. Hilar nodes may also be involved (see Fig. 2.30), often asymmetrically, unlike sarcoidosis in which symmetrical enlargement of the hilar nodes is usual, though not invariable. The massive enlargement of nodes may cause compression of adjacent structures, particularly the superior vena cava with consequent obstruction. Involvement of the thymus and the lymph-nodes in the internal mammary chains in the superior mediastinum may give rise to retrosternal masses (Fig. 8.7). This occurs most frequently in young patients with nodular sclerosing Hodgkin's disease which is often associated with cervical node involvement. Calcification of lymph-nodes in Hodgkin's lymphoma occurs only after treatment with cytotoxic drugs or radiotherapy.

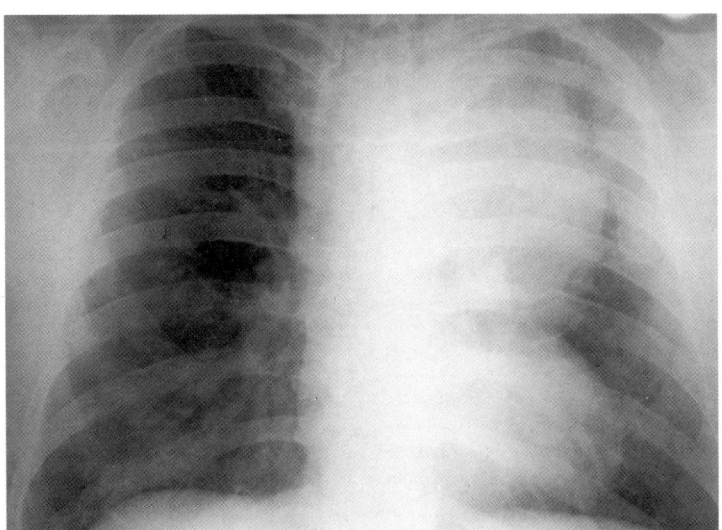
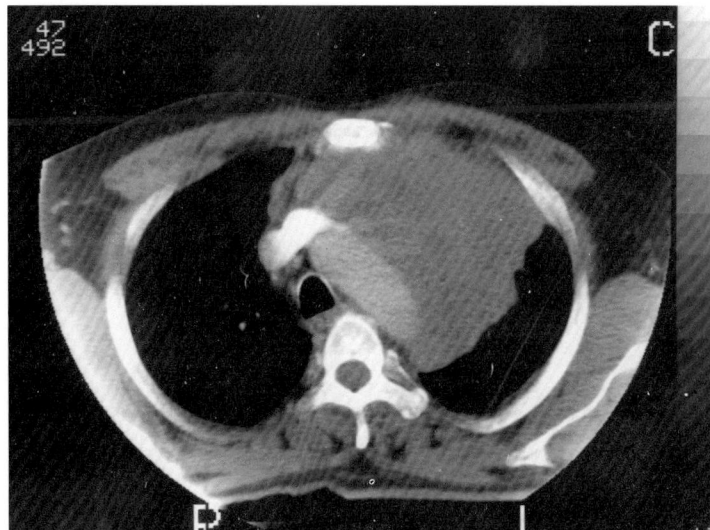

Fig. 8.7 Hodgkin's disease, frontal radiograph and CT scan. A large left sided superior mediastinal mass is present. The computed tomogram showed this extending across the mid line in front of the superior vena cava and lying to the left and in front of the aortic arch which is displaced to the right with the trachea. Biopsy revealed the mass to be due to Hodgkin's disease.

Non-Hodgkin's lymphoma may affect any of the mediastinal nodes and the diagnosis can only be made by histological examination. Frequently the intrathoracic manifestations are only one part of a widespread generalized disease. A higher incidence of non-Hodgkin's lymphoma, particularly the histiocytic variety, occurs in patients who are immunosuppressed or immunodeficient.

In leukaemia, mediastinal and hilar node enlargement is the commonest intrathoracic feature and is more common in lymphocytic leukaemia than in the myeloid type. Pleural effusion and pulmonary infiltration are less frequent than node enlargement.

Metastatic carcinoma

One of the commonest causes of mediastinal lymph-node enlargement is metastatic involvement by carcinoma of the bronchus (Fig. 8.8). Sometimes the primary lesion is difficult to detect in the lungs or is very small, in spite of a large mediastinal mass. Symptoms arise from pressure on surrounding structures, cough and dyspnoea being the commonest. Facial swelling due to obstruction of the superior vena cava and phrenic nerve and recurrent laryngeal nerve paralysis also occur. The detection of hilar and mediastinal nodes for staging of carcinoma of the bronchus is of utmost importance in management and treatment. Metastases from other primary malignant tumours include carcinoma of the upper intestinal tract, oesophagus, prostate, breast and kidney.

Other causes

Other causes of lymphadenopathy include sarcoidosis (see Fig. 2.29 and chapter 6) and silicosis (see chapter 7), in which calcification may occur in the rims of the nodes, so-called 'eggshell' calcification. Enlarged nodes are also seen in berylliosis, and in an unusual form of benign hyperplasia in which a solitary mass is present (Castleman's disease).

Bronchogenic cysts

The majority of bronchogenic cysts are situated adjacent to the trachea or one of the major airways (Fig. 8.9). They are lined with bronchial mucosa and contain liquid mucoid material. Rarely there is a communication with the bronchial tree when a fluid level may be seen within the cyst on the chest radiograph. They rarely produce symptoms

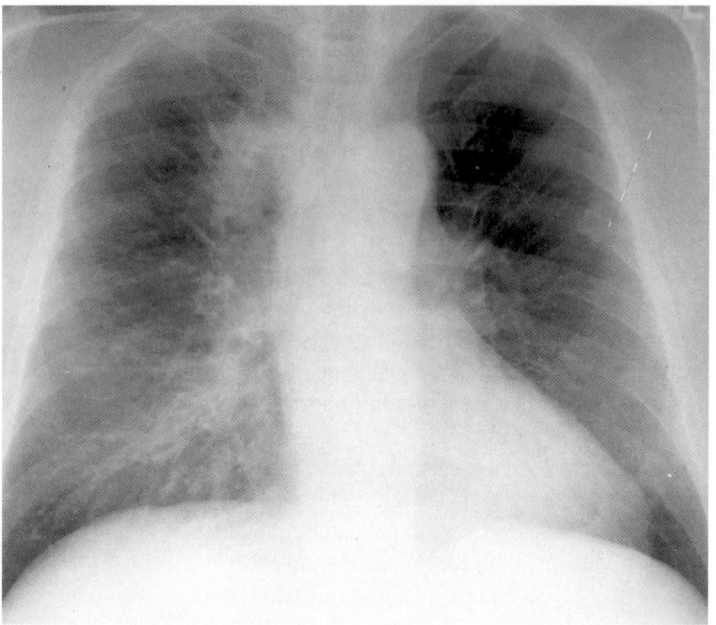

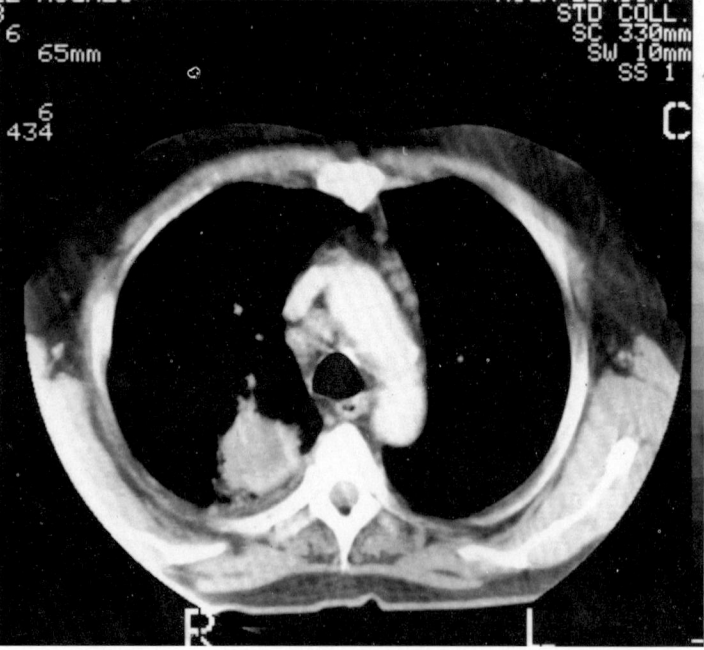

Fig. 8.8 Squamous cell carcinoma in the right upper lobe. The frontal chest radiograph shows a lesion in the lung together with some enlargement of nodes at the right hilum and in the right paratracheal region. The CT scan shows nodes greater than 1cm between the trachea and SVC and also to the left of the aortic arch confirming extensive mediastinal lymph node involvement.

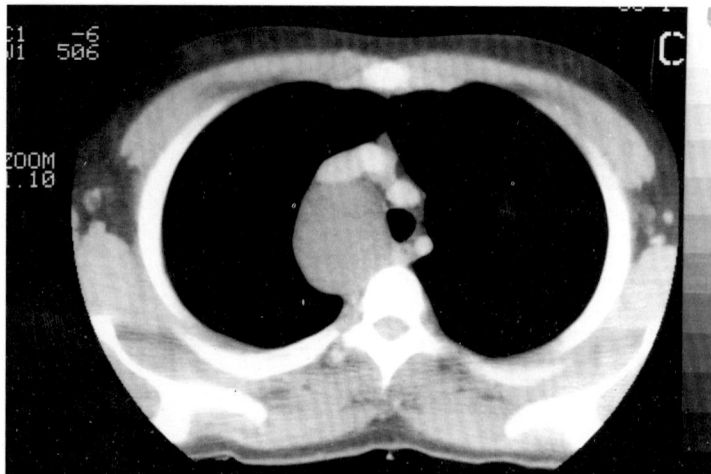

Fig. 8.9 Bronchogenic cyst. Radiographs showed a clearly defined opacity on the right side of the trachea. In the CT scan the density of the contents is that of fluid.

but may become infected in which case they can increase rapidly in size and produce symptoms not only of the infection but also from compression of adjacent airways. Radiologically they are seen as smooth, clearly defined masses adjacent to the trachea or main bronchi. Widening of the carina may be present — similar to that seen due to an enlarged left atrium with which a cyst may be confused.

Pleuropericardial cysts

These cysts almost never cause symptoms, nor do they become infected; they are usually chance findings on routine chest radiographs. They may communicate with the pericardium and are thought to be developmental in origin arising from errors in differentiation of coelomic cavities. Radiologically the cysts are smooth, round or oval, projecting from the heart border (see Fig. 2.37). Sometimes they are found in the interlobar fissures and on the diaphragm and they are frequently found in the anterior cardiophrenic angle. They commonly range from 3–8cm in diameter and contain clear fluid.

Lipoma

The mediastinum normally contains a variable amount of fat, and lipomas may occur in any part. They often reach a great size before symptoms occur and are frequently a chance finding on the radiograph (see chapter 2). They may be seen on plain radiographs to be of low density, but this is readily demonstrable by CT (see Fig. 2.36). Generalized lipomatosis of the mediastinum may occur as a complication of steroid therapy. Lipomas in the lower mediastinum should be differentiated from diaphragmatic hernias, which may contain omental fat. Bowel may be demonstrated within such a hernia either by CT or a barium meal and follow-through examination (see Fig. 2.41).

Duplication cysts of the oesophagus

Similar to bronchogenic cysts but rarer, duplication cysts of the oesophagus are developmental cysts arising from the foregut. They occur adjacent to the oesophagus, with which they may communicate (Fig. 8.10), and are lined with oesophageal, gastric or even intestinal mucosa.

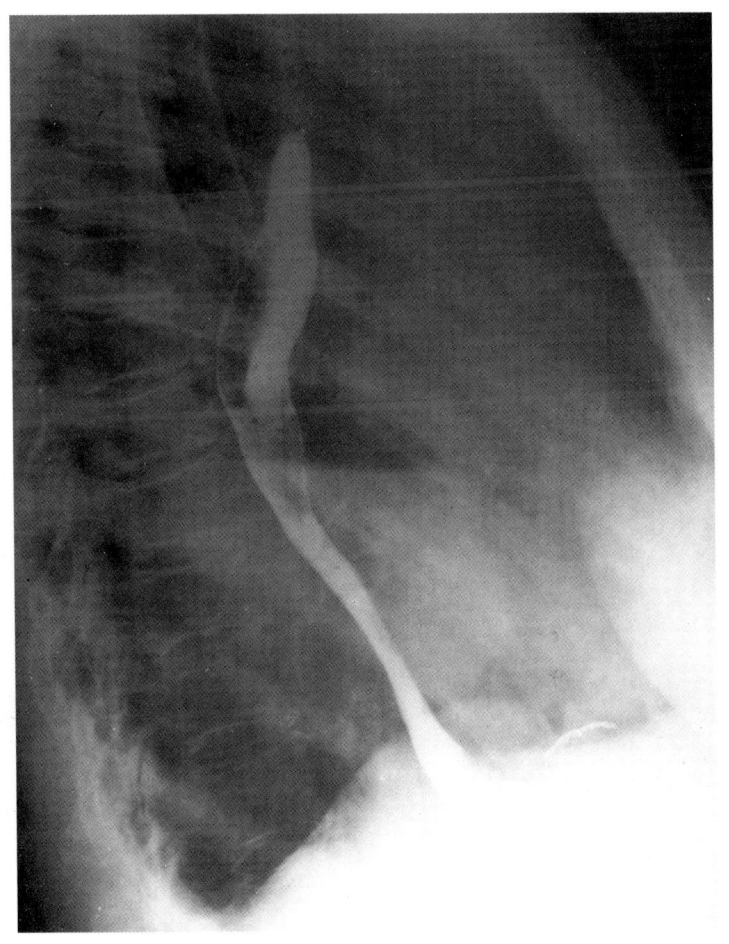

Fig. 8.10 Foregut cyst. Lateral chest radiograph with barium in the oesophagus. The cyst which had an air fluid level lay close to the right side of the lower half of the oesophagus. Though the cyst did not fill with barium there was a communication with the oesophagus which permitted air to get into it.

Neuroenteric cysts

These cysts are also developmental cysts of the foregut and arise as a result of failure of complete separation of the endoderm from the notochordal plate during embryonic development; they are lined by both gastrointestinal and neural elements. They occur in the posterior mediastinum adjacent to the oesophagus and are usually connected to the meninges by a stalk, and occasionally to the gastrointestinal tract below the diaphragm. Communication to the gastrointestinal tract may be patent and allow the cyst to be filled by gas. Because of the connection with the meninges defects in the upper dorsal vertebrae are frequently present (Fig. 8.11). Very rarely this communication is patent and cerebrospinal fluid from the subarachnoid space may be found in the cyst. The communication can be demonstrated by myelography.

Aneurysms of the aorta

Aneurysms of the aorta may be saccular or fusiform.

Ascending aorta: aneurysms of this portion of the thoracic aorta bulge forwards and to the right, rarely to the left (Fig. 8.12). They may erode the back of the sternum and anterior ends of the ribs and costal cartilages.

Arch of aorta: aneurysms here displace adjacent structures, such as the trachea and main bronchi, backwards and to the right causing compression and erosion. As a result such patients complain of 'brassy' cough, dyspnoea and haemoptysis. Left recurrent laryngeal paralysis may occur causing a hoarse voice. These aneurysms and aneurysms of the head and upper limb arteries may bulge upwards into the superior mediastinum as far as the thoracic inlet (see Fig. 2.38).

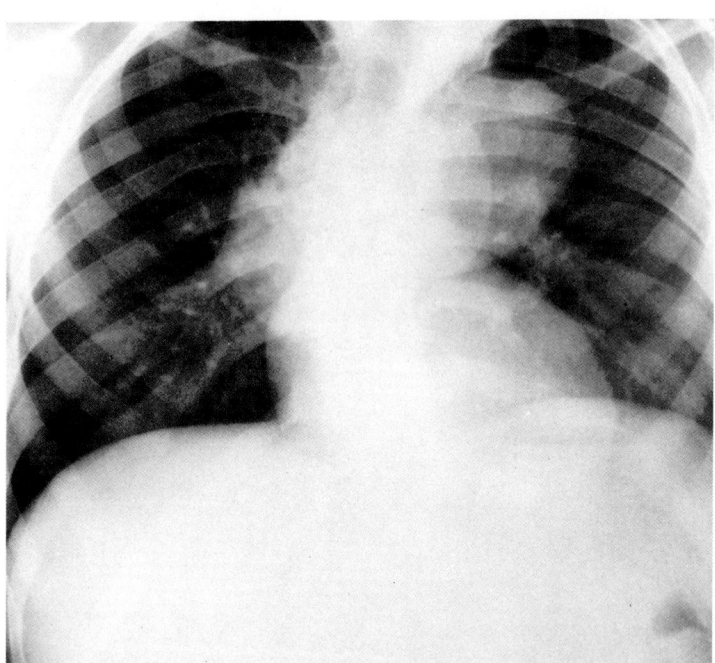 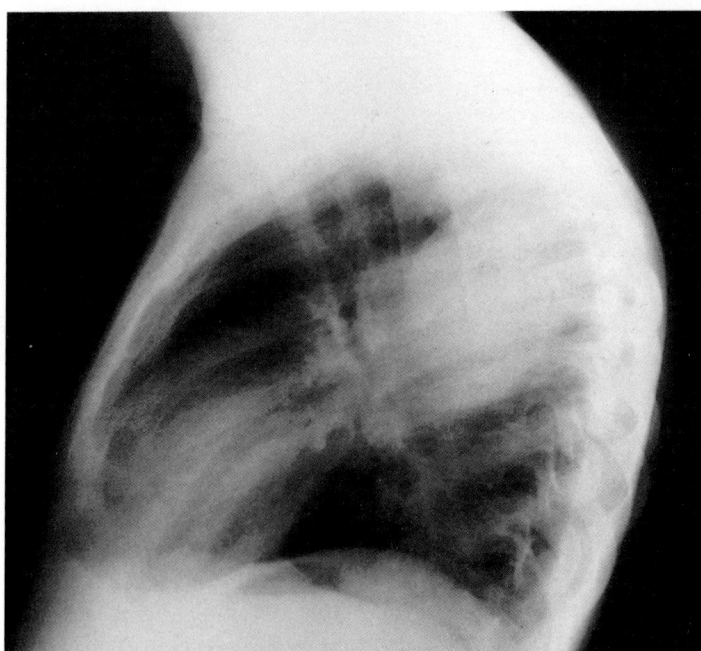

Fig. 8.11 Neuroenteric cyst. Left and right, radiographs of a child with a lobulated cyst on either side and in front of the spine which has numerous defects causing a mid dorsal kyphosis.

Descending aorta: aneurysms of this section of the aorta bulge to the left and forwards. They erode the adjacent vertebrae and compress the left lung into which they may rupture (see Fig. 2.39).

The possibility that a mass in the mediastinum close to the aorta from which it cannot be separated on a chest radiograph might be an aneurysm should always be borne in mind, particularly before a biopsy is attempted. Computed tomography with contrast enhancement or aortography will quickly show the true nature of the lesion. Calcification in layers may be visible on plain radiography in the wall of an aneurysm.

Tumours of the oesophagus

Carcinoma is the commonest tumour of the oesophagus. The presenting symptom is dysphagia. The tumour is usually of insufficient size to be visible on a plain chest radiograph when discovered, though it may cause deformity of the posterior mediastinal line, or the azygo-oesophageal recess. On computed tomography the mass can be identified and its limits in the mediastinum defined. Carcinoma of the oesophagus has a poor prognosis.

Benign tumours are rare, but when they occur they may be very large before discovery and dysphagia is a late symptom. Leiomyoma is the commonest type, but fibromas,

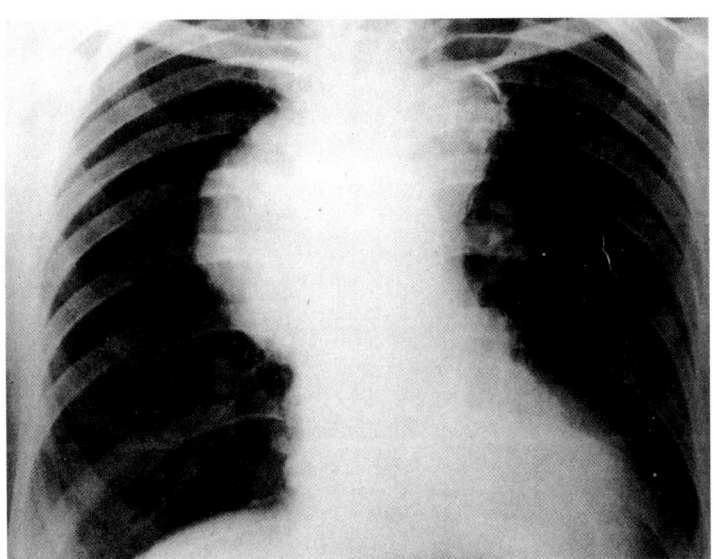

Fig. 8.12 Aneurysm of the ascending aorta. The plain radiograph shows a soft tissue mass which was closely related to the anterior aspect of the ascending aorta bulging forwards and to the right. Heavy calcification is noted in the aorta. The aortogram shows a widened ascending aorta with partial filling of the aneurysm just proximal to the arch. The remainder of the aneurysm is filled with thrombus.

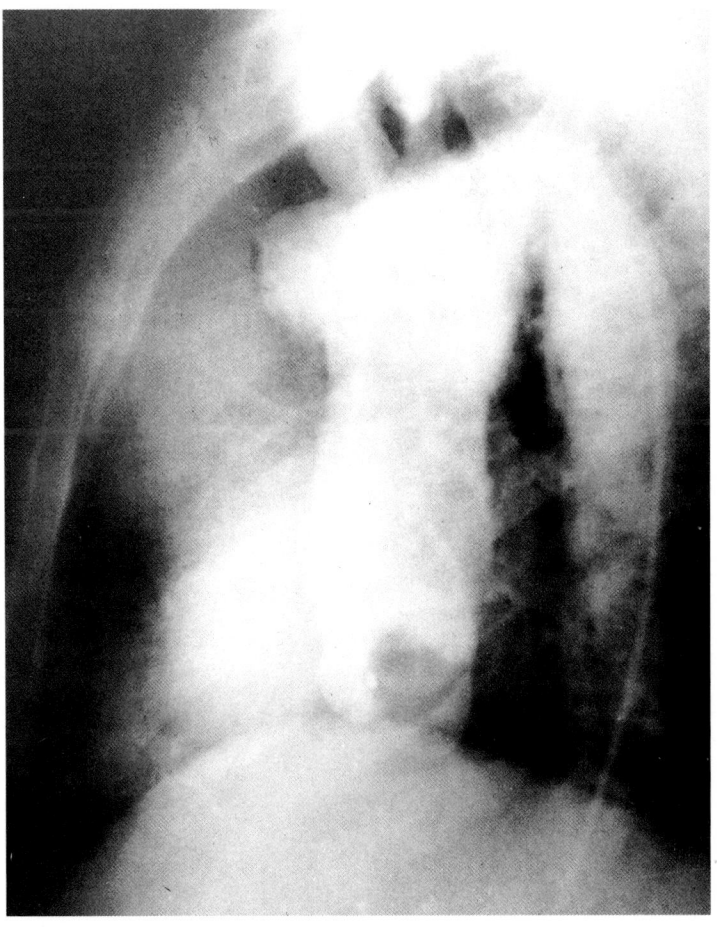

lipomas and hamartomas occur. Projection of the tumour into the lumen of the oesophagus may cause a large polypoid mass to be formed within the lumen on a relatively small stalk. The mass is frequently detected on a plain chest radiograph to the right and in front of the descending aorta and filling the azygo-oesophageal recess (Fig. 8.13).

Neurogenic tumours

Neurogenic tumours are second only to retrosternal thyroid in frequency amongst the mediastinal masses. They include neurofibroma (from the nerve sheath), neurilemmoma (from the sheath of Schwann), ganglioneuroma (from the sympathetic ganglia), ganglioneuroblastoma (usually malignant), neuroblastoma (highly malignant) and paraganglioma (phaechromocytoma and chemodectoma).

Neurofibromas and neurilemmomas mostly arise from the intercostal nerves and rarely from the vagus and phrenic nerves. Neurofibromas may be part of generalized neurofibromatosis (Von Recklinghausen's disease). They appear as smooth, round or oval masses usually in the angle between the vertebral body and the posterior ends of the ribs (Fig. 8.14). The ribs may show evidence of pressure, splaying and erosion caused by the tumour and there may be widening of the intervertebral foramen, particularly if there is an intraspinal component of the tumour.

These tumours also occur along the course of the intercostal nerves in the chest wall and appear then as extrapleural masses on the chest radiograph. Ganglioneuromas occur along the sympathetic chain, as do neuroblastomas; they lie more anteriorly than neurofibromas, along the side of the vertebral body, and appear as paravertebral smooth oval masses with a broad mediastinal base on chest radiographs. Punctate calcification may be visible within the tumours.

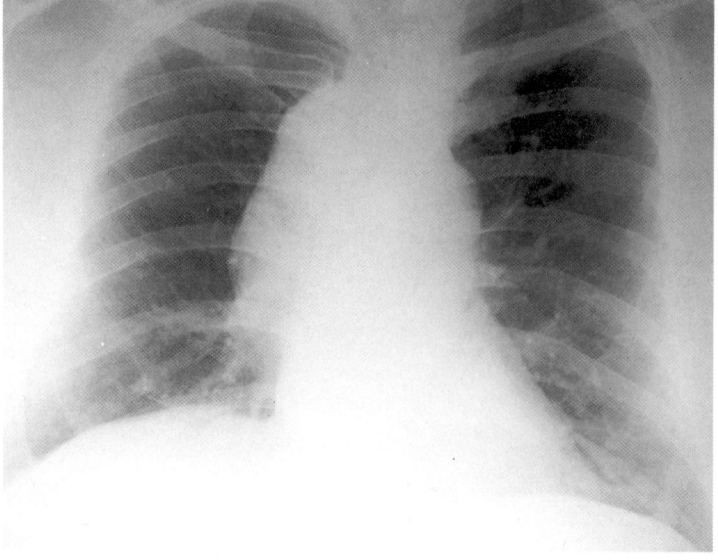

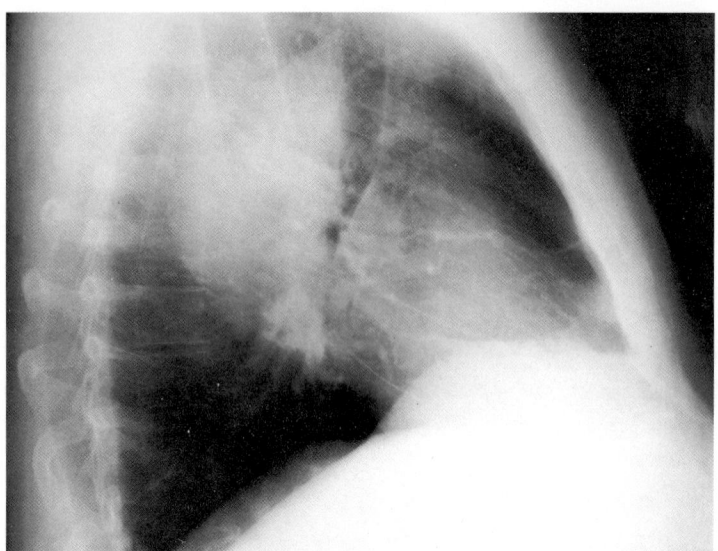

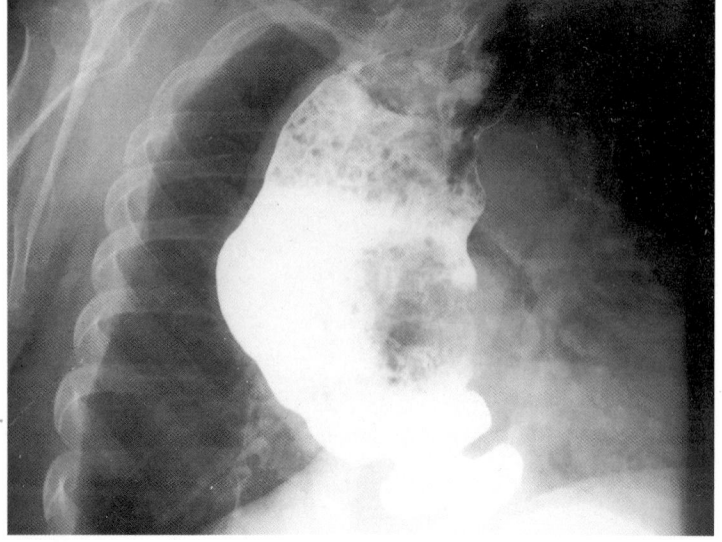

Fig. 8.13 Leiomyoma of the oesophagus. Top and middle, chest radiographs. A large mass is seen in the posterior mediastinum displacing the trachea and main bronchi forward. The mass bulges to the right from the level of the thoracic inlet to the level of the right dome of the diaphragm. Bottom, a barium swallow shows a very large intraluminal filling defect in the oesophagus. The tumour was a pedunculated leiomyoma. The patient had very few symptoms with only occasional dysphagia.

Meningocoele

This rare cause of a posterior mediastinal mass is due to herniation of the meninges through the intervertebral foramen. The appearances of the lesion are similar to neurofibroma with a smooth round paravertebral mass at any level of the thoracic spine. The lesion often causes enlargement of the intervertebral foramen and may be associated with a thoracic scoliosis. Vertebral and rib anomalies are often associated and the lesion may occur in association with generalized neurofibromatosis. It is important to recognize this lesion before a surgical resection of what is thought to be a neurofibroma is undertaken.

The meningocoele may be demonstrated by myelography or by computed tomography, when a connection with the spinal canal can be seen.

Extra-medullary haematopoesis

This is a rare cause of a posterior mediastinal mass. The mass consists of haematopoetic tissue and is associated usually with some form of chronic haemolytic anaemia. The lesion most commonly presents as a lobulated paravertebral mass or masses in the lower part of the thorax (Fig. 8.15).

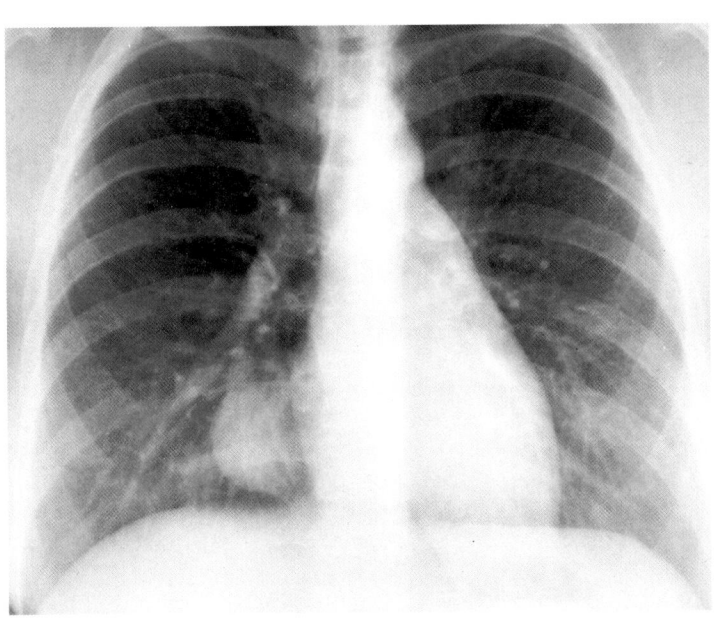

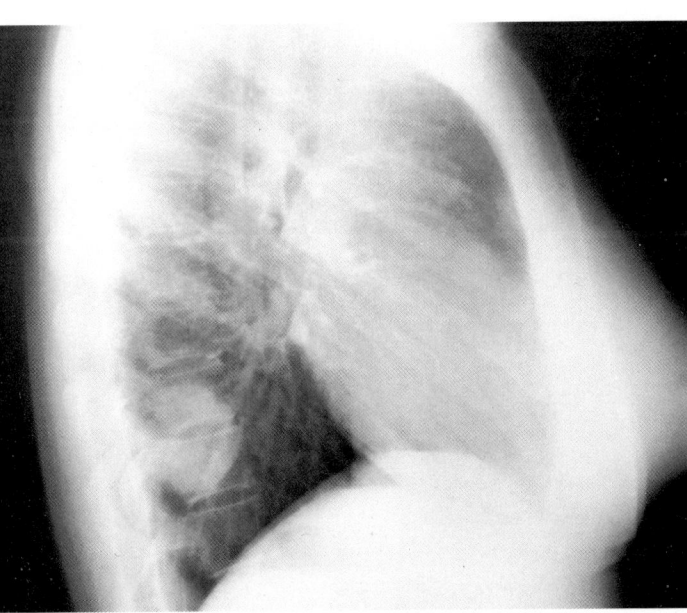

Fig. 8.14 Paravertebral neurofibroma, chest radiographs. A smooth round mass is seen in the right paravertebral gutter. There is slight splaying of the adjacent ribs but no other evidence of bone erosion and no widening of the intervertebral foramen.

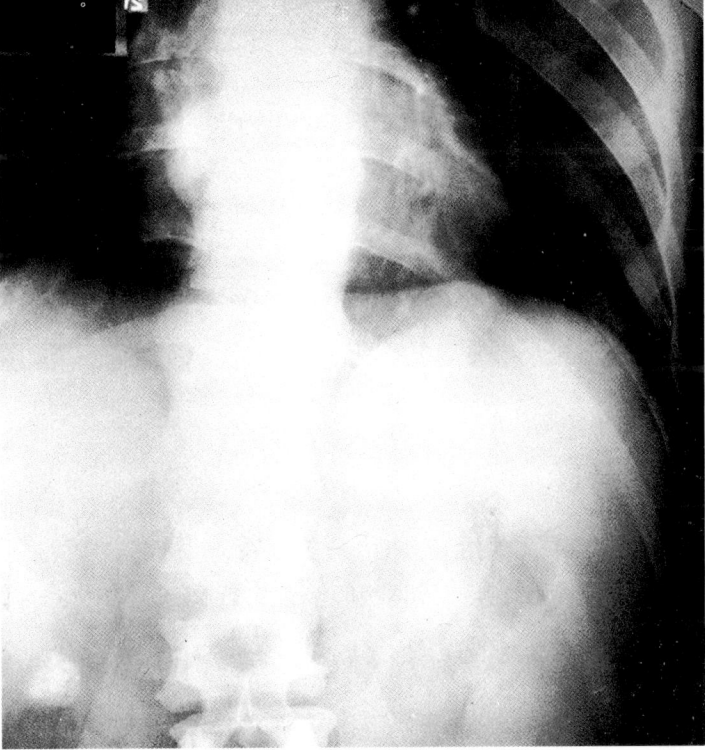

Fig. 8.15 Extramedullary haematopoesis. This radiograph of the upper abdomen and lower thorax in a patient with haemolytic anaemia shows marked splenomegaly and bilateral paravertebral swellings at the level of the diaphragm due to extramedullary haematopoesis.

Tumours of the spine

Tumours of the spine and posterior aspects of the ribs may invade the posterior mediastinum and paravertebral gutter (Fig. 8.16).

Superior mediastinum

Tumours occurring commonly in the superior mediastinum include retrosternal thyroid, enlarged lymph nodes, bronchogenic cysts (see Fig. 2.18) and aneurysms of the aorta and head and neck vessels.

Mediastinitis

Acute mediastinitis

The commonest cause of acute infection of the mediastinum is perforation of the oesophagus which may occur after instrumentation, biopsy, foreign body impaction or may be spontaneous associated with severe vomiting. Occasionally acute mediastinitis results from spread of infection of soft tissues of the neck and the spine. Infected mediastinal cysts may also cause acute mediastinitis. Patients present with severe central chest pain, which may radiate to the arms, fever and leukocytosis. When the infection is the result of rupture of the oesophagus, gas may be seen in the mediastinum and this may spread into the soft tissues of the neck. Acute infection may form abscesses in the mediastinum (Fig. 8.17) which may rupture into the pleura, the bronchi or the oesophagus.

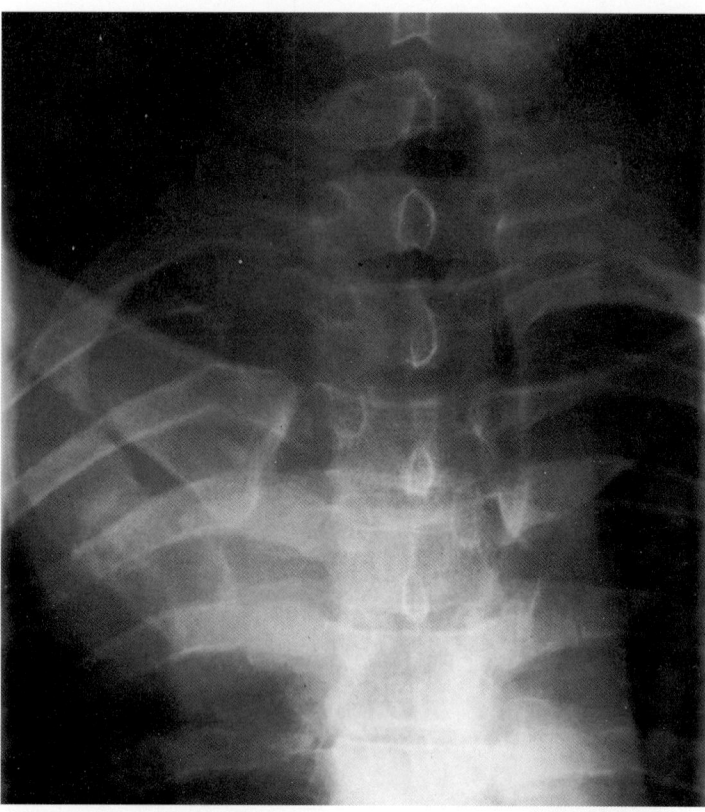

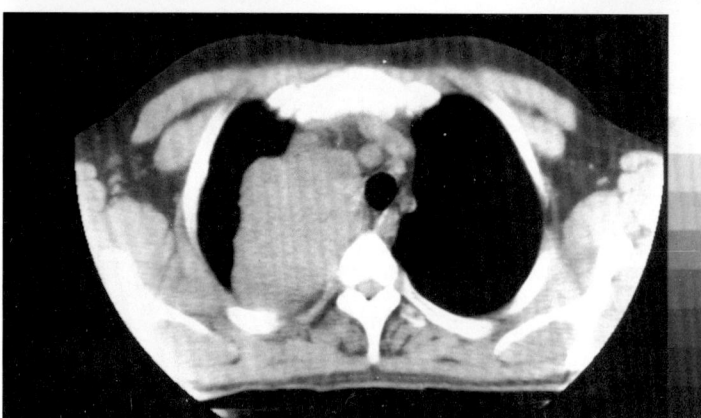

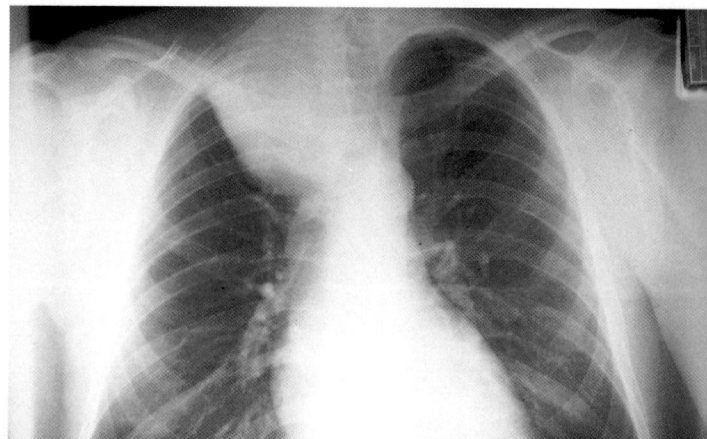

Fig. 8.16 Giant cell tumour of rib. The chest radiograph shows a mass on the right side of the upper mediastinum displacing the trachea slightly to the left. A film of the dorsal spine shows destruction of the medial end of the right second rib. The head and neck of the rib are missing. They should lie just below the transverse process of the vertebra which is intact. The CT scan shows the mass extending forwards on the right side of the mediastinum.

Chronic mediastinitis — fibrosing mediastinitis

Chronic infection of the mediastinum occurs in tuberculosis and histoplasmosis secondary to chronic mediastinal lymphadenitis, and occasionally following infection of the spine. The infection usually invades the upper mediastinum and is associated with considerable fibrosis. In many cases of fibrosing mediastinitis the cause is not found. It may be associated with similar fibrosing conditions in other parts of the body such as retroperitoneal fibrosis, pseudotumour of the orbit, sclerosing cholangitis and Riedel's thyroiditis. Retroperitoneal fibrosis and fibrosing mediastinitis has been reported following injection of methysergide, a drug used in the treatment of migraine. The superior mediastinum is most commonly involved though the fibrosis may extend down to invade the pericardium. Symptoms of superior vena caval obstruction are the commonest presentation, occurring in one-half of cases. The mediastinum is usually widened (Fig. 8.18). A tumour-like mass of fibrous tissue may be present. In addition to the superior vena cava and innominate veins involvement of the aorta, pulmonary arteries and veins, oesophagus and the airways by constricting fibrosis can occur. Spread of the fibrous tissue into the pleura and lungs is occasionally seen. The diagnosis is made by biopsy as differentiation from malignant infiltration cannot otherwise be made.

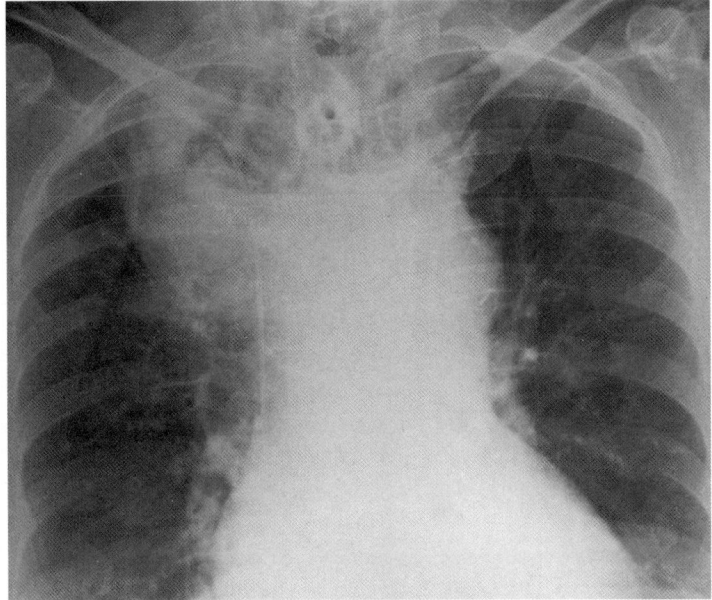

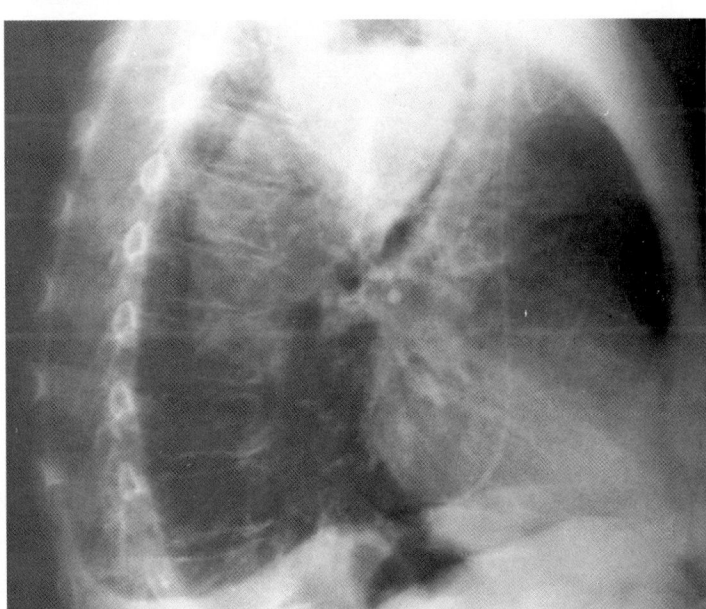

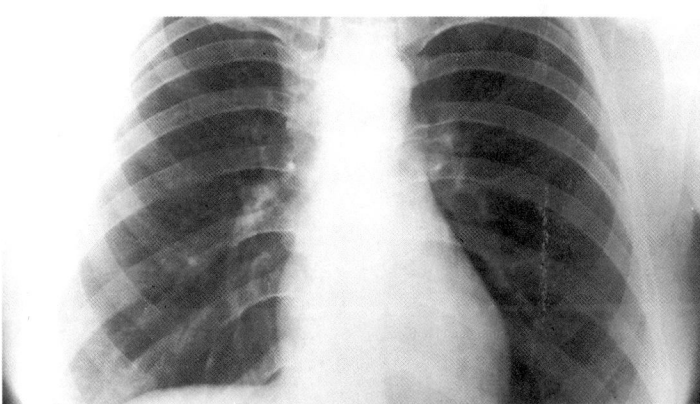

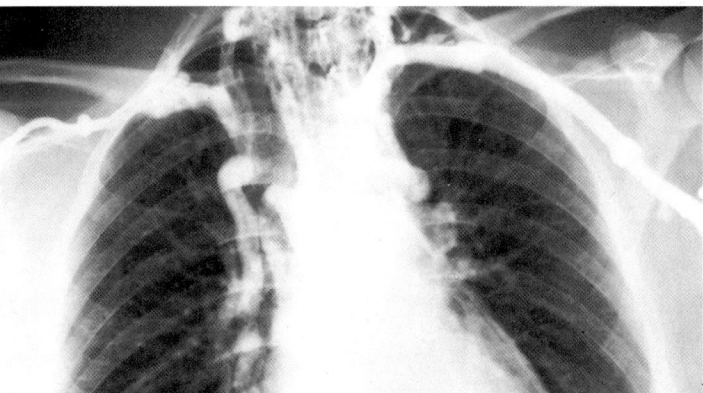

Fig. 8.17 Acute mediastinitis. Following oesophagoscopy the patient became ill with fever, chest pain and surgical emphysema in the neck. Tracheostomy was performed. The radiographs show an abscess has developed in the upper mediastinum behind the trachea which is compressed and displaced forward. There is surgical emphysema in the neck. The patient died. A perforation of the oeosphagus in the neck was discovered at post-mortem leading to an abscess which extended down into the mediastinum.

Fig. 8.18 Fibrosing mediastinitis. The patient presented with obstruction of the superior vena cava. The frontal radiograph shows slight widening of the superior mediastinum due to distension of the collateral veins. A venogram shows no filling of the innominate veins or SVC. There is filling of the azygos and hemiazygos veins; a large right internal mammary vein and the pericardio-phrenic vein on the left.

Pneumomediastinum

Air or gas in the mediastinum may result from trauma (see chapter 9), rupture of the oesophagus (see above), spread upwards of retroperitoneal or peritoneal gas, or spontaneously. Spontaneous pneumomediastinum is rare in adults and occurs most frequently in new born infants. The gas almost certainly arises from the rupture of alveoli in or near the hilum of one of the lungs and tracks from there into the tissue planes of the mediastinum and then into the soft tissues of the neck. Apart from the neonatal period, spontaneous pneumomediastinum is associated with asthmatic attacks, spontaneous pneumothorax, fibrosing conditions of the lungs (such as fibrosing alveolitis), diabetes and parturition. In the last two it appears to be related to prolonged vomiting and prolonged rise in the intra-alveolar pressure associated with labour. In neonates one-third of cases of spontaneous pneumomediastinum give a clear history of aspiration. The condition is also frequently associated with neonatal respiratory distress syndrome. On the chest radiograph, linear and band-like dark lines indicating gas are seen in the mediastinum under the pleura, around the heart, thymus, great vessels and on each side of the trachea passing upwards into the neck (Fig. 8.19). In infants, large quantities of gas may be seen anteriorly outlining the thymus, which is displaced to the right, and pneumopericardium may also be present. Adults, though they may have central chest pain, usually do not suffer respiratory embarrassment as the gas passes freely into the neck, but in some instances, and particularly in infants, the accumulation of gas in the mediastinum causes dyspnoea, obstruction of venous return, tachycardia and hypotension. The gas, if under pressure, may rupture into the pleura and cause pneumothorax.

Mediastinal Haematoma

Trauma is the commonest cause of haemorrhage into the mediastinum (see chapter 9). The second most common

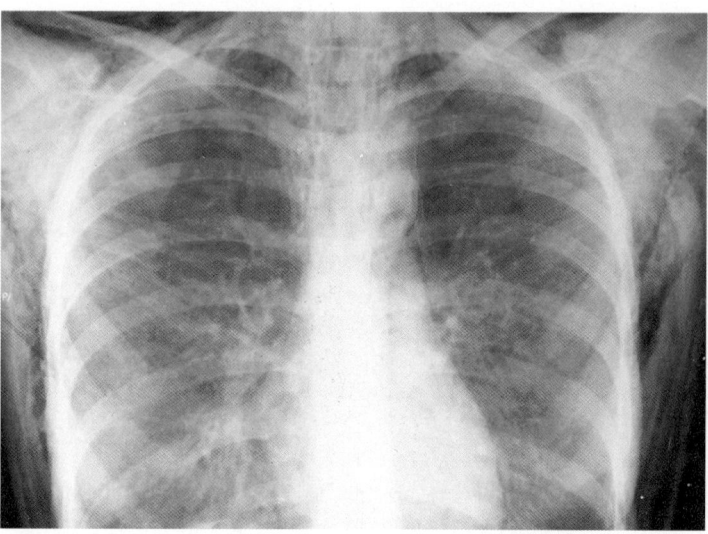

Fig. 8.19 Pneumomediastinum. Associated with a severe attack of asthma. This chest radiograph shows extensive surgical emphysema in the chest wall and neck. Note also the air raising the pleura on the diaphragm around the heart and along the aorta. Linear streaks due to air are seen in the upper mediastinum either side of the trachea and vessels.

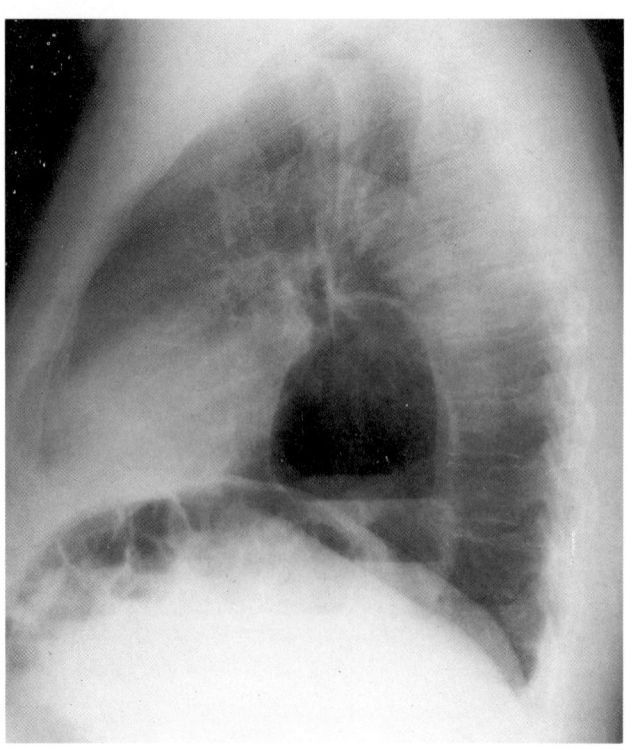

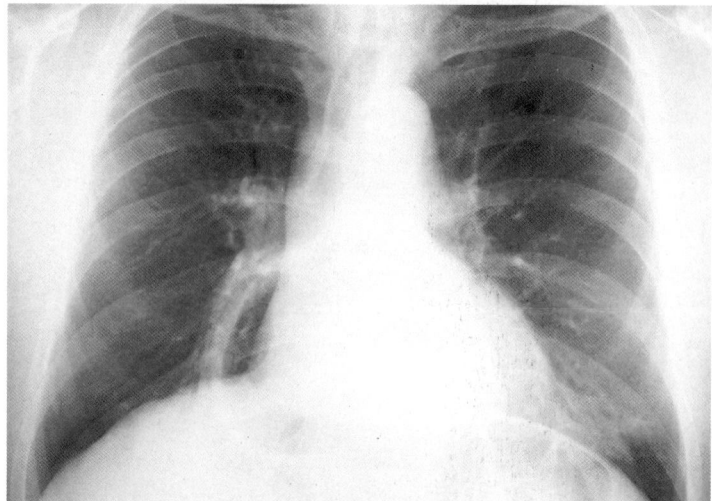

Fig. 8.20 Hiatus hernia and pharyngeal diverticulum. Left and right, radiographs showing a large gas containing viscus which is the major part of the stomach, with fluid levels behind the heart. The stomach has rotated on its long axis after passing into the chest through the diaphragmatic hiatus. In addition an air/fluid level is seen in an opacity in the posterior part of the mediastinum at the thoracic inlet. A barium swallow showed this to be due to a pharyngeal diverticulum.

cause is dissecting aneurysm of the aorta, though other aneurysms may rupture into the mediastinum and cause similar appearances. Bleeding may occasionally be spontaneous, sometimes associated with blood coagulation disorders. The chest radiograph shows widening of the mediastinum, frequently around the aortic arch. Blood may rupture into the pleura and cause haemothorax and may track into the hilum of a lung, usually the left, causing perihilar shadowing and segmental collapse. The superior vena cava may become obstructed.

Oesophageal Disorders

Tumours of the oesophagus are described above under tumours of the mediastinum but there are several disorders of the oesophagus which may cause opacities on the chest radiograph and therefore are discussed here because they enter into the differential diagnosis of other lesions of the mediastinum.

Achalasia of the cardia

Dilatation of the oesophagus may be caused by benign or malignant strictures but is rarely of sufficient magnitude to be apparent on a chest radiograph. In achalasia of the cardia however, in which there is neuromuscular disorder, the oesophagus is frequently greatly dilated and shows as an elongated opacity along the length of the mediastinum on a plain chest radiograph (see Fig. 5.9). Patients complain of dysphagia, regurgitation of food and cough. Sometimes there is no history of oesophageal symptoms, the condition being discovered on a chest radiograph perhaps taken because of recurrent chest infection. On barium examination, the oesophagus is dilated (usually containing undigested food), the cardia is narrow and has a beak-like appearance, opening only occasionally and there is an absence of peristaltic 'stripping' waves in the oesophagus. An air fluid level is frequently present in the oesophagus in the upper part of the mediastinum. The well known sign of absence of a gastric air bubble is not totally reliable as gas is occasionally seen in the stomach even in severe achalasia. Recognized complications of achalasia include recurrent chest infections, lipoid pneumonia and carcinoma of the oesophagus.

Diverticulum of the oesophagus
Pharyngeal (Zenker's) diverticulum
Pharyngeal diverticulum may extend from the neck down into the upper part of the mediastinum. An air fluid level may be seen in the para-oesophageal mass in the upper mediastinum (Fig. 8.20). The diverticulum fills with contrast medium on a barium swallow examination.

Traction diverticulum
This lesion is usually due to fibrosis, following tuberculosis or histoplasmosis, pulling on the oesophagus and forming a diverticulum. Depending on the size of the neck of the diverticulum it will either contain air alone or have an air fluid level. Traction diverticula usually occur in the upper mediastinum.

Pulsion diverticulum
This is due to congenital weakness in the wall of the oesophagus and usually occurs in the lower mediastinum.

Hiatus hernia
Weakness of the oesophageal hiatus permits the upper part of the stomach to herniate into the lower mediastinum. This may be intermittent and only demonstrable on a barium study with the patient tilted head downwards in the Trendelenberg position or it may be constant and visible as a ring opacity behind the heart, often with a fluid level on a plain chest radiograph (Figs 8.20 and 8.21). Patients with hiatus hernia have variable symptoms. The reflux of gastric contents which is associated with a loss of normal sphincter mechanism at the cardia when it lies in the chest may cause oesophagitis with pain and discomfort. Benign stricture of the oesophagus may then result from the continued regurgitation of gastric fluid into the oesophagus.

Systemic sclerosis
Systemic sclerosis may affect the oesophagus. At first there is some loss of motility with mild dilatation; later reflux oesophagitis and hiatus hernia may occur giving rise to oesophageal stricture.

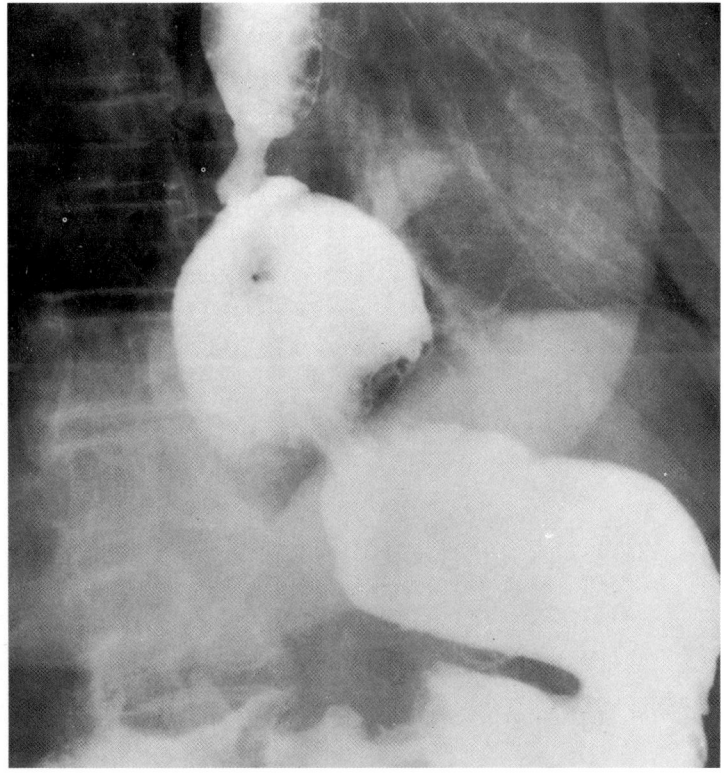

Fig. 8.21 Hiatus hernia. Barium meal showing a hernia with free gastro-oesophageal reflux in the supine position. Some localised narrowing of the oesophagus is present just above the cardia due to oesophagitis.

9

Chest Injuries

Trauma to the chest is often of great importance though unfortunately frequently not recognized because head injuries, fractures of limbs and superficial wounds distract attention from injury to vital organs within the thoracic cage. The thoracic cage provides considerable protection against injury to the intrathoracic organs though in children, where the ribs are more pliable, protection is less. Injuries may be due to blunt or penetrating trauma. Penetrating wounds are often accompanied by the introduction of foreign material and bacteria so that not only are there the direct effects of trauma but also the complications of infection. Thus gunshot wounds and stab wounds are frequently followed by lung abscesses, empyema, acute mediastinitis etc.

The basic investigation for chest trauma is the frontal chest radiograph. This should if possible be taken in the erect position, though in seriously injured patients this may not be possible. Interpretation of radiographs taken with the patient supine is more difficult. Such lesions as pleural effusions and pneumothorax may be difficult to appreciate as they collect at the back and front of the chest respectively in the supine position. Radiological investigation with computed tomography (CT), arteriography etc. may be necessary to diagnose and show the extent of injury to the thoracic organs.

Ribs and Chest Wall

Contusion of the chest wall and fractures of ribs and the sternum, though painful, are not usually of serious clinical consequence. Fractures may occur anywhere in the ribs but the common site is along the postero-lateral aspects of the sixth to the ninth ribs; this is also the commonest site for stress fractures due to coughing (Fig. 9.1). Fractures to the first three ribs are an indication that there has been severe trauma to the chest and a careful search for evidence of rupture of the trachea and bronchi and of the aorta should then be made. Fractures of the lower three ribs may be associated with injury to the spleen, liver or kidneys. With fractures of the ribs there is frequently an extra-pleural haematoma causing an extra-pleural opacity on the radiograph, best seen on tangential views of the ribs.

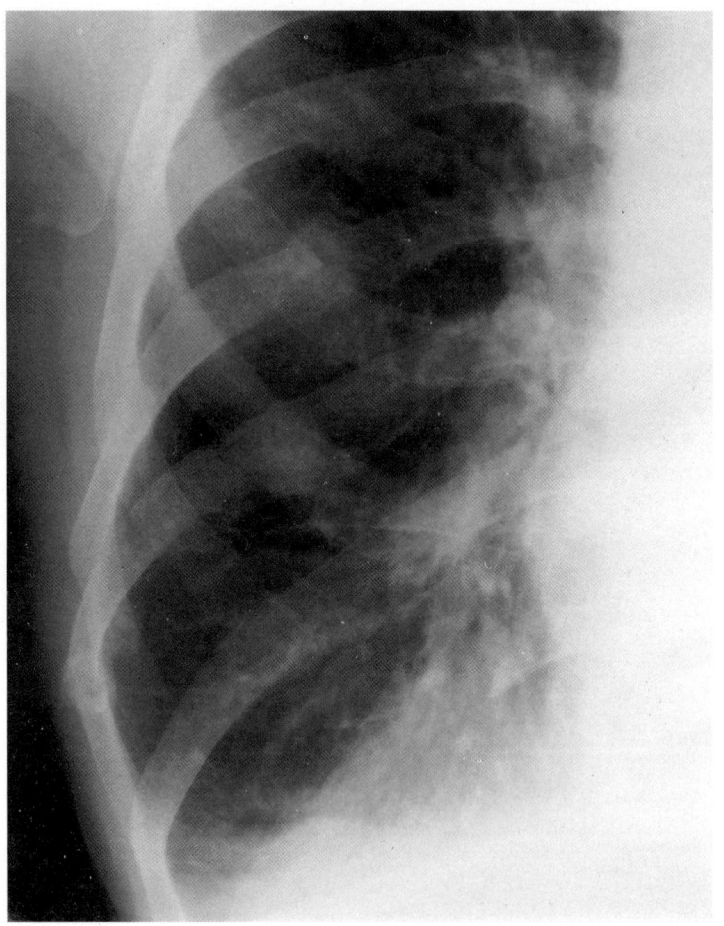

Fig. 9.1 Fractures of the seventh, eighth and ninth ribs with abundant callus due to coughing in a patient with chronic bronchitis.

Blows to the front of the chest may cause a fracture of the sternum — this will not be visible on the frontal radiograph and lateral views and tomography may be necessary to demonstrate the break.

Complications of fracture of the ribs include pneumothorax, pleural effusions, haemothorax and a flail segment ('stove-in chest'). Occasionally, surgical emphysema in the chest wall can be seen without any evidence of pneumothorax. However, puncture of the lungs must have occurred to produce the surgical emphysema and a pneumothorax may develop later. Where there are multiple fractures of ribs then a segment of the chest wall may lose its rigidity and show visible paradoxical movement on respiration (Fig. 9.2).

Pleura

Pneumothorax

Penetrating injuries or puncture of the lung by fractured ribs may cause pneumothorax. The importance of recognition of this complication is that it may lead to tension pneumothorax where the intra-pleural pressure becomes so great that the lungs are compressed and the mediastinum so shifted that cardiovascular embarrassment occurs leading to cardiac arrest and death. It is particularly important to recognize a pneumothorax if it is necessary to intubate the patient and give intermittent positive pressure respiration or a general anaesthetic as these may convert a

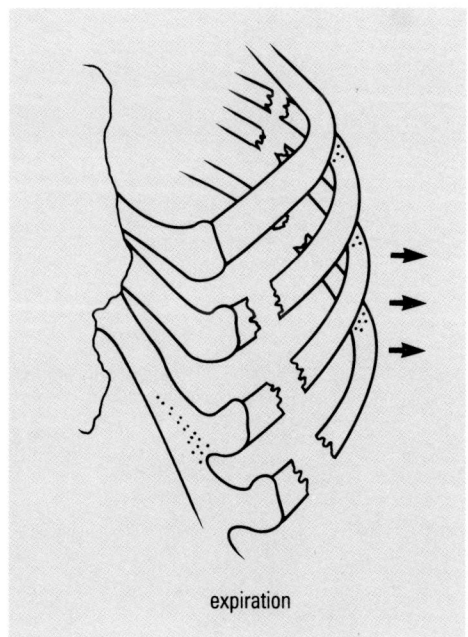

expiration

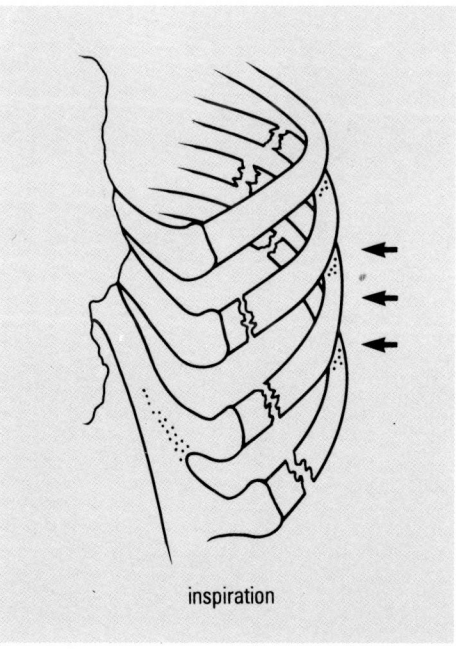

inspiration

Fig. 9.2 Diagram showing a flail segment (stove-in chest) moving paradoxically on respiration.

simple pneumothorax into a tension pneumothorax (Fig. 9.3). When a pneumothorax is present a line due to the visceral pleura is seen on the chest radiograph running parallel to the chest wall. This line may be more easily seen on a radiograph taken on expiration rather than inspiration. Between the line of the chest wall no lung markings (vessels) can be identified (Fig. 9.4). The lung which is collapsing as a result of the pneumothorax does not become more dense until the pneumothorax is very large. With a small pneumothorax a reduction in ventilation of the lung causes a vasoconstriction and the lung vessels diminish, thus the overall density of the collapsing lung is unaltered. However, if there is contusion of the lung, infection or pulmonary oedema, the lung will become more dense and the pneumothorax more readily seen. If the radiograph is taken with the patient supine, the air in the pleura may collect anteriorly and appear as a radio-

lucent area outlining the heart border or the anterior aspect of the diaphragm (Fig. 9.5). If possible a film in the lateral decubitus position or a lateral view with the beam horizontal should be obtained to confirm the pneumothorax if it is not possible to obtain a film in the erect position.

Haemothorax and pleural effusion

Blood cannot be distinguished from effusion on a chest radiograph but is found on aspiration. Haemorrhage into the pleural space usually results from a tear of the lung and pleura or from damage to an intercostal vessel and is a frequent accompaniment of traumatic pneumothorax and of penetrating wounds of the chest wall. Fluid in the pleura accumulates in the classical manner when the patient is erect — in the costophrenic sulcus rising in the axilla and posteriorly. Occasionally it only collects below the lung

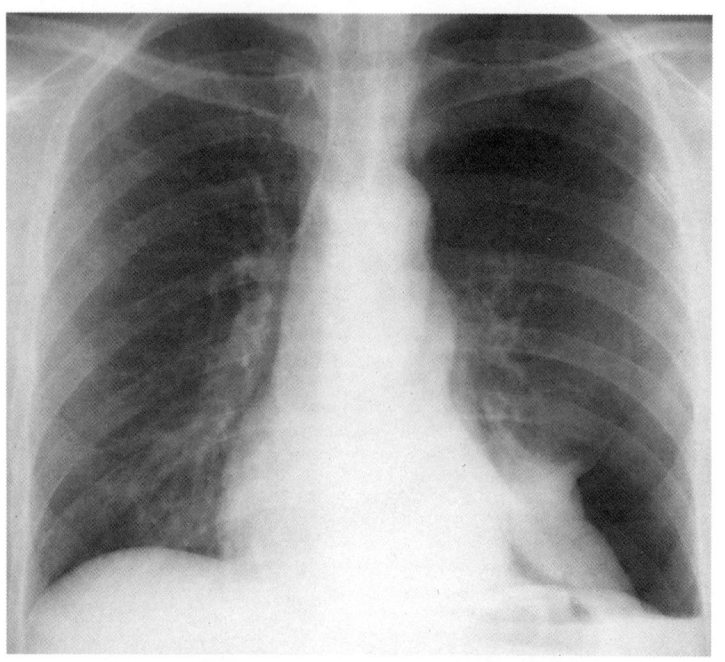

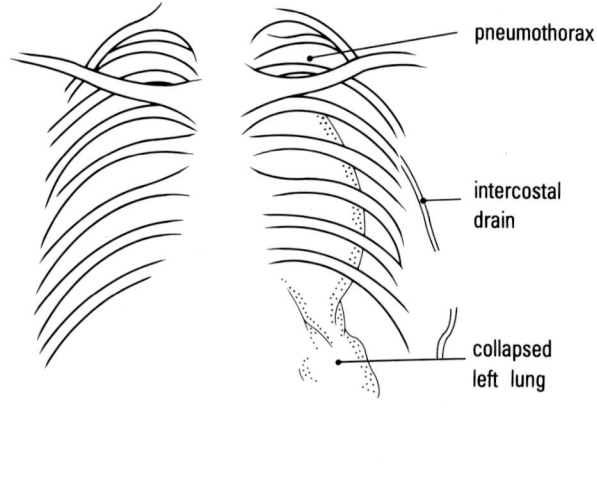

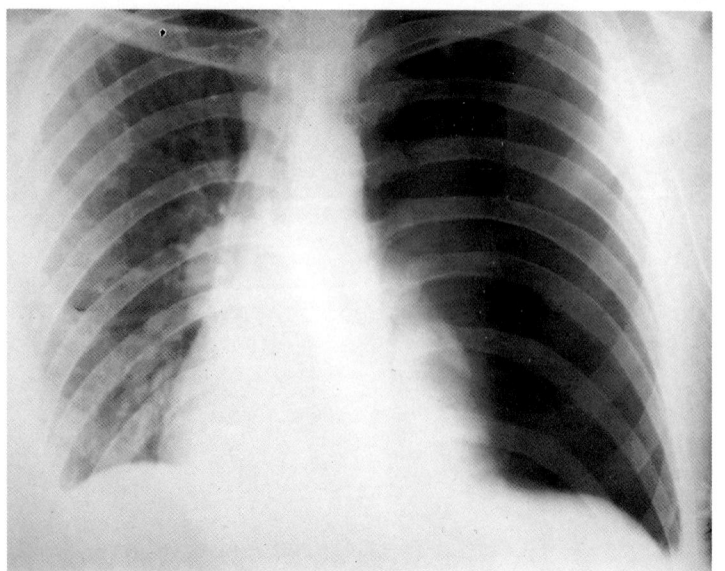

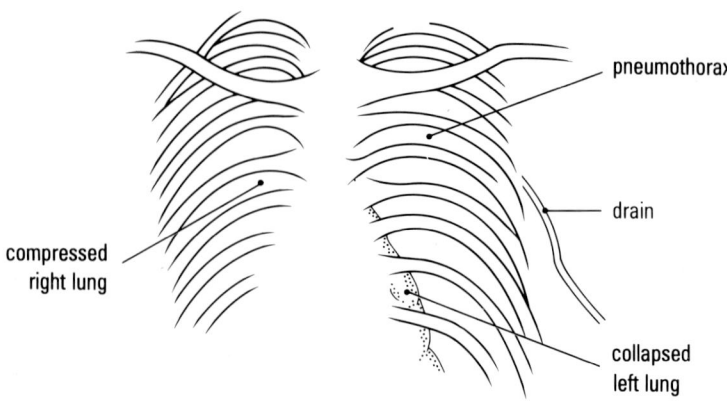

Fig. 9.3 (a) A simple pneumothorax becoming (b) a tension pneumothorax, because of displacement of the intercostal drainage tube seen in the left axilla.

between the lower lobes and the diaphragm. This sub-pulmonary collection of fluid may be difficult to recognize particularly on the right side where there is no gastric air bubble to outline the undersurface of the diaphragm. It should be suspected when there is an apparent elevation of the diaphragm on an erect frontal radiograph (see Chapter 7). If the patient is supine the fluid will collect posteriorly and appear on the chest radiograph as a homogeneous increase in density. A radiograph in the lateral decubitus position may be necessary to show the effusion.

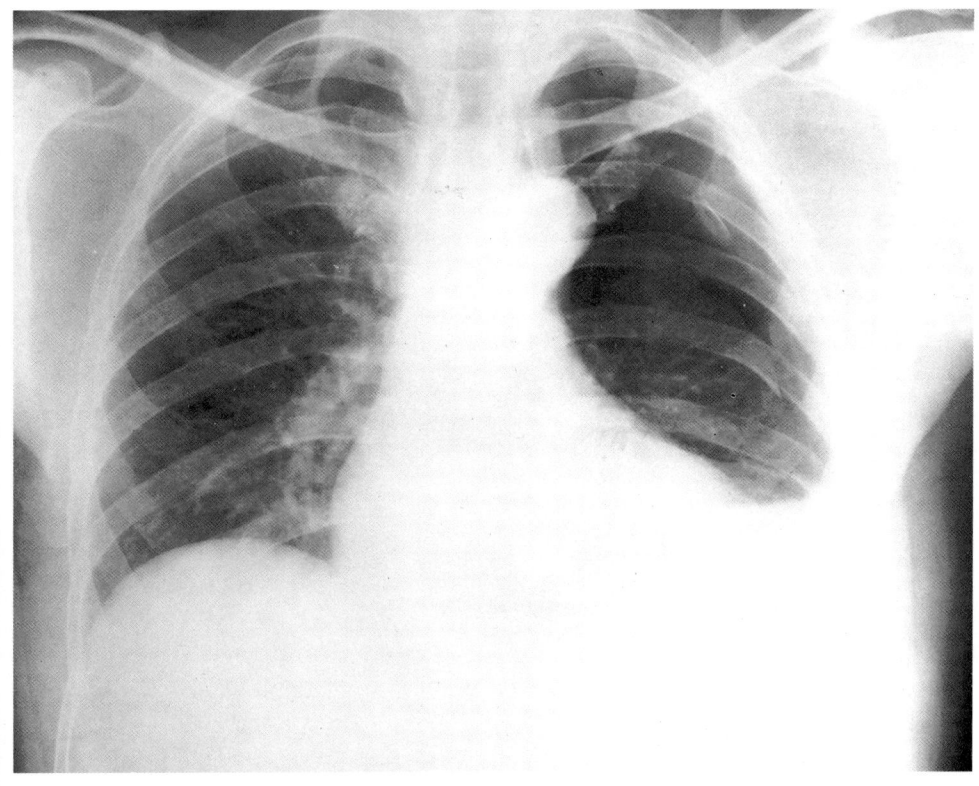

Fig. 9.4 Erect frontal radiograph showing multiple fractures of the left ribs and a hydropneumothorax with a fluid level above the left dome of the diaphragm.

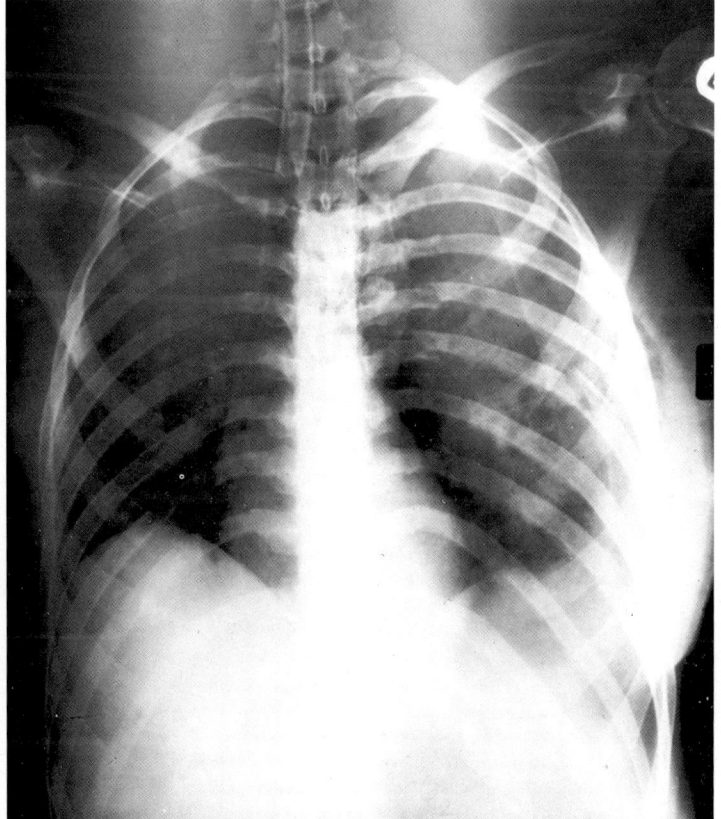

Fig. 9.5 Supine frontal radiograph in a severely injured patient. Fractures of the left, third to ninth ribs are present and there is a left hydropneumothorax. Note the air to the left of the heart and the lung edge running about 1 inch parallel to the chest wall above the diaphragm. Note also a little surgical emphysema in the chest wall. As the patient was being ventilated, this pneumothorax became a tension pneumothorax shortly after this examination was performed.

The Lung

Contusion

Bruising of the lung develops within a few hours of injury, usually on the side of the trauma but sometimes in the opposite lung as a contre-coup injury. It appears on the chest radiograph as ill-defined, non-segmental, non-homogeneous opacification of the lung (Fig. 9.6). It may increase over the first 24 hours but then gradually clears over the next few days so that by one week complete resolution has usually occurred.

Laceration of the lung

A tear of the lung may result from penetrating or blunt trauma. In the latter, shearing forces cause tears into which there is bleeding and an intra-pulmonary haematoma forms — such haematomas may be single or multiple. At first they are usually ill-defined because of surrounding contusion but as time passes they form clearly-defined round or elliptical radiographic opacities (Fig. 9.7). These lesions may cavitate and develop air fluid levels or they may form clearly defined intra-pulmonary cysts — either air or fluid containing.

Fat embolism

Though not necessarily a result of trauma to the chest an injured person usually with a fracture of the legs or pelvis, may suffer from embolization of fat into the lungs and also into the systemic system. If not severe, the chest radiograph may be normal but at about 48 to 72 hours widespread fine nodular opacification of the lungs may occur, sometimes with confluent patchy areas of consolidation (Fig. 9.8). The opacities are due to small fat particles in the alveolar capillaries leading to extensive intra-alveolar haemorrhages. This damage to the alveolar capillaries may cause the adult respiratory distress syndrome (ARDS) which may lead to death.

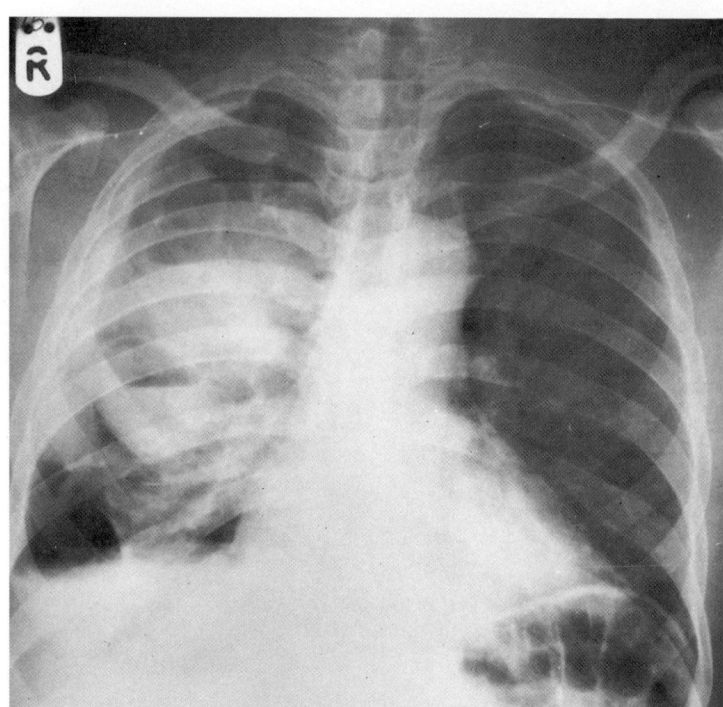

Fig. 9.7 Multiple lacerations of the right lung with haematomas following a road traffic accident. Several of the right ribs are broken including the upper three.

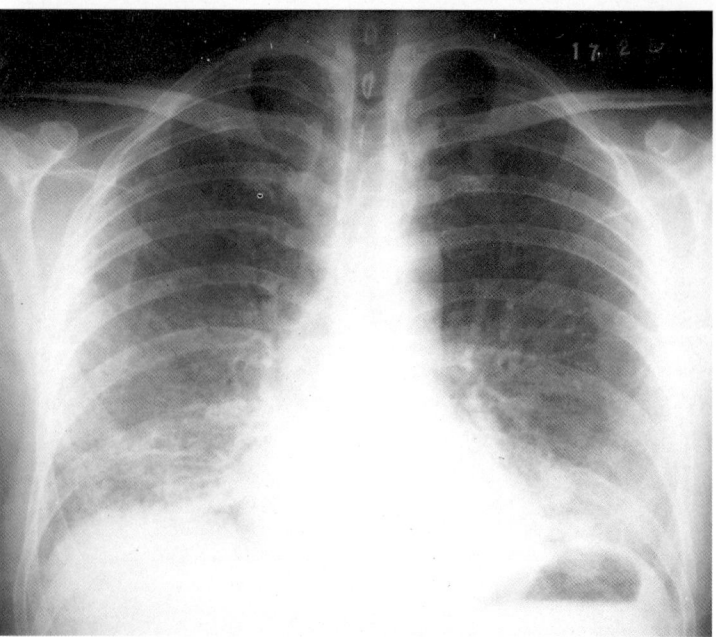

Fig. 9.8 Fat embolism. Chest radiograph. Fine nodular opacities have developed in the lung three days after severe trauma causing fractures of the femur and pelvis.

Fig. 9.6 A radiograph showing extensive contusion of the left lung. There are fractures of both first ribs.

Inhalation

Inhalation of blood, vomit, foreign material (both fluid and solid) and foreign bodies frequently occurs in the severely injured. Obstruction of the airways leads to pulmonary collapse (Figs 9.9 and 9.10). Later infection with pneumonia and abscesses may complicate the clinical and radiological picture, particularly if early aspiration and removal of foreign material is not undertaken.

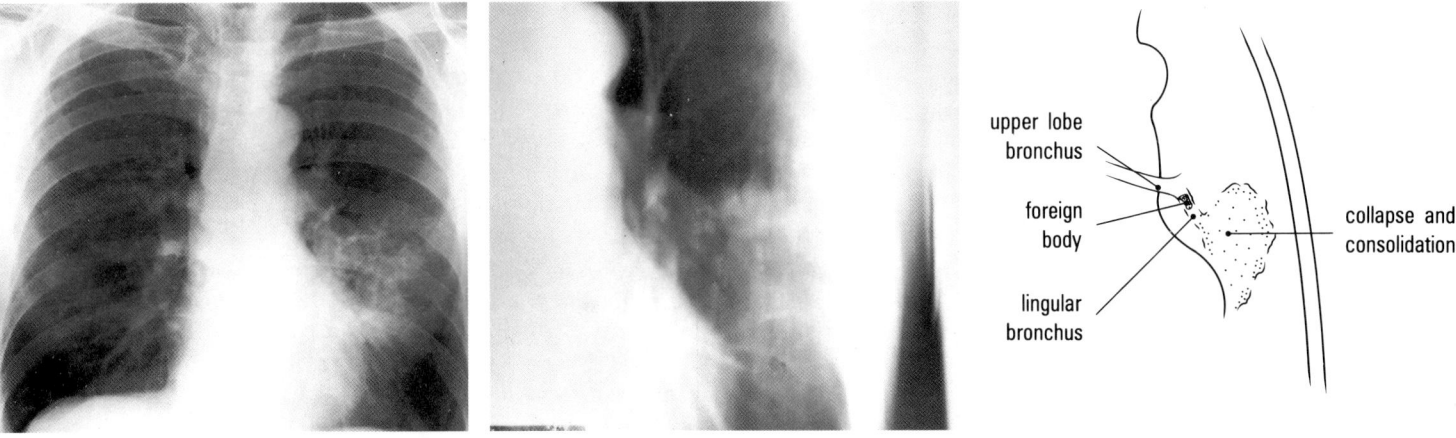

Fig. 9.9 Foreign body. (a) An area of collapse and consolidation is seen in the lingula. (b) A tomogram shows an opaque foreign body, a piece of mutton bone, in the lingular bronchus.

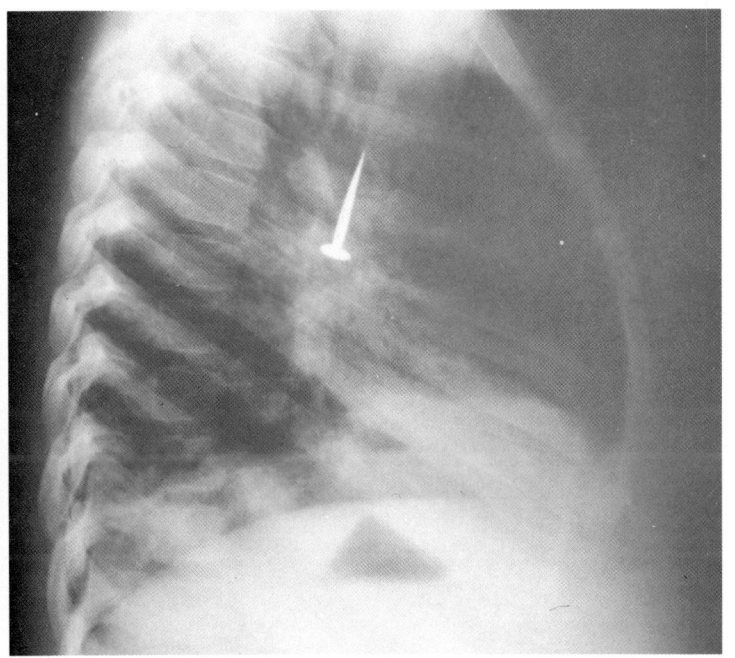

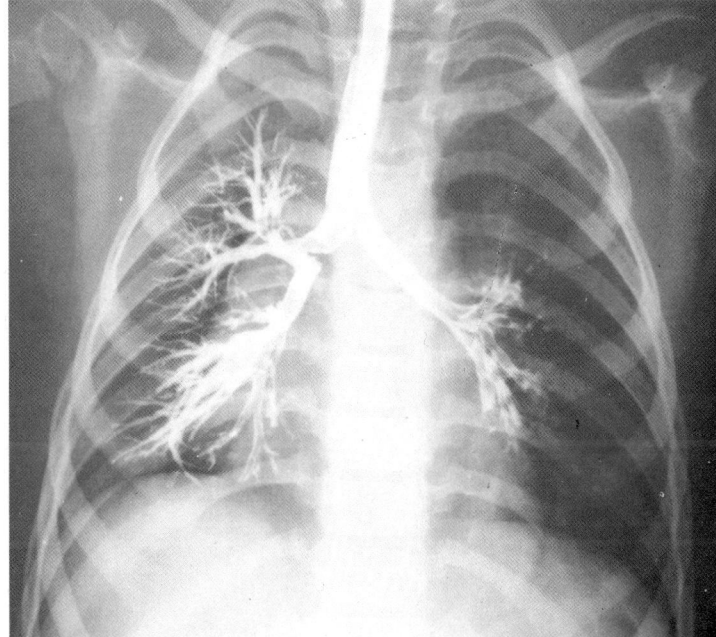

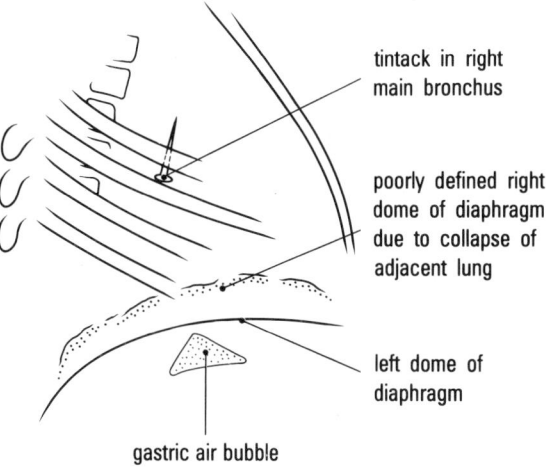

Fig. 9.10 Lateral radiograph and bronchogram of a child. A metallic foreign body, a tintack, is seen obstructing the right intermediate bronchus and causing collapse of the right middle and lower lobes. Bronchography after removal of the tintack shows a residual localized stenosis of the bronchus at the site of impaction.

Shock lung
(adult respiratory distress syndrome — ARDS)

This serious complication of trauma is due to the breakdown of the integrity of the alveolar–capillary membrane allowing leakage of fluid, serum and blood into the alveoli and interstitium of the lung. Symptoms generally start about 48 hours after injury. The damage to the alveolar–capillary membrane causes respiratory failure which nearly always precedes the onset of radiographic change by some 12 hours. The chest radiograph may then show in both lungs patchy ill-defined areas of homogeneous density which may become confluent (Fig. 9.11). An air bronchogram is frequently present and the appearances are those of patchy consolidation. These areas, over the next 24 hours, may increase in extent so that the areas become confluent. The lung becomes stiff and assisted ventilation is usually required to maintain oxygenation. If resolution is slow fibrous elements are laid down and the radiograph develops a reticular pattern or later a honeycomb pattern indicating extensive fibrosis.

Radiation pneumonitis

Extensive therapeutic radiation may cause considerable pulmonary damage. Response of the tissues however is variable and depends on several factors. The larger the irradiated volume the greater the effects. A dose of less than 20 Gy (2000 rads) is unlikely to cause any damage to the lungs. Chemotherapeutic drugs such as bleomycin and cyclophosphamide potentiate the effect of radiation and corticosteroids suppress it.

The acute phase of pneumonitis does not usually commence until two to three months after the completion of radiotherapy. There is sometimes a pleural effusion. The chest radiograph shows increasing opacification of the irradiated area of lung often with a sharp edge correspond-

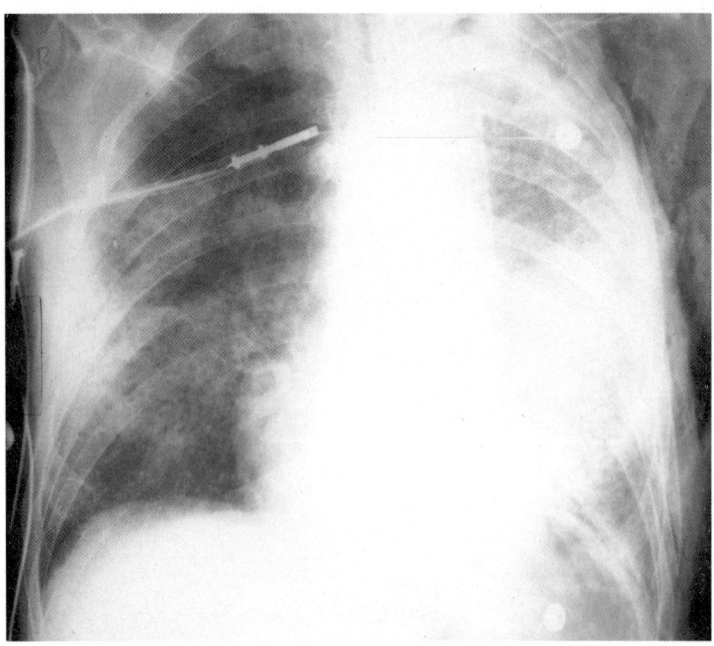

Fig. 9.11 Shock lung. Five days following left upper lobectomy. Diffuse opacification of both lungs due to alveolar exudate has occurred. The appearances on the left are complicated by postoperative changes including surgical emphysema in the chest wall. An endotracheal tube is present as the patient is being ventilated.

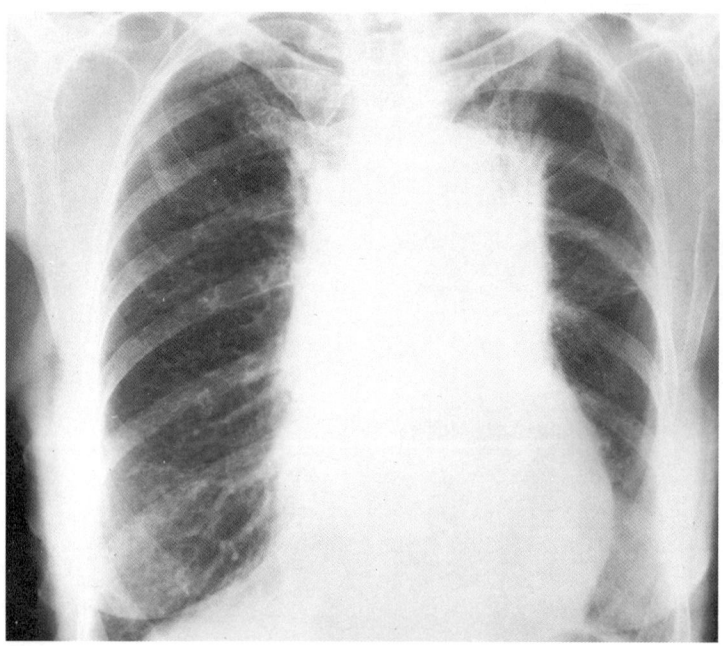

Fig. 9.12 Radiation pneumonitis. A radiograph showing dense pulmonary consolidation with an air bronchogram visible in the upper part of the left side of the irradiated area.

ing to the edge of the radiation port. This area of lung becomes consolidated and an air bronchogram is often visible (Fig. 9.12).

In the chronic phase, symptoms decrease unless the volume of lung affected is sufficient to cause respiratory embarrassment. Fibrosis of the affected lung occurs and this may progress for up to two years. The chest radiograph may then show a dense area of shrunken fibrotic lung.

The Trachea and Main Bronchi

Damage to the trachea occurring from endotracheal intubation is usually slight and of no consequence but prolonged intubation, especially with a cuffed tube, can lead to pressure ulceration of the tracheal mucosa which may heal by fibrosis and stricture formation (Fig. 9.13).

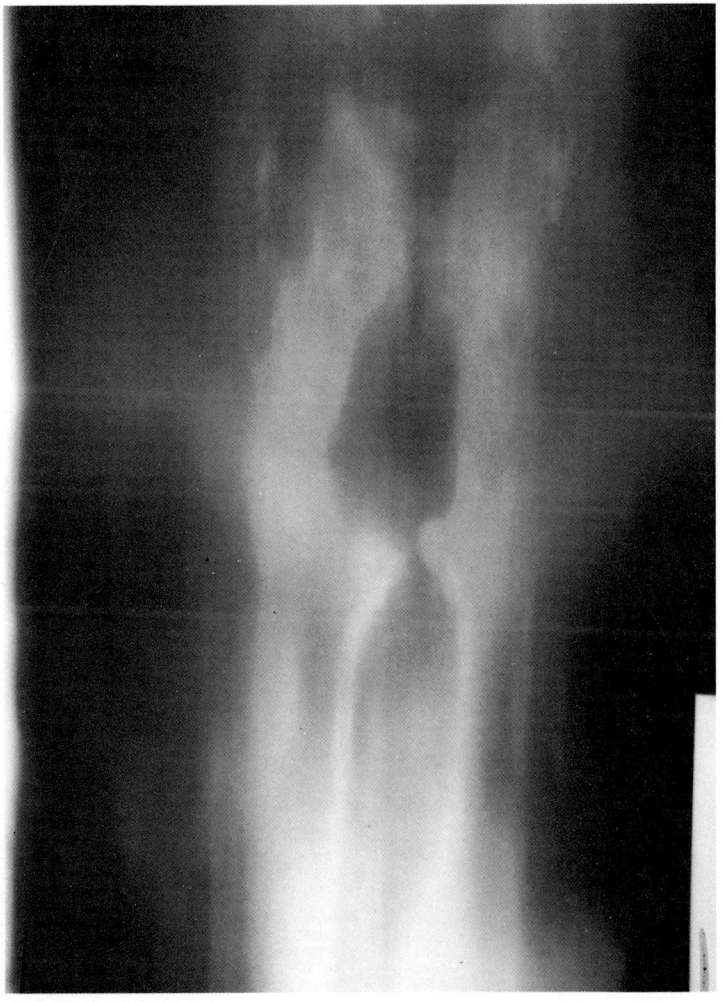

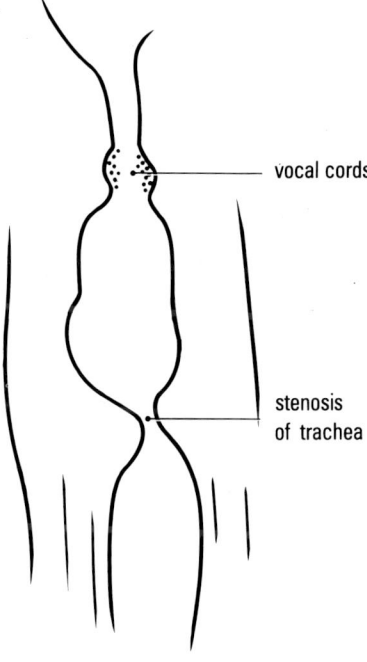

Fig. 9.13 A tomogram showing stenosis of the trachea following prolonged intubation.

Trauma to the chest may cause a tear or rupture of the trachea or main bronchi. A rupture may totally encircle the airway so that there is separation of the ends or a tear may be incomplete and not involve all the layers of the wall. The trachea in the neck may be damaged by blunt or penetrating trauma though in the thorax blunt trauma is usually responsible. In fifty percent of cases of rupture of the trachea or main bronchi, fractures of the first three ribs are present.

Recognition of damage to the airway will frequently depend on the chest radiograph. The commonest finding is pneumothorax, though in at least one-third this is not present and pneumomediastinum is the only early feature (Fig. 9.14) (see chapter 8). The air may track upwards into the soft tissues of the neck and subcutaneous surgical emphysema may become palpable. Collapse of the lung may occur though this complication may be late and result from neglecting surgical repair of a ruptured bronchus — such lack of intervention leads to a stricture of the airway (Fig. 9.15). Rupture of the airway should be suspected on the radiograph and confirmed by bronchoscopy.

Aorta and its Main Branches

Rupture of the aorta is a severe complication of both blunt and penetrating trauma and is the commonest cause of death in chest injury. In post-mortem cases the ascending aorta just above the aortic valve is affected by chest trauma much more frequently than in those who survive, in ninety-five percent of whom the tear is at the isthmus and insertion of the ligamentum arteriosum. It is commonly accepted that the cause is due to sudden deceleration of the body making the heart, lungs and ascending aorta move rapidly forward. This injury is commonly the sequel to an automobile accident but has also been reported following other forms of trauma such as falls from a height, air crashes, falls from horses and blows to the trunk from blunt objects. Immediate death is the commonest outcome but ten to twenty percent survive over one hour. In those who survive the tear involves the media and intima, the adventitia remaining intact. As the adventitia is not totally impervious to blood, bleeding occurs into the mediastinum to a variable degree (Fig. 9.16). Rupture of this remaining layer may occur at any time especially as blood pressure recovers after the initial shock of injury. Because the condition is treatable by immediate surgery, its recognition is of great importance.

Progressive widening of the upper mediastinum after an injury may be due to venous haemorrhage but because it may follow a rupture of the aorta, aortography should be undertaken. CT may show an aneurysm and a large tear but is unlikely to show small tears. When more widely available, magnetic resonance imaging and endo-oesophageal ultrasound may become the methods of choice as the aorta

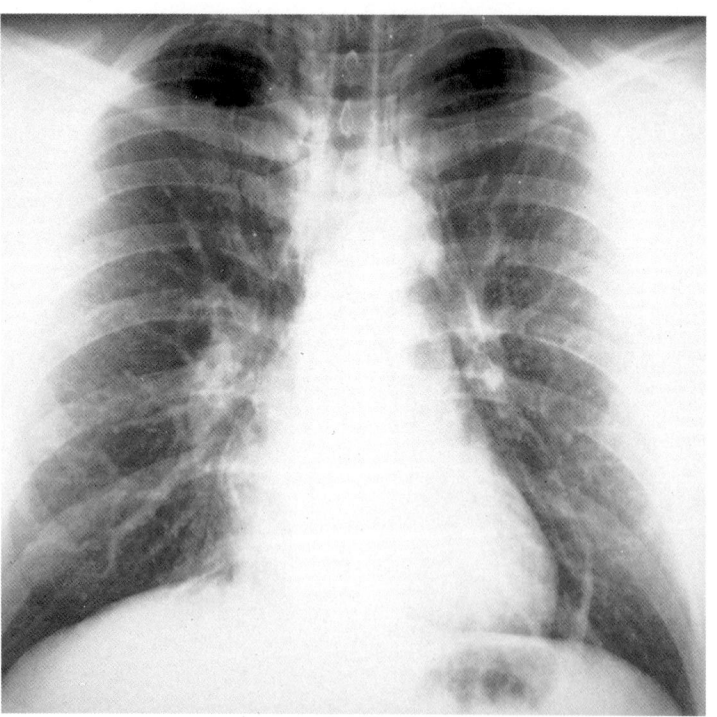

Fig. 9.14 Rupture of the trachea. Air in the mediastinum outlining the heart, trachea and vessels has resulted from a tear in the lower trachea in this patient following a road traffic accident. He had a fracture of both legs and the pneumomediastinum was at first overlooked. He subsequently developed a pneumothorax and collapse of the left lung.

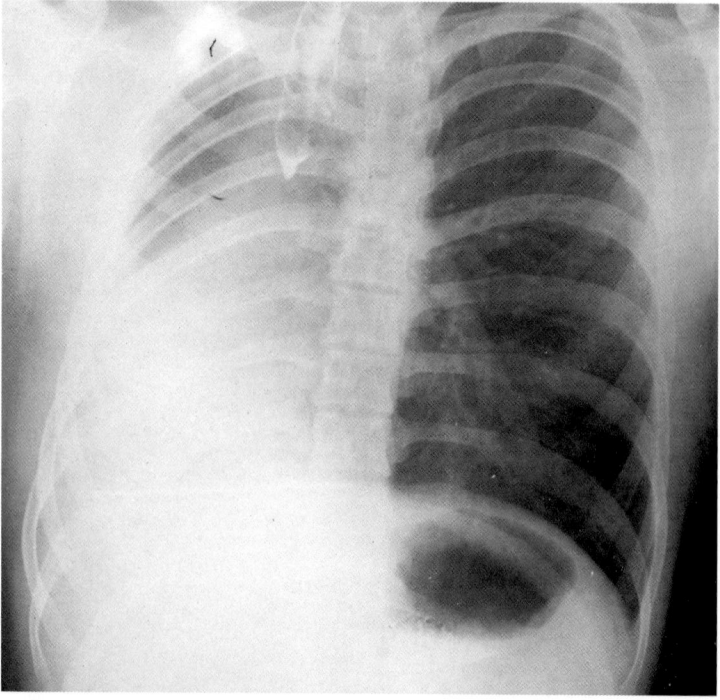

Fig. 9.15 Total collapse of the right lung as a result of a stricture of the right main bronchus following rupture. This patient had had severe trauma with rupture of the spleen and liver and multiple fractures. Repair of the bronchus was not performed. Frontal radiograph with contrast medium in the trachea and right main bronchus which is totally occluded near its origin.

is well displayed by these methods. In addition to progressive widening of the mediastinum, the chest radiograph may show loss of definition and outline or increase in size of the aortic knuckle. The left main bronchus may be displaced downwards. Blood may track into the hilum of the left lung and cause perihilar shadowing. It may burst through into the pleural space, almost invariably on the left side, causing a haemothorax. A useful early radiological sign of ruptured aorta is the appearance of an extra-pleural opacity at the left apex, an apical cap, due to blood tracking along the course of the left subclavian artery (Fig. 9.17). Angiographically, all that may be seen is a

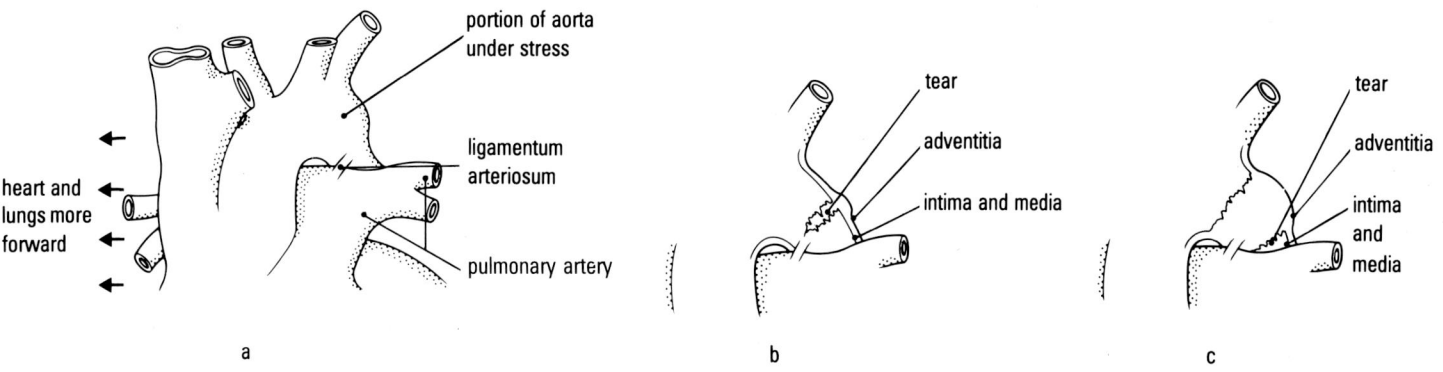

a

b

c

Fig. 9.16 Diagram of aortic rupture. (a) Mechanism of tear of the isthmus. (b) Partial tear. (c) Complete tear.

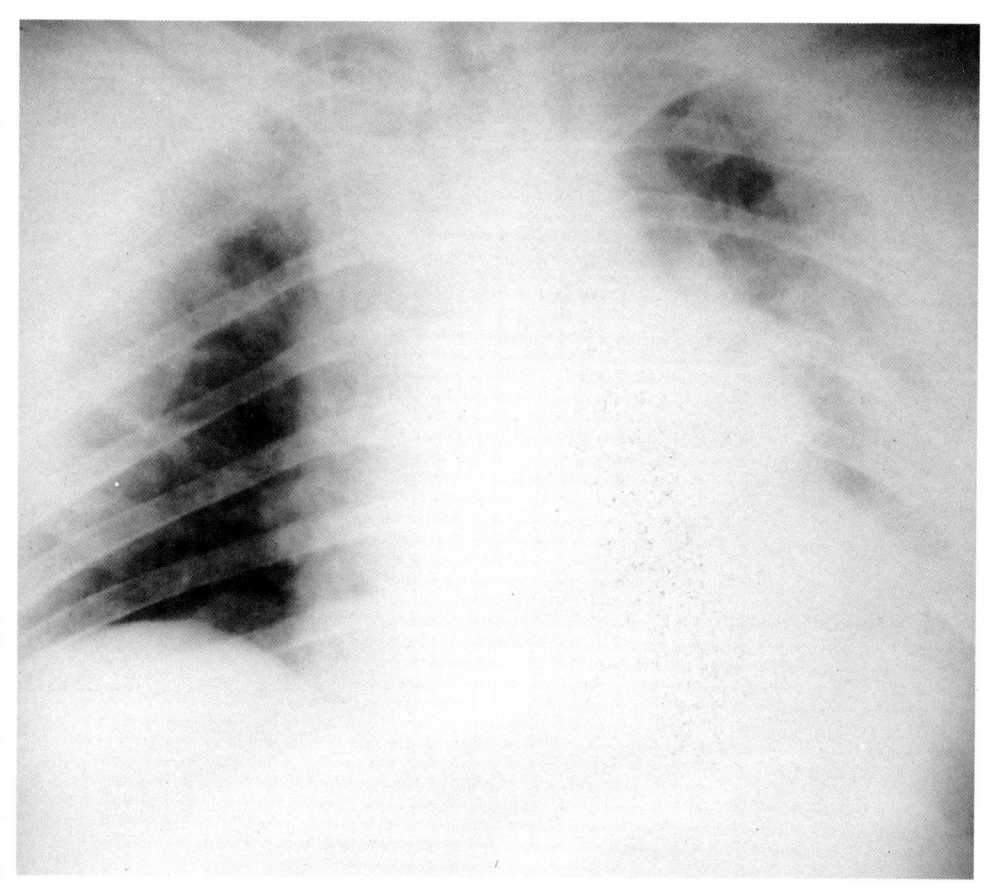

Fig. 9.17 Rupture of the aorta. Three hours after an automobile accident, this radiograph with the patient supine shows widening of the mediastinum, loss of definition of the aortic knuckle, a left apical cap and blood in the left perihilar region.

small break in the outline of the aorta and a flap of intima within the lumen, usually at the isthmus (Fig. 9.18). If there is complete transection of the aorta, the intima and media retract so that a smooth fusiform aneurysm is seen, at the ends of which the torn intimal flaps may be visible (Fig. 9.19). As time goes on, a saccular aneurysm may form causing a large mediastinal mass displacing adjacent structures. Calcification in the wall of the aneurysm commonly develops in those patients who survive.

A tear or avulsion of the right innominate artery or left subclavian artery is usually associated with a fall on the shoulder, trauma similar to that causing avulsion of the brachial plexus. The radiological features are similar to those of rupture of the aorta but there is absence or reduction of the radial pulse on the affected side. The diagnosis is made angiographically (Fig. 9.20). Such tears

may result in aneurysms of the great vessels arising from the aorta.

The Oesophagus

Traumatic perforation of the oesophagus is caused almost entirely by instrumentation, though penetrating wounds of the thorax can rarely cause damage. Spontaneous or post-emesis rupture occurs most frequently in the lower third of the oesophagus but trauma due to instrumentation most frequently occurs at the upper end in the post-cricoid region outside the thorax. However, in perforation of the cervical oesophagus, fluid and food leak into the soft tissues and track downwards into the upper mediastinum causing acute mediastinitis and abscess formation (see Chapter 8).

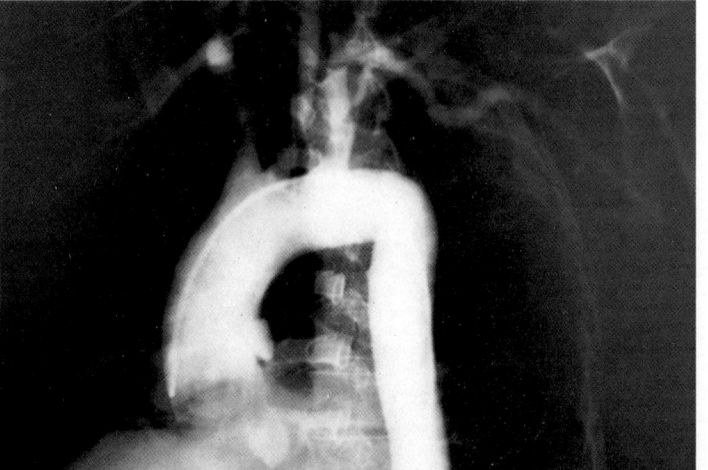

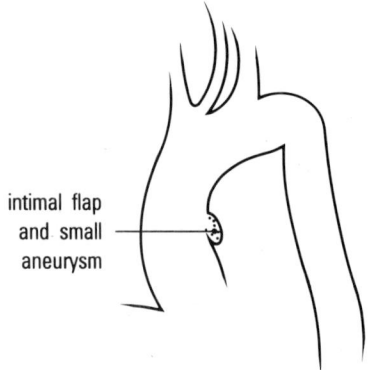

Fig. 9.18 Partial tear of the aorta. This arteriogram shows a small tear in the less common site, the ascending aorta. A small flap of intima has been raised by the tear.

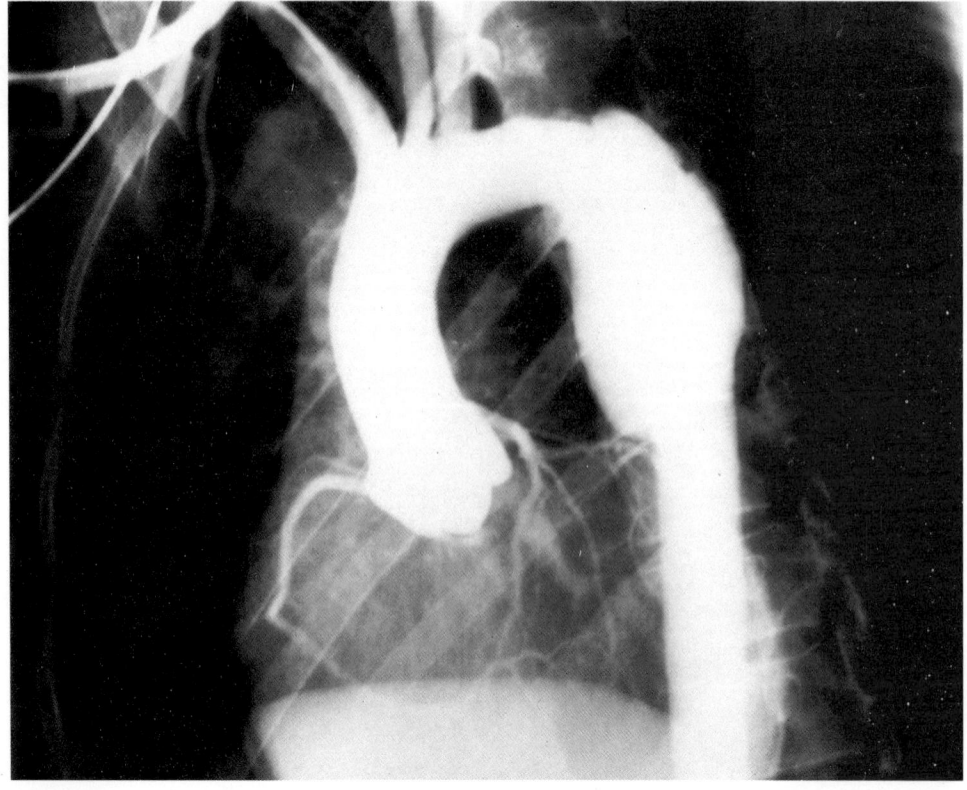

Fig. 9.19 Arteriogram of a complete tear of the aorta at the common site, the isthmus, showing the characteristic fusiform swelling of the aorta.

The Thoracic Duct

A frequent cause of rupture of the thoracic duct is surgery, usually operations on the aorta or oesophagus. The duct may be injured by manipulation in this region giving rise to leak of chyle into the mediastinum. The collection of chyle usually ruptures into the pleura producing chylothorax, though this may take several days to develop.

Other causes of rupture of the thoracic duct include penetrating injuries such as gunshot wounds and stab wounds and rarely blunt trauma such as road traffic accidents. Because of its position, injury to the duct in the lower part of the chest usually produces right sided chylothorax, and injury in the upper part of the chest, as during repair of coarctation of the aorta, causes left sided chylothorax (see Fig. 7.11).

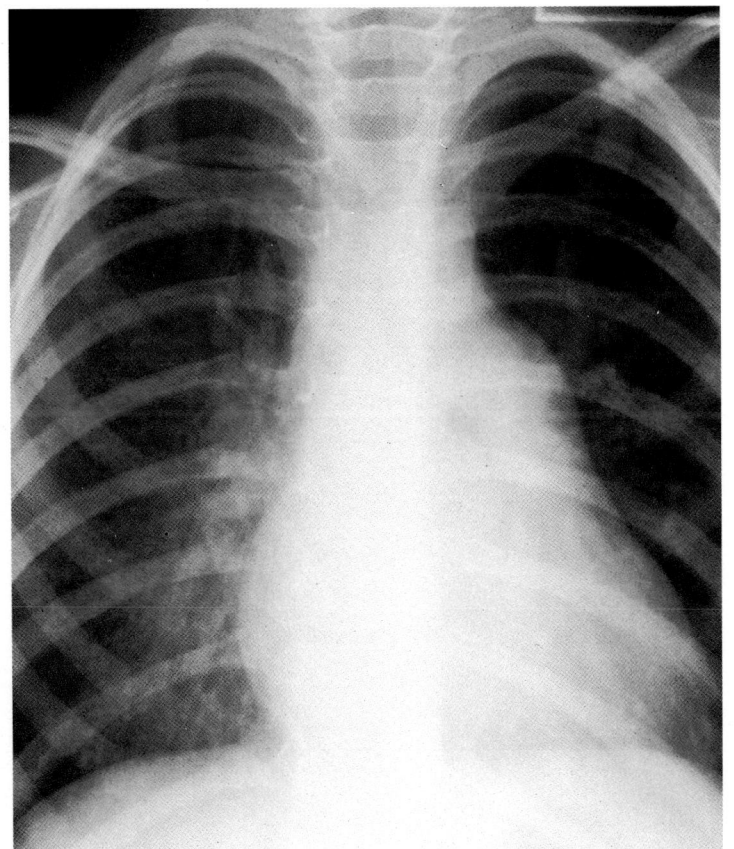 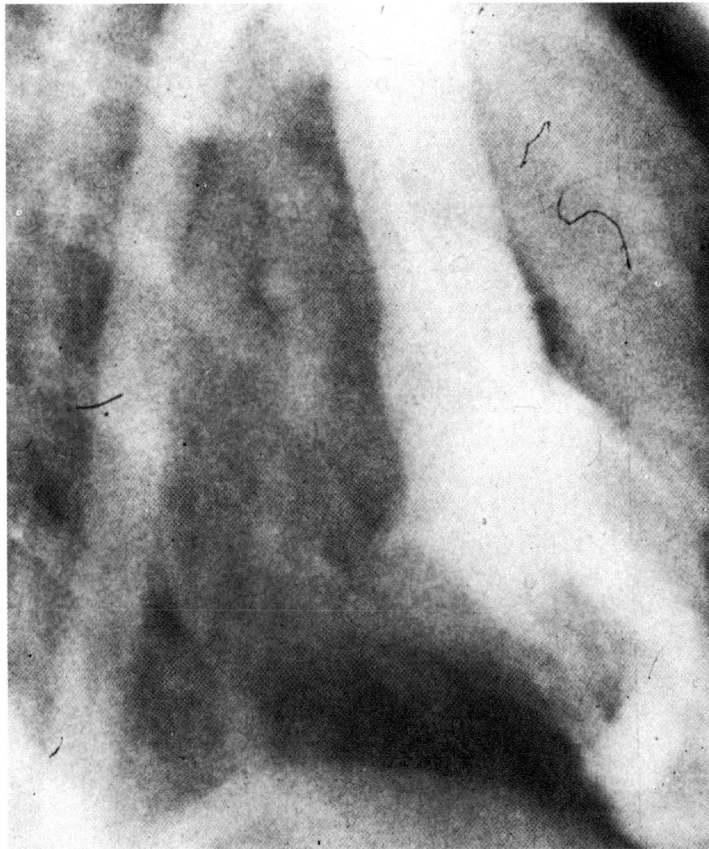

Fig. 9.23 Ventricular septal defect due to trauma. Severe trauma to this child caused acute heart failure. (a) Chest radiograph showed an enlarged heart and pulmonary plethora. A previous chest radiograph, a few months before, had been normal. (b) Left ventricular angiogram showed an aneurysm at the apex of the ventricle and a ventricular septal defect. Contrast is seen passing into the right ventricle in front of the left ventricle during systole.

INDEX

A

achalasia, 70, 133
actinomycetes, 69–70
actinomycosis, 33
adenoid cystic carcinoma (cylindroma), 55
adult respiratory distress syndrome (ARDS), 142
allergens and haptens, 100–11
allergic disorders
  asthma, 80
  bronchopulmonary aspergillosis, 80, 81–2
  Churg–Strauss syndrome, 83
  cryptogenic pulmonary eosinophilia, 83
  extrinsic allergic alveolitis (EAA), 84–5
  polyarteritis nodosa, 84
alveolar cell carcinoma, 27, 50–2
alveolar microlithiasis, 102
alveolar proteinosis, 95
alveolitis
  extrinisic allergic, 84–5
  fibrosing, 100
amyloid nodule 28
aorta
  aneurysm of, 40–1, 126–7
  injury to, 144–6
    rupture, 144–6
  unfolding of, 20
aortography, normal, 19
apical radiography, normal, 8, 9
arteriovenous fistula, 32, 94
arthritis, rheumatoid, 29, 104–5
asbestosis, 109
  pleural calcification, 115
aspergilloma, 71–2
aspergillosis, bronchopulmonary, 80–2
Aspergillus, 30
  pneumonia, 72, 73
aspiration penumonia, 70
asthma, 80
azygos lobe, 21

B

bacterial pneumonia, 66–7
barium swallow, normal, 10, 11
Behçet's syndrome, 106
Blastomyces dermatitidis, 74

blastomycosis, 75
Bochdalek hernia, 43
bronchi
  bronchial gland tumours, 54–5
  bronchiectasis, 63
  bronchiolar cell carcinoma, 27, 50–2
  bronchitis, chronic, 60
  bronchogenic cyst, 31, 60, 124
  bronchography, normal, 15–17
  bronchopulmonary aspergillosis, 80, 81–2
  carcinoid tumours, 31, 54

bronchi cont.
  carcinoma of, 33, 46–50, 124
    computerized tomography, 51–2
    rupture of, 144
bubonic plaque, 67
bullous lung disease, 61–2

C

calcification
  in inflammatory masses, 27–31
  pleural, 114, 115
Candida, 72, 73
carcinogens, lung cancer and mesothelioma, 110
carcinoid tumours, 31, 54
carcinoma, 35
  adenoid cystic, 55
  alveolar cell (bronchiolo-alveolar cell), 27, 50–2
  bronchial gland, 54–5
  of the bronchus, 33, 46–50, 124
  cavitating, 47
  of the hilum, 36
  metastatic, 124
  oat cell, 46
  of the oesophagus, 127
  presenting as pneumonia, 70–1
  squamous cell, 29, 35, 124
  vertebrae, 51
cardiomyophathy, pulmonary hypertension, 93
cavitating carcinoma, 47
chest wall, 117–8
  injuries, 136–7
  tumours, 25
chickenpox pneumonia, 68
chlamydial pneumonia, 68
chlorine, pulmonary oedema caused by, 108
chronic thromboembolism, 90
Churg–Strauss syndrome, 83
chylothorax, 112, 113
coal miner's pneumonconiosis, 47
Coccidioides immitis 74
coccidioidoma, 75
coccidioidomycosis, 75
companion shadows, 21
computerized tomography (CT)
  bullous lung disease, 62
  fibrosing alveolitis, 100
  lung tumours, 50–2
  normal, 12–15
cryptococcoma, 74
Cryptococcus neoformans, 73
cryptogenic fibrosing alveolitis (CFA), 99–100
cryptogenic pulmonary eosinophilia, 83
cystic fibrosis, 64
cysts
  bronchogenic, 31, 124
  dermoid, 38, 121
  hydatid, 32
    ruptured, 30
  mediastinum, 121–30